CIRCULATORY AND RESPIRATORY
MASS TRANSPORT

CIRCULATORY AND RESPIRATORY MASS TRANSPORT

A Ciba Foundation Symposium

Edited by
G. E. W. WOLSTENHOLME
and
JULIE KNIGHT

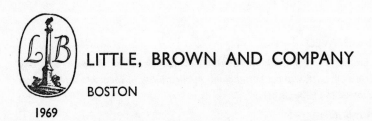

LITTLE, BROWN AND COMPANY

BOSTON

1969

First published 1969

Containing 101 illustrations

Standard Book Number 7000 1390 3

Contents

CONTENTS

Membership

Symposium on Circulatory and Respiratory Mass Transport, held 16th–18th July, 1968

C. G. Caro	⎱ Chairmen	Department of Aeronautics, Physiological Flow Studies Unit, Imperial College of Science and Technology, London
M. J. Lighthill	⎰	Imperial College of Science and Technology, London
B. Altshuler		Institute of Environmental Medicine, New York University Medical Center, New York
G. A. Brecher		Department of Physiology, University of Oklahoma Medical Center, Oklahoma City
A. C. Burton		Department of Biophysics, University of Western Ontario, London, Ontario
G. Cumming		Department of Medicine, Queen Elizabeth Hospital, Birmingham
C. N. Davies		London School of Hygiene and Tropical Medicine, London
L. E. Farhi		Department of Physiology, State University of New York, Buffalo, New York
M. A. Floyer		Medical Unit, The London Hospital, London
A. C. Guyton		Department of Physiology and Biophysics, University of Mississippi Medical Center, Jackson, Mississippi
N. A. Lassen		Department of Clinical Physiology, Bispebjerg Hospital, Copenhagen
S. G. Mason		Department of Chemistry, McGill University, Montreal
J. Mead		Department of Physiology, Harvard University School of Public Health, Boston, Massachusetts
E. W. Merrill*		Department of Chemical Engineering, Massachusetts Institute of Technology, Cambridge, Massachusetts
D. C. F. Muir		National Coal Board, Edinburgh
P. R. Owen		Department of Aeronautics, Imperial College of Science and Technology, London
J. R. Philip		CSIRO Division of Plant Industry, Canberra
J. Piiper		Max-Planck Institut für Experimentelle Medizin, Göttingen

* Contributed *in absentia*

MEMBERSHIP

E. M. Renkin   Department of Physiology and Pharmacology, Duke University Medical Center, Durham, North Carolina

P. G. Saffman   Department of Fluid Mechanics, California Institute of Technology, Pasadena, California

D. L. Schultz   Department of Engineering Science, University of Oxford

J. T. Stuart   Department of Mathematics, Imperial College of Science and Technology, London

M. G. Taylor   Department of Physiology, University of Sydney

J. B. West   Department of Medicine, Royal Postgraduate Medical School, London

The Ciba Foundation

The Ciba Foundation was opened in 1949 to promote international cooperation in medical and chemical research. It owes its existence to the generosity of CIBA Ltd, Basle, who, recognizing the obstacles to scientific communication created by war, man's natural secretiveness, disciplinary divisions, academic prejudices, distance, and differences of language, decided to set up a philanthropic institution whose aim would be to overcome such barriers. London was chosen as its site for reasons dictated by the special advantages of English charitable trust law (ensuring the independence of its actions), as well as those of language and geography.

The Foundation's house at 41 Portland Place, London, has become well known to workers in many fields of science. Every year the Foundation organizes six to ten three-day symposia and three to four shorter study groups, all of which are published in book form. Many other scientific meetings are held, organized either by the Foundation or by other groups in need of a meeting place. Accommodation is also provided for scientists visiting London, whether or not they are attending a meeting in the house.

The Foundation's many activities are controlled by a small group of distinguished trustees. Within the general framework of biological science, interpreted in its broadest sense, these activities are well summed up by the motto of the Ciba Foundation: *Consocient Gentes*—let the peoples come together.

Preface

THE idea of a symposium on physiological flow processes was first suggested to the Director of the Ciba Foundation by Dr. Colin Caro, Director of the Physiological Flow Studies Unit at Imperial College, London, in February 1967. The interdisciplinary nature of the proposed meeting made it exactly the type of project through which the Foundation feels that it can contribute to biological and medical advance, and the suggestion was readily taken up. In the following months the details of the symposium were worked out during consultations between Mr. A. V. S. de Reuck for the Foundation, and Dr. Caro and Professor James Lighthill of Imperial College.

The purpose of this symposium was that of the Physiological Flow Studies Unit itself: to bring together physical scientists and physiologists concerned with flow processes in the body in order to make possible a collaborative approach to problems of physiological transport. The Foundation invited a small group of specialists (finally numbering twenty-three members) which nevertheless spanned a range of scientific disciplines that was probably wider than at any of its previous symposia. The meeting was held in July 1968, and this volume contains the formal papers and the discussions arising from them.

The editors are most grateful to the participants for their ready cooperation which has made possible the early publication of the book; they would particularly like to thank Dr. Caro for his generous help and advice, which continued long after the meeting itself.

Inevitably several intended participants were unable to come to the meeting; among them we especially note Professor E. W. Merrill, of the Massachusetts Institute of Technology, who nevertheless provided us with a research film (and has contributed *in absentia* to this volume), and Professor G. I. Barenblatt of the Institute of Mechanics, Moscow State University, who at the last moment was unable to attend.

CHAIRMAN'S INTRODUCTION

C. G. CARO

THIS is an interdisciplinary symposium on mass transport in the circulatory and respiratory systems. We are naturally pleased to learn that it is the most extensively interdisciplinary symposium that the Ciba Foundation has arranged. Further self-congratulation would however be inappropriate, because physical scientists have for centuries made contributions in physiology, and collaboration between physical scientists and physiologists is in no sense a phenomenon exclusive to this decade or century. But at the present time we seem to be witnessing, quite apart from the general growth of science, collaboration on a scale previously unimaginable. We suspect that this process is still in its infancy and that there is much more still to come from collaboration between these groups of scientists.

We have an ambitious programme; that of covering more than is perhaps normally tackled in a meeting of this kind. We are discussing problems in three fields—the physiology of blood and blood vessels, the interstitial fluid and spaces, and the respiratory system. The title of the symposium, "Mass Transport", indicates that we shall be considering the free and forced convective motion of materials in these systems. This title seems to have caused a little confusion. We gather that several applications were received to join the symposium from people properly engaged in mass transport!

We shall be discussing the properties of physiological fluids and analysing various flow processes, including the characteristics and influences of the boundaries or media through which flow occurs. There was initially some attempt to concentrate on passive as opposed to active phenomena, but we are studying physiology and so, appropriately, there will be consideration both of active and of passive processes.

To undertake these tasks there is an international representation of physiologists and physical scientists. The physiologists may be particularly interested in one or more fields, but all possess more than a little knowledge of physical principles underlying their work. The physical scientists have independently, or in collaboration, worked on physiological problems. Nevertheless there may be difficulties in communication in a meeting of this sort. We hope therefore that particular care will be taken to present ideas in terms

1

which are generally comprehensible, so that they can be manipulated across disciplinary boundaries. With this objective achieved we have confidence that the proceedings may add not only to physiological knowledge but also to the lustre of interdisciplinary collaboration.

We have one other task, and that a most pleasurable one, of thanking Dr. Wolstenholme and the Ciba Foundation for setting up this meeting.

SECTION I
MASS TRANSPORT IN TISSUE SPACES

INTERSTITIAL FLUID PRESSURE–VOLUME RELATIONSHIPS AND THEIR REGULATION

ARTHUR C. GUYTON

Department of Physiology and Biophysics, University of Mississippi School of Medicine, Jackson, Mississippi

UNTIL recently it was believed almost universally by physiologists that the normal interstitial fluid pressure is slightly positive with respect to atmospheric pressure in essentially all parts of the body. This belief was based primarily on so-called "needle pressure" measurements—that is, measurements of the pressure that must be applied to fluid in a hypodermic needle to cause fluid flow into the tissues. Yet, there were many disquieting features to this belief, such as the observation by McMaster (1941) nearly thirty years ago that fluid is very slowly absorbed into tissues from the tip of a minute syringe needle when the pressure in the needle is exactly equal to atmospheric pressure. Also, nearly forty years ago Krogh, Landis and Turner (1932) pointed out that tissue oedema does not occur until the venous pressure is raised to about 15 mm. Hg, thus indicating that the body has a significant safety factor against oedema. According to our conventional understanding of tissue fluid dynamics, such a rise in venous pressure should increase interstitial fluid pressure by approximately 12 mm. Hg, which should in turn cause extreme oedema. Likewise, it is common knowledge that the colloid osmotic pressure of the plasma proteins must fall to less than one-half normal before generalized systemic oedema will occur.

Also, if all the interstitial fluid were freely mobile, a tremendous quantity of fluid should be available to move into the circulatory system whenever the capillary pressure falls very low. Yet Wang and co-workers (1947) and Ingraham and Wiggers (1945) demonstrated that this is the case in haemorrhaged animals only when they have been allowed to drink water until the time of haemorrhage. Here again it appears that the quantities of extra fluid available in the tissue spaces that can readily be given up to the circulating blood are much less than our previous understanding of tissue fluid has led us to believe.

A simple way to explain all these findings would be to assume that the tissues are normally compacted together and that the amount of fluid present in the interstitial spaces is only that amount bound in some way in the tissues or required to fill the minute interstices between the cells and extracellular

4

elements. Furthermore, it might be assumed that there is some mechanism which continually attempts to remove interstitial fluid, thereby causing a subatmospheric pressure in the interstitial fluid spaces. In partial support of such a concept have been many measurements, made over the past sixty years or more, of subatmospheric pressure in special spaces of the body, such as a normally negative pressure in the intrapleural space (Agostoni, Taglietti and Setnikar, 1957), in the pericardial space (E. H. Wood, personal communication), in the joint spaces (Bauer, Ropes and Waine, 1940), and in the epidural space (Heldt and Moloney, 1928). All these are areas in which the tissues are protected from collapse caused by atmospheric pressure pressing on the outside of the body. Consequently, it might be assumed that some absorbing force common to all of these spaces could be causing the negative pressure.

THE CAPSULE METHOD FOR MEASURING INTERSTITIAL FLUID PRESSURE

With this background in mind, we wished to determine whether or not the needle method does indeed measure interstitial fluid pressure accurately or whether some other method for measuring interstitial fluid pressure might give different results. To do this, we developed three new methods for measuring interstitial fluid pressure, as follows (Guyton, 1963, 1965b).

First, we implanted a hollow capsule, perforated by many small holes, into tissues and left the capsule until all healing had occurred. Then the pressure was measured in the cavity of the capsule by inserting a needle to its centre or by leaving a catheter in the cavity and measuring the pressure through the catheter.

Second, we implanted a small piece of almost any type or shape of plastic into the tissues, and later penetrated the skin with a needle so that the flat surface of the needle lay on the surface of the plastic where a fine layer of fluid exists, thereby allowing measurement of pressure in this fine layer of fluid.

Third, we elevated the skin by any mechanical means, thereby pulling fluid into the area underneath the elevation. This fluid was held in this area for hours to days, and the equilibrated pressure was measured in the impounded fluid through a curved needle.

The pressures measured by all these methods have been negative with respect to atmospheric pressure in essentially all normal tissues. In subcutaneous tissue the pressure measures an average of −6 to −7 mm. Hg by all three different methods. However, the pressure measured by the perforated capsule is far more stable over a period of hours and days than are the pressures measured by the other two methods. Furthermore, the capsule pressure responds within a few minutes to changes in interstitial fluid pressure, which allows dynamic studies (Guyton, 1963).

Most often we have used capsules with a diameter of about 15 mm. and perforated by approximately 150 1-mm. holes. About four weeks is required for complete healing of the surgical wound, and by that time typical connective tissue has grown through the perforations to line the cavity with about 1 mm. thickness of tissue. T-1824 dye injected into the cavity was shown to move freely between the cavity and the surrounding tissue spaces, proving that the fluid in the cavity is not in some special encysted state (Guyton, 1963). In addition, when two capsules are implanted approximately 30 mm. apart, elevation of the pressure in one capsule to a supra-atmospheric pressure always causes very rapid movement of fluid from this capsule into the capsule where pressure is still subatmospheric (Guyton, Scheel and Murphree, 1966). The pressure in the second capsule rises within a few seconds to approach that in the first capsule.

COMPARISON OF CAPSULE PRESSURE MEASUREMENTS AND NEEDLE PRESSURE MEASUREMENTS

We have used many different procedures to alter the dynamics of fluid exchange at the capillary membrane when determining whether or not the capsule method is capable of recording predicted changes in interstitial fluid pressure (Guyton, 1963, 1965b; Guyton, Scheel and Murphree, 1966; Guyton et al., 1966). For instance, in one series of animals the venous pressure was raised to a level of 40 to 60 mm. Hg in the leg of a dog, and the interstitial fluid pressure was measured in an implanted capsule. Pressure was also measured by the usual needle technique. The capsule pressure was initially −7 mm. Hg but rose extremely rapidly for the first 30 minutes, then progressively more slowly for the next few hours. The needle pressure measured about +2 mm. Hg at the beginning of the experiment and still measured +2 mm. Hg at the end of three hours. Thus, the interstitial fluid pressure as measured by the capsule method changed, as would be predicted, while the needle pressure measurements failed to change at all.

As another example, the colloid osmotic pressure of the plasma was changed suddenly by intravenous infusion of concentrated dextran solution. The capsule measurements of interstitial fluid pressure showed an immediate drop (within three minutes) in the negative pressure of the tissues, indicative of tissue dehydration. On the other hand, pressures measured by the needle technique actually rose, which is opposite to the effect that would be expected.

TISSUES IN WHICH NEGATIVE INTERSTITIAL FLUID PRESSURES HAVE BEEN MEASURED

Capsules have been implanted in muscle, retroperitoneal spaces, lungs and kidneys, in addition to subcutaneous tissues all over the body (Guyton, 1963; Meyer, Meyer and Guyton, 1968). Pressures in the muscles have averaged about −5 mm. Hg, in the retroperitoneal space approximately the same as in the subcutaneous space, and in the lungs as low as −16 mm. Hg but usually between −3 and −10 mm. Hg. Pressures in the kidneys have been almost exactly equal to atmospheric pressure, sometimes slightly below and sometimes slightly above (C. Ott, unpublished observations).

EFFECT OF OEDEMA ON INTERSTITIAL FLUID PRESSURE

In making more than a thousand measurements of interstitial fluid pressure in the subcutaneous tissues of dogs, we have observed an almost invariable rule: so long as the tissues are normal, the measured capsule pressure is sub-atmospheric, while any degree of oedema whatsoever, caused either by inflammation or by generalized interstitial fluid oedema, is associated with a

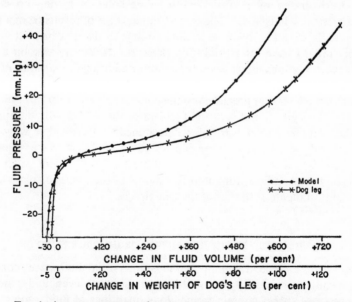

FIG. 1. Average pressure–volume curve (×—×) of the interstitial fluid space measured in the leg of the dog contrasted with the pressure–volume curve (dots) of a tissue model composed of a rubber bag stuffed with water-filled balloons and cotton fibres. (Reprinted with permission from Guyton, 1965a.)

pressure greater than atmospheric pressure (Guyton, 1963, 1965a). To state
this another way, the atmospheric pressure level is the dividing line between
the non-oedematous state and the oedematous state. A positive pressure in
the interstitial spaces causes these spaces to balloon outward and to fill with
fluid, while pressures less than atmospheric pressure are associated with
compaction of the tissues, which is the normal state.

PRESSURE–VOLUME CURVE OF THE INTERSTITIAL SPACES

To understand better the dynamics of interstitial fluid volume changes, the
pressure–volume curve of the interstitial spaces, illustrated by the curve through
the crosses in Fig. 1, was determined in the following manner (Guyton, 1965a).
Capsules were implanted in the lower hind legs of dogs, and later each leg
was removed from the body, with a tourniquet placed around its cut end.
The leg was weighed continuously on a balance while the interstitial spaces
were either dehydrated by perfusion of the blood vessels with concentrated
dextran solution having a colloid osmotic pressure of approximately 100 mm.
Hg or overhydrated by perfusion with saline solution having no colloid
osmotic pressure whatsoever. The curve is an average of results from a series
of animals, showing that increase in fluid volume of tissues causes at first an
extremely rapid rise in interstitial fluid pressure. However, as soon as this
pressure reaches atmospheric level, tremendous additional quantities of fluid
in the leg cause very little additional rise in pressure until the weight of the leg
reaches about 60 per cent greater than the control value. From this point on,
the skin of the leg becomes very tight and pressure rises rapidly once again.

Pressure–volume curves were also determined in three other ways with
results generally the same as those illustrated in Fig. 1. The curve passing
through the dots was recorded from a rubber bag stuffed with water-filled
balloons and cotton, illustrating that this model of the tissues displays a type
of curve almost identical to that of the true tissues.

FLOW OF FLUID IN TISSUES—MOBILE OR IMMOBILE FLUID?

One of the obstacles to accepting that most interstitial fluid spaces normally
have a negative pressure is the well-known fact that even under normal
conditions these spaces contain tremendous quantities of fluid—some 12 to
20 per cent of the body weight, as indicated by sodium space, inulin space,
thiocyanate space, and other space measurements. Therefore a question
that must be resolved is: how could so much fluid be present in the tissue

spaces without causing a positive fluid pressure? A possible answer to this
is that the fluid is in an entrapped and non-mobile state. We therefore studied
the degree of mobility of the fluid in the tissue spaces. To do this, we implanted
two perforated capsules approximately 30 mm. apart in subcutaneous tissue,
and measured the conductance (or resistance) for movement of fluid from one
of these to the other (Guyton, Scheel and Murphree, 1966). Fig. 2 illustrates

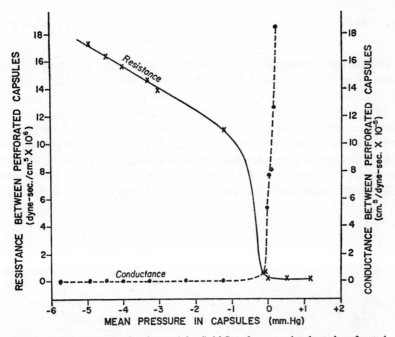

FIG. 2. Conductance (and resistance) for fluid flow from one implanted perforated
capsule to another located 30 mm. away, illustrating the tremendous increase in
conductance when the interstitial fluid pressure rises from subatmospheric pressure
level to supra-atmospheric pressure level. (Reprinted with permission from Guyton,
Scheel and Murphree, 1966.)

the effect on this conductance (or resistance) of changing the interstitial fluid
pressure (mean pressure in the capsules). Note that conductance was almost
nil so long as the interstitial fluid pressure was less than atmospheric pressure.
On the other hand, at the very moment that the interstitial fluid pressure rose
to greater than atmospheric pressure, fluid began to move with great rapidity
from one capsule to another, the conductance increasing suddenly about
10,000-fold.

These studies demonstrated that even the slightest increase of interstitial pressure above atmospheric pressure causes much very mobile interstitial fluid to accumulate. Yet, no such mobility exists for the large mass of fluid normally present in the tissue spaces. Therefore, we must suggest that the fluid normally in the tissues is almost entirely in a trapped state such as in a hyaluronic acid gel, or combined with collagen or other elements of the tissue, or held in very minute spaces between the compacted solid or semi-solid elements of the tissues.

EFFECT OF INTERSTITIAL FLUID PRESSURE ON MOVEMENT OF FLUID THROUGH THE CAPILLARY MEMBRANE

The Starling hypothesis of an equilibrium state across the capillary membrane originated with Starling's observation (1896) that plasma proteins exert a colloid osmotic pressure. However, three other elements also important to the hypothesis were never measured by Starling; these are interstitial fluid colloid osmotic pressure, capillary pressure, and interstitial fluid pressure. Landis (1927) demonstrated the importance of capillary pressure on movement of fluid through the capillary membrane, and others have demonstrated the importance of interstitial fluid colloid osmotic pressure (Sterling, 1951; Wasserman, Joseph and Mayerson, 1956). Yet it still remained to be demonstrated that changes in interstitial fluid pressure also affect movement of fluid

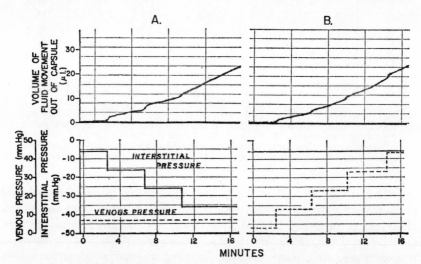

FIG. 3. Movement of fluid through the tissue capillary membrane caused by (A) progressive decrease of interstitial fluid pressure to more negative values and (B) progressive increase in venous pressure to more positive values. (Reprinted with permission from Guyton et al., 1966.)

through the capillary membrane. Using the capsule procedure we have been able to do this (Guyton *et al.*, 1966). Fig. 3A illustrates the results from such an experiment. A special apparatus was built to measure rate of fluid movement from the tissue into the cavity of a capsule; this rate is indicated by the slope of the curve in the figure. Note that when the capsule pressure was decreased by pulling fluid out of the cavity of the capsule, fluid began to flow out of the tissue into the cavity. Each time the capsule pressure was lowered by 10 mm. Hg, the rate of flow increased almost exactly proportionately. Fig. 3B shows the effect in the same animal of holding the interstitial pressure constant but raising the venous pressure (and consequently the capillary pressure) in steps. These experiments demonstrate that the fourth element in Starling's hypothesis, interstitial fluid pressure, plays almost exactly the same quantitative role in movement of fluid across the capillary membrane as does capillary pressure, except that it acts in the opposite direction.

ESTIMATIONS OF FUNCTIONAL CAPILLARY PRESSURE

The newer methods for measuring interstitial fluid pressure have provided a means of estimating the "functional capillary pressure" of the tissues—that is, the average mean pressure in the capillaries tending to force fluid outward through the capillary membrane. Landis (1927) made most of his capillary pressure measurements in large arterial or large venous capillaries, and many people have used an average of these two measurements as the average functional capillary pressure. Among many reasons for doubting the validity of this are the following. First, most capillaries of the body remain closed most of the time, and the pressure in these is probably much nearer venular pressure than arteriolar pressure. Second, the venous capillaries are much more extensive and larger in size than are the arterial capillaries. Third, the permeability coefficient for venous capillaries is considerably greater than that for arterial capillaries. All these factors weight the mean functional capillary pressure much more toward the venous end of the capillary than toward the arterial end.

By using values that we have measured for (1) interstitial fluid pressure, (2) colloid osmotic pressure of tissue fluid taken from capsules, and (3) plasma colloid osmotic pressure, it has been possible to calculate the fourth value in the Starling equilibrium equation, capillary pressure. Thus, in a large series of dogs we have found the average plasma colloid osmotic pressure to be approximately 20 mm. Hg, the interstitial fluid colloid osmotic pressure as measured or calculated from the intracapsular protein to be about 4 mm. Hg, and the interstitial fluid pressure to be about −7 mm. Hg. Putting these values together we can calculate that for an equilibrium state to occur at the capillary membrane, the mean functional capillary pressure of the tissues would have to be approximately 9 mm. Hg. This is an incredibly low value in comparison with the value of 22 to 25 mm. Hg that has been assumed for many years on the basis of Landis's measurements. In the human being, in which the colloid osmotic pressure is approximately 8 mm. Hg greater than in the dog, one can make similar calculations and derive a capillary pressure of approximately 17 mm. Hg. J. Prather, in our laboratories, has been reassessing this problem, measuring all these values simultaneously in the same animal under many different conditions. He finds a calculated mean functional capillary pressure of approximately 10 mm. Hg, this value remaining relatively constant even in such states as inflammatory oedema (unpublished observations). Obviously, this calculated value does not take into account the possibility of a non-equilibrium state at the capillary membrane. Indeed, the very fact that fluid flows away from tissues by way of the lymph channels indicates that there is not an equilibrium state at the capillary membrane. Yet, data from many sources indicate that the pressure drop across the capillary membrane caused by the non-equilibrium state is probably less than 1 mm. Hg under normal conditions. Therefore, these calculations of mean functional capillary pressure deserve further serious attention.

MECHANISM CAUSING THE NORMALLY NEGATIVE INTERSTITIAL FLUID PRESSURE

At present we have only a hypothesis for the mechanism that causes the normally negative interstitial fluid pressure, but there are good reasons for believing that it does function continually in the tissues. First, if the functional capillary pressure is as low as the above calculations lead one to believe, the colloid osmotic pressure of the plasma could create a highly negative pressure in the interstitial spaces simply as the result of osmotic absorption of fluid out of the spaces. However, for such osmotic absorption to occur, there must be some additional mechanism to keep the protein concentration in the interstitial fluid spaces at a very low level. Since only very slight lymph flow is required for this purpose, it is completely reasonable to believe that the lymphatic pump is the responsible mechanism. In support of this are observations from several laboratories that negative pressures can develop in peripheral lymphatic channels (Allen, 1938; Blocker et al., 1959). Also, in our own studies of interstitial pressure in the leg of the dog, we have found that immobilizing the leg for only a few hours causes a progressive rise of the pressure from its very negative value of −7 mm. Hg up to about −2 mm. Hg. Then return of activity of the leg causes the pressure to begin falling again, sometimes as much as several mm. per hour, this effect presumably resulting from return of effectiveness of the lymphatic pump.

PHYSICAL ANALYSIS OF FORCES THAT TEND TO MOVE FLUID THROUGH MEMBRANE PORES

Fig. 4 shows an analysis of the different forces affecting fluid movement through the pores of different tissue membranes. Much of this analysis is obvious but certain points require attention.

The centre of the analysis represents the capillary, and on either side of this is the interstitial space. To the right, a cell is placed in the interstitial space, and to the very far right is the skin. In the left side of the analysis the cell is replaced by a gelatinous mass which is supposedly present in the interstitial spaces.

To follow this analysis, let us start at the capillary membrane. This shows two types of forces acting at the capillary membrane, osmotic forces and hydrostatic forces, and the values given in this diagram are approximately those that we have calculated for a human being. The osmotic forces are based on plasma and interstitial fluid protein measurements, and the interstitial fluid hydrostatic force, −7 mm. Hg, is the value that we have measured

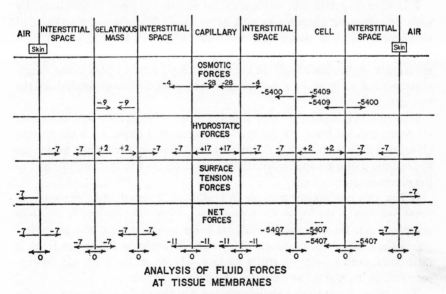

ANALYSIS OF FLUID FORCES
AT TISSUE MEMBRANES

FIG. 4. Analysis of forces that cause movement of fluid through pores in tissue membranes. All forces are expressed as mm. Hg.

in perforated capsules. Thus, the functional hydrostatic pressure of the human capillary is calculated to be +17 mm. Hg.

At the cell membrane we assume that there is a +2 mm. Hg hydrostatic pressure inside the cell, and that this is balanced by a slightly greater osmotic pressure inside the cell than that in the interstitial spaces. Obviously, the values inside the cell are completely unknown, but +2 mm. Hg has been chosen because it is approximately equal to the "total tissue pressure" which will be discussed later. At the skin it is shown that surface tension in the pores of the skin provides a force to balance the negative pressure in the interstitial space and therefore to prevent suction of air into the spaces.

To the left in the analysis the gelatinous mass is shown to exert a colloid osmotic pressure to pull fluid out of the interstitial spaces into the gel. Such an effect for gels is well known (Glasstone, 1946). The quantitative value given in the analysis is the amount required to give a state of equilibrium.

Note especially that the forces at all of the different membranes balance out to be zero, as shown at the bottom of the figure. This is the necessary criterion for equilibrium.

PHYSICAL ANALYSIS OF MECHANICAL FORCES AT THE TISSUE MEMBRANES

It is often forgotten that mechanical forces can be caused in the tissues by solid or semi-solid elements as well as by fluid. Therefore, the analysis of mechanical forces in tissues is entirely different from the analysis of fluid movement through the pores of membranes. Mechanical forces cause actual movement of the tissue itself, in contrast to fluid forces which cause simple movement of molecules through membranes. Fig. 5 gives an analysis of the mechanical forces.

Note that in this analysis three different types of forces must be considered: (1) compressional forces of the solid and semi-solid elements of the tissues, (2) tensional forces of different tissues, and (3) hydrostatic forces. Note that hydrostatic (but not osmotic) forces are common both to this analysis and to the previous one.

Before this mechanical analysis is explained in detail, it is necessary to point out that all the forces are represented as pressures. Actually the solid compressional forces represent intense force at the minute contact points where the solid elements touch. However, it is assumed that the force is distributed evenly over the entire surface. Therefore, the force can be represented, by averaging the force per unit area, as pressure.

To explain this analysis I shall again begin at the capillary and move to the right in Fig. 5. Hydrostatic forces act on both sides of the capillary membrane,

+17 mm. Hg pressure inside and −7 mm. Hg outside, making a total hydro-static pressure gradient across the membrane of 24 mm. Hg. Opposing this are capillary wall tensional force and solid compressional force from outside the capillary. The tensional force is caused by stretch of the capillary wall itself and can be represented as a pressure equal to approximately −15 mm. Hg acting toward the centre of the capillary. The compressional force exerted

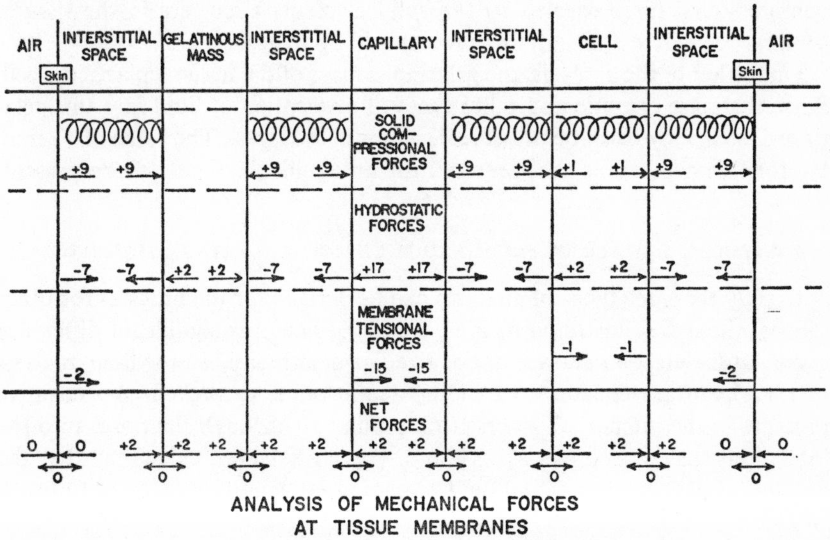

ANALYSIS OF MECHANICAL FORCES
AT TISSUE MEMBRANES

FIG. 5. Analysis of mechanical forces tending to displace tissue interfaces. All forces are expressed as mm. Hg.

on the outside of the capillary by solid tissues is estimated as approximately +9 mm. Hg. This represents the transmission of pressure through the tissues by the solid components of the tissues rather than by the fluid component. The value of +9 mm. Hg is the amount calculated to be necessary to establish equilibrium when the interstitial fluid pressure is −7 mm. Hg and the total tissue pressure as measured by an inflated balloon in the tissue is +2 mm. Hg, the normal value. Note at the bottom of the figure that the pressures across the capillary membrane show a net value of zero so that a state of mechanical equilibrium exists.

At the cell membrane, one also has all three forces: solid compressional forces on the outside of the cell, hydrostatic forces on both sides of the cell membrane, and cell membrane tensional force. The membrane tensional and intracellular compressional forces are shown to be almost zero, because of measurements made by Cole (1932). The fluid forces are the same as those shown in Fig. 4 for the fluid forces across the cell membrane. And the solid compressional force on the outside of the cell is the same as that on the outside of the capillary. Here again the net forces across the cell membrane add up to zero, so that a state of mechanical equilibrium exists.

At the skin one has the negative interstitial fluid pressure of −7 mm. Hg, a force caused by curvature of the skin (about 2 mm. Hg), and the same compressional force exerted by the solid elements elsewhere in the tissues, +9 mm. Hg. Here again all these forces add up to zero.

On the left of the analysis, the gelatinous mass of the tissue replaces the cell. Since there are osmotic and other types of absorption of fluid into this gelatinous mass, a hydrostatic pressure develops in the mass. The value of +2 mm. Hg for this pressure is that required for an equilibrium state to be present.

PHYSICAL ANALYSIS OF FLUID AND MECHANICAL FORCES IN THE LUNGS

Exactly the same types of analyses can be derived for the lungs as for other tissues; these are illustrated in Figs. 6 and 7. The only significant difference occurs at the alveolar surface of the alveolar membrane. In the fluid analysis of Fig. 6, surface tension force acting at the pores to prevent the negative pressure in the interstitial spaces from pulling air through the pores into the interstitial spaces is shown as −19 mm. Hg. It has been calculated that the amount of negative interstitial fluid pressure that would be required to break

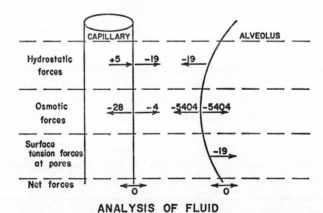

ANALYSIS OF FLUID
FORCES IN LUNGS

Fig. 6. Analysis of forces tending to cause movement of fluid through the pores of membranes in the lung. All forces are expressed as mm. Hg.

the surface tension at the pores of the alveolus would be more than 100,000 mm. Hg (Guyton and Lindsey, 1959).

In the mechanical analysis of Fig. 7 the concave curvature of the alveolus causes a negative force to be applied to the alveolar membrane, tending to

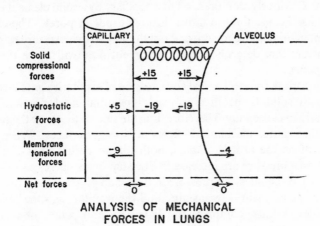

ANALYSIS OF MECHANICAL
FORCES IN LUNGS

FIG. 7. Analysis of mechanical forces tending to cause displacement of interfaces in the lung. All forces are expressed as mm. Hg.

pull it toward the alveolus. This is the well-known surface tension and elastic tension effect which tends to cause collapse of the alveolus.

THE CONCEPTS OF INTERSTITIAL FLUID PRESSURE, SOLID TISSUE PRESSURE AND TOTAL TISSUE PRESSURE

If one accepts the fact that forces can be transmitted through tissues both by fluid and by solid or semi-solid tissue elements, then it is immediately apparent that the total mechanical forces acting at any given interface in the tissues will equal the fluid forces only when absolutely no contact points exist between the solid or semi-solid tissue elements. In normal tissues there are many such contact points, so that the forces exerted by the fluids of the tissues cannot possibly be equal to the total force exerted at any given interface in the tissues. For this reason, we must derive new terminology to describe the different types of forces that can develop at tissue interfaces. The analyses of Figs. 4 to 7 demonstrate the principles upon which such terminology can be based. From these, one can see that pressures can be transmitted through tissues by two principal means; by way of the fluids and by way of the solid and semi-solid elements. This gives rise to two different types of pressure, (1) "interstitial fluid pressure" and (2) "solid tissue pressure". The additive effect of both of these together equals the total pressure that occurs at any given tissue interface, and this can be called simply "total tissue pressure".

It is very important to recognize the distinction between the different types of tissue pressure because they have different physical significance within the tissues. Obviously, compression of a capillary by a solid element of a tissue cannot in itself cause fluid to move through capillary pores. Therefore, it is only the interstitial fluid pressure and not the solid tissue pressure nor the total tissue pressure that determines whether or not fluid will move through the capillary pores.

When one speaks of mechanical compression of capillaries or of larger blood vessels, both solid tissue pressure and interstitial fluid pressure can act mechanically to cause this. Therefore, it is the sum of these, or the *total tissue pressure*, that causes mechanical effects at tissue interfaces. When a blood pressure cuff on the arm is inflated, both the interstitial fluid pressure and the solid tissue pressure are increased. The sum of the increases in these two pressures will be equal to the pressure in the blood pressure cuff; therefore the pressure in the cuff will be transmitted all the way through the tissue to the blood vessels to cause compression. It is very important not to make the mistake of thinking that all of this pressure is transmitted from the blood pressure cuff to the blood vessels simply by way of fluid in the interstitial spaces. Indeed, we have been able to show by capsule pressure measurements that only a fraction of the pressure exerted on the outside of the skin is transmitted through the tissues by way of the fluid.

An especially important feature of solid tissue pressure is that theoretically it is one of the major factors determining the shapes of cells and other tissue elements. This is because solid tissue pressure is calculated to be about +9 mm. Hg, which is sufficient to cause compaction of the cells, thus making the cells conform to the available spaces.

Finally, one can ask the question, what is measured by the needle pressure method? When fluid is injected into a tissue from the tip of a needle it is necessary to displace tissue, creating a space that is no longer a normally compacted tissue space. Furthermore, an interface exists until this fluid is absorbed, and the pressure in the fluid must be sufficient to balance all other pressures at this interface. Therefore, this pressure should be equal to *total tissue pressure*, or about +2 mm. Hg in most tissues. This is approximately the pressure measured by the needle method (Burch and Sodeman, 1937; Wells, Youmans and Miller, 1938). Essentially the same principles hold for tissue pressures measured by inflating blood vessels (Kjellmer, 1964), rubber tubes or rubber balloons in tissues, all of which theoretically give an indication of total tissue pressure, not interstitial fluid pressure.

SUMMARY

Experiments have indicated in many different ways that the interstitial fluid pressure is negative with respect to atmospheric pressure, rather than positive as has always been assumed. Normally the tissue cells and intra-cellular elements appear to be compacted against each other, and the fluid in the intercellular spaces is mainly immobile, perhaps bound in the gel of the ground substance. In oedematous states the pressure is positive and free fluid can be moved easily and rapidly through the spaces. Analyses of the forces that cause (a) movement of fluid through pores in tissue membranes and (b) mechanical movement of tissue interfaces demonstrate that two basic types of pressure occur in tissues. These are (1) pressure caused by fluid in the tissue spaces, which can be called "interstitial fluid pressure", and (2) pressure caused by the solid and semi-solid elements of the tissues, which can be called "solid tissue pressure". The sum of these two is equal to the "total tissue pressure". It is the interstitial fluid pressure that tends to cause movement of fluid through pores in tissue membranes, while it is total tissue pressure that tends to cause collapse of blood vessels.

REFERENCES

AGOSTONI, E., TAGLIETTI, A., and SETNIKAR, I. (1957). *Am. J. Physiol.*, **191**, 277–282.
ALLEN, L. (1938). *Am. J. Physiol.*, **123**, 3–4.
BAUER, W., ROPES, M. W., and WAINE, H. (1940). *Physiol. Rev.*, **20**, 272–312.
BLOCKER, T. G., Jr., SMITH, J. R., DUNTON, E. F., PROTAS, J. M., COOLEY, R. M., LEWIS, S. R., and KIRBY, E. J. (1959). *Ann. Surg.*, **149**, 884–897.
BURCH, G. E., and SODEMAN, W. A. (1937). *J. clin. Invest.*, **16**, 845–850.
COLE, K. S. (1932). *J. cell. comp. Physiol.*, **1**, 1–9.
GLASSTONE, S. (1946). *Textbook of Physical Chemistry*, pp. 1258–1263. New York: Van Nostrand.
GUYTON, A. C. (1963). *Circulation Res.*, **12**, 399–414.
GUYTON, A. C. (1965a). *Circulation Res.*, **16**, 452–460.
GUYTON, A. C. (1965b). *Invest. Ophthal.*, **4**, 1075–1084.
GUYTON, A. C., and LINDSEY, A. W. (1959). *Circulation Res.*, **7**, 649–657.
GUYTON, A. C., PRATHER, J. W., SCHEEL, K., and McGEHEE, J. (1966). *Circulation Res.*, **19**, 1022–1030.
GUYTON, A. C., SCHEEL, K., and MURPHREE, D. (1966). *Circulation Res.*, **19**, 412–419.
HELDT, T. J., and MOLONEY, J. C. (1928). *Am. J. med. Sci.*, **175**, 371–375.
INGRAHAM, R. C., and WIGGERS, H. C. (1945). *Am. J. Physiol.*, **144**, 505–512.
KJELLMER, I. (1964). *Acta physiol. scand.*, **62**, 31–40.
KROGH, A., LANDIS, E. M., and TURNER, A. H. (1932). *J. clin. Invest.*, **11**, 63–95.
LANDIS, E. M. (1927). *Am. J. Physiol.*, **82**, 217–238.
McMASTER, P. D. (1941). *J. exp. Med.*, **73**, 85–108.
MEYER, B. J., MEYER, A., and GUYTON, A. C. (1968). *Circulation Res.*, **22**, 263–271.
STARLING, E. H. (1896). *J. Physiol., Lond.*, **19**, 312–326.

STERLING, K. (1951). *J. clin. Invest.*, **30**, 1228–1237.
WANG, S., OVERMAN, R. R., FERTIG, J. W., ROOT, W. S., and GREGERSON, M. I. (1947). *Am. J. Physiol.*, **148**, 164–173.
WASSERMAN, K., JOSEPH, J. D., and MAYERSON, H. S. (1956). *Am. J. Physiol.*, **184**, 175–182.
WELLS, H. S., YOUMANS, J. B., and MILLER, D. G., Jr. (1938). *J. clin. Invest.*, **17**, 489–499.

DISCUSSION

Burton: It would be interesting to have a comparable analysis of hydrostatic forces in plants, where there is a far greater spread of values. There is of course the difference that the plant cell wall is rigid and able to sustain a very large pressure difference across it whereas animal cells are deformable and have elasticity.

Guyton: Scholander has compared hydrostatic pressures in animal tissues and plants (Scholander, P. F., Hargens, A. R., and Miller, S. L. [1968]. *Science*, **161**, 321–328). He concludes that the situations are qualitatively the same but about three orders of magnitude different quantitatively. Several thousand mm. Hg negative pressure occur in plants, whereas we find negative pressures of the order of 0 to − 10 mm. Hg in animal interstitial fluid.

Philip: Professor Guyton's Fig. 4 (p. 13) is puzzling at first glance. We see, for example, the "osmotic forces" in the interstitial space assigned two values, − 4 and − 5,400. Evidently this dualism arises from the fact that the reflection coefficients appropriate to the capillary wall are quite different from those for the cell membrane. This seems to lead to some formal difficulties in treating this system as a thermodynamic continuum in the way discussed on p. 41 of my paper. This has proved fruitful in the soil–plant–atmosphere system; but a rather more elaborate formalism along the lines of the thermodynamics of irreversible processes may be needed here.

Burton: Professor Guyton, what exactly is the crucial difference which causes the needle with its drop of fluid to measure what you call the total tissue pressure, and the capsule to measure what you call fluid pressure?

Guyton: It is essentially a matter of time. When a needle is inserted into a tissue and a drop of fluid is injected, the fluid balloons out against the tissues so that the pressure measured is the total tissue pressure. If sufficient time is allowed, the drop will be absorbed, but practically no one using this method ever allows enough time. They may allow 60 seconds but 30 minutes are often needed for even a small volume of fluid to be absorbed. If a needle is left inserted for 30 minutes or more the recorded pressure finally goes negative. Yet each time the tissue moves physically, the pressure goes still further negative as if there were a ball-valve action; therefore the needle method is an unreliable one for measuring normal tissue pressure. If the needle method is used carefully, as in P. D. McMaster's work referred to in my paper ([1941]. *J. exp. Med.*, **73**, 85–108), absorption of fluid into the tissue from the needle can be observed. The difference is really in the grossness of the technique.

Saffman: Do you still measure the same fluid pressure if you use different fluids in the needle?

Guyton: It makes no difference when the capsule technique is used, because osmotic pressure is not involved along the measuring catheter, only hydrostatic pressure. If the fluid in the capsule is entirely changed, the measurement is not affected.

Cumming: Presumably the manometer is filled with liquid right up to the capsule?

Guyton: There is a liquid-filled connexion all the way from the centre of the capsule to the manometer. We frequently pull capsular fluid at a rate of about $0 \cdot 1$ ml./hr. into the catheter until capsular fluid fills the whole manometric system, and we still measure the same negative pressure.

Cumming: Have you made histological studies of the tissues surrounding the capsule after implantation?

Guyton: Yes. It is typical fibrous tissue.

Cumming: Could elastin and fibrin be attached to the capsule and pulling outwards?

Guyton: Even if such tissue did pull outwards, it would make no difference if there are open spaces through the capsule perforations. And we showed that there are open spaces, by demonstrating movement of fluid from one capsule to another.

Caro: What happens to the pressure if you measure it over a long period in a small piece of isolated blood vessel?

Guyton: In order to see whether fluid would be absorbed? I don't know; and I am not sure whether this has been done.

Caro: You have shown that granulation tissue develops when you implant capsules.

Guyton: Yes, but there are other methods for measuring tissue pressure in which you do not get granulation tissue, such as Scholander's method and two other methods that I referred to in my paper.

Floyer: Experiments of ours (unpublished observations) confirm completely Professor Guyton's findings. The following experiment seems to suggest that the negative pressure is not an artefact of the capsule, but is a true reading of extra-vascular tissue pressure. A capsule was implanted into the subcutaneous tissue (we have done this in both rat and man) and was left two or three months before any measurements were made. Capsule pressure was then measured by inserting a fine needle; another needle was placed in the subcutaneous tissue near the capsule. A reading could be obtained from the needle in the tissue only if a small amount of fluid was injected to form a small "bleb". At first the tissue needle pressure recorded was about $+ 3$ mm. Hg, whereas the capsule pressure was $- 4$ to $- 6$ mm. Hg. The tissue needle pressure gradually fell (over about 20 minutes) and seemed to be approaching asymptotically to the level in the capsule, but when it reached about $- 1$ mm. Hg the needle level started to swing wildly and we could not obtain a valid reading below this.

We have also done some studies on the protein content of the fluid in the capsule, both in rats and in two human volunteers. In a group of rats, the intra-capsular pressure and the protein content of the fluid was measured at weekly intervals after insertion of the capsule. One week after implantation the protein content of the fluid was very similar to that of plasma, but after six weeks it had fallen to about one-third of this concentration; the albumen/globulin ratio had increased to about twice that of plasma. Pressure readings followed the same pattern; one week after encapsulation the pressure was positive ($+ 2$ to $+ 3$ mm. Hg) but after six weeks the level had reached a steady value of $- 4$ to $- 6$ mm. Hg. Very similar results were obtained in man.

We have also studied the effect of posture on capsule pressure in man. A capsule was inserted subcutaneously in the abdominal wall about 30 cm. below the level of the heart. We wished to obtain simultaneous readings of capsule pressure and venous pressure at the same level, but as the subjects had no subcutaneous vein near the capsule we used instead an arm vein held at the same level. (This probably gave a higher reading than one would obtain from a vein in the abdomen, on account of the "waterfall" up to the neck and down into the heart.)

When the subject was tilted from the reclining to the erect posture, the capsule pressure fell by 1–2 mm. Hg, although the venous pressure at the level of the capsule rose by 20 mm. Hg. The capsule pressure remained steady even though the subject remained standing for 20 minutes. We would like to study the effect of posture further, and hope to be able to implant a capsule in the leg of a volunteer near a vein in which pressure can be measured.

Burton: Why does the capsule pressure go down as one stands up?

Floyer: I imagine that it is due to reflex vasoconstriction. When one stands up the baroceptor mechanism constricts the subcutaneous arterioles and this lowers the tissue pressure. One also sees a sudden fall in capsule pressure after intravenous injection of noradrenaline; presumably the arterioles constrict and lower the capillary pressure, and hence the tissue pressure.

Davies: What is the effect of the pressure reduction in a capsule implanted into the lung on the interstitial tissue of the lung? Does it cause a steady flow of fluid from the surface of the alveoli into the lung tissue?

Guyton: We presume so, but the answer is strictly theoretical. We have implanted single capsules (ranging from 0·75 cm. to 1·5 cm. in diameter) in the lungs of dogs, and the average pressure for about 30 implants was − 4 mm. Hg. If we eliminate the infected and oedematous capsules, the average recorded pressure was about − 7 or − 8 mm. Hg. In six instances we had beautiful implants with practically no growth of tissue around the capsules, and the pressures were − 12 to − 16 mm. Hg.

Davies: The capsules are obviously very large compared with an alveolus, of which the average diameter in a dog is 100 μm. Does the capsule become wrapped in fibrous tissue?

Guyton: Yes. Even a good implantation in the lungs has 1–1·5 mm. fibrous tissue around it.

Davies: Are you really measuring the interstitial fluid pressure in the lung?

Guyton: Fluids move through the spaces of the fibrous tissues quite readily, and we assume that the fluids in the spaces are in contact with the interstitial spaces in the lungs. (We feel more certain of this with subcutaneous implantations than with intrapulmonary ones.) In the lungs it is possible that we are dealing with fibrous tissue that has bronchiolar rather than pulmonary vasculature because of the tendency for repaired tissues in the lungs to be invaded by bronchiolar blood vessels. Therefore, we are not quite sure what we are dealing with in the lungs, but we do get negative pressure readings.

Davies: If your interpretation is correct for the leg one could argue that the same is true of the lung.

Guyton: One could also expect even more negative interstitial fluid pressure in the lung than elsewhere, because the capillary pressure is lower; this may be why we record lung interstitial fluid pressures as low as − 16 mm. Hg in a few animals. This is much lower than we ever record in other tissues.

Cumming: This would accord with the clinical observations of the resorption of pleural exudates.

West: The relevant capillary pressure in the lung will depend on the part of the lung where you implant the capsule, being lowest at the top and highest at the bottom of the lung. One would expect a difference in interstitial pressure from the top of the lung to the bottom, and we have some indirect evidence of this, based on the distribution of blood flow in excised dog lungs (Hughes, J. M. B., Glazier, J. B., Maloney, J. E., and West, J. B. [1968]. *J. appl. Physiol.*, in press).

The distinction Professor Guyton makes between total tissue pressure and fluid tissue pressure makes good sense for the pressure in the intrapleural space of the lung. I. Setnikar and E. Agostoni ([1962]. *Proc. int. Union Physiol. Sci.*,

2

1, 281–286) pointed out that two pressures can be distinguished there; the mechanical pressure which holds the lung inflated, and the pressure due to the absorption of fluid, the Starling equilibrium pressure. There is evidence that the latter pressure is more negative than the former, just as in systemic tissues the interstitial fluid pressure may be much less than the total tissue pressure. The pressure around the larger blood vessels in the lung—the extra-alveolar vessels—may be thought of in the same way. There is the mechanical pressure which tends to hold open the vessels rather as the static recoil pressure in the intrapleural space holds the lung open, and a more negative interstitial fluid pressure due to the absorption of fluid in the perivascular space.

Guyton: Investigators working in respiratory physiology tend to accept our approach very readily, being already familiar with the same problems in the pleural spaces. We have made a similar analysis for the lung to that for the other tissue spaces of the body (p. 16 and Figs. 6 and 7 of my paper).

Burton: The interstitial fluid space in the normal lung is extremely small, and in such a small reservoir the slightest movement of water changes the osmotic pressure in that space enormously, so that the lung is a very different situation from that of the Starling–Landis hypothesis in the peripheral vessels.

Guyton: I don't think so. Measurements of sodium space indicate an interstitial fluid content of about 20 per cent of the lung mass (Taylor, A. E., Gaar, K., and Guyton, A. C. [1966]. *Am. J. Physiol.*, **211**, 66–70).

Burton: Furthermore, I am not sure that one should assume an equilibrium of the osmotic forces across the alveolus, as you indicate in Fig. 6 (p. 16). There is suggestive but not conclusive evidence that rather than water vapour being lost from the alveoli to the respiratory tract, water is being gained by the tissues from the alveoli. This is based on the study of temperatures down the respiratory tract, which are indices of the amount of evaporation occurring (Armstrong, H. G., Burton, A. C., and Hall, G. E. [1958]. *J. Aviat. Med.*, **29**, 593–597). Your calculation is valid if you assume an equilibrium, but we may not have an exact equilibrium and the lungs may be gaining water from the upper respiratory tract, contrary to the usual textbook statements.

Guyton: Just as Starling's equilibrium in the capillary has to take into account the fluid that becomes lymph, we have to consider the net exchange of fluid in the lung. One can calculate from available data that the amount of non-equilibrium at the peripheral capillary due to lymphatic flow is normally less than $0 \cdot 5$ mm. Hg, so that one can usually ignore it. However, in oedema this factor may be as great as 5 or 6 mm. Hg. Likewise, it is probable that net movement of water through the alveolar membrane is normally insufficient to alter alveolar membrane dynamics significantly. Yet anaesthesiologists have observed severe oedema in patients who breathe supersaturated air.

THEORY OF FLOW AND TRANSPORT PROCESSES IN PORES AND POROUS MEDIA

J. R. PHILIP

CSIRO Division of Plant Industry, Canberra, Australia

FOR the purposes of this interdisciplinary meeting I wear a hat labelled "nine parts fluid-mechanician,† one part physiologist"; and what I shall attempt is to discuss some fluid-mechanical aspects of flow and transport processes in pores and porous media, and to relate these to some concepts of flow and transport of interest in physiology. Demands of rigour, brevity, and interdisciplinary communicability all conflict; and I have chosen here to develop my topic in a qualitative and relatively unmathematical way which may irritate some fluid-mechanicians, but be acceptable to some physiologists.

THE FLOW OF INCOMPRESSIBLE NEWTONIAN FLUIDS

The general equation describing the isothermal flow of an incompressible Newtonian fluid is known in English-speaking countries as the Navier-Stokes equation. Its basic ingredients are, essentially, Newton's Second Law of Motion, supplemented by Newton's hypothesis of fluid friction that the shearing stress is directly proportional to the rate of strain (Newton, 1687)‡. It may be written

$$\partial U/\partial t + (U \cdot \nabla) U = -\nabla \Phi + \nu \nabla^2 U \qquad (1)$$

Here U is the vector flow velocity, t is time, ν is the kinematic viscosity, and Φ is the potential defined by (2):

$$\Phi = P/\rho + \Omega \qquad (2)$$

where P is the fluid pressure, ρ the fluid density, and Ω the potential of the external or "body" forces.

Equation (1) was developed by Navier (1823) and later by Poisson (1831). The subsequent derivation by Saint-Venant (1843) and Stokes (1845) is the one accepted today.

† There is perhaps a place for a term more specific than "rheologist". "Fluid-mechanic" has an ambiguous plural. The slightly archaic "mechanician" (Onions, 1959) is available and avoids ambiguity.

‡ "Resistentiam, quae oritur ex defectu lubricitatis partium Fluidi, caeteris paribus, proportionalem esse velocitati, qua partes Fluidi separantur ab invicem."

In view of incompressibility, equation (1) is supplemented by the continuity requirement

$$\nabla \cdot U = 0 \tag{3}$$

A particular physically realizable flow is then represented by the solution of the system (1), (3) subject to the appropriate (physically realizable) initial and boundary conditions. We return to the matter of the boundary conditions later.

It is useful to recognize a special class of fluid motions, which we shall designate *exactly linear*. For such flows the "inertia terms"

$$(U \cdot \nabla) U \equiv 0 \tag{4}$$

so that equation (1) reduces to the linear form

$$\partial U / \partial t = -\nabla \Phi + \nu \nabla^2 U \tag{5}$$

with a very great simplification in the mathematics. Exactly linear flows include some quite complicated fluid motions (e.g. Taylor, 1923; Kovásznay, 1948), but the only ones which concern us here are steady flows parallel to the generators of cylinders of general (not necessarily singly-connected) cross-section.

We shall be concerned also with what might be termed *conditionally linear* flows, for which the "inertia terms" are, in general, non-zero but are negligibly small relative to the terms on the right of equation (1). It is easily shown that a flow is conditionally linear provided the appropriate Reynolds number, ul/ν, is small enough. Here u and l signify, respectively, a velocity and a length characteristic of the motion. Conditionally linear steady flows (*Stokes flows* in normal usage) thus obey the equation

$$\nu \nabla^2 U = \nabla \Phi \tag{6}$$

it being understood that the Reynolds number of the motion is "small" in an appropriate sense. On the other hand *exactly linear* steady flows obey equation (6) unconditionally.†

The study of Stokes flows seems to be regarded by many fluid-mechanicians as a disreputable practice, if not an outright perversion. One of our colleagues (Saffman, 1967) writes of low Reynolds number hydrodynamics as "a dull, pedestrian subject in which a great deal of work produces little of scientific interest". This poor opinion of Stokes flow studies arises in part from their patent inadequacy in dealing with fluid motions (especially in two dimensions)

---

† There remains, of course, the requirement that the flow be hydrodynamically stable; but this need not detain us in the context of the flows to be discussed here.

around finite obstacles in effectively infinite flow regions. When obstacle and flow region are of comparable dimensions, however, this objection has no substance; and Stokes flows are highly relevant to the problems of pores and porous media which concern us here. I can only hope you find my development of this theme not too pedestrian.

Most treatments of flow and transport processes in pores and porous media are built around Poiseuille's Law and Darcy's Law. It is of some interest to consider the history of these laws and to interpret them in relation to the Navier-Stokes equation.

Poiseuille's Law

Poiseuille's Law for the steady laminar flow of a fluid in a straight circular cylindrical tube may be written

$$q = -\frac{\pi a^4}{8\nu}\frac{d\Phi}{dx} \tag{7}$$

where q is the flux, a is the radius of the tube, and $d\Phi/dx$ is the potential gradient.

Equation (7) (with the quantity $\pi/8\nu$ treated simply as a constant) was proposed as an experimentally based empirical law by the engineer Hagen (1839) and independently by the physiologist Poiseuille (1840). A well-known physiology reference work states that Poiseuille's Law "underlies the science of hydrodynamics". This, perhaps, puts the cart before the horse, but much credit is due to Poiseuille for the precision of his experiments.

The Poiseuille flow is, of course, exactly linear and obeys equation (6). The story of the recognition of (7) as the appropriate solution of (6) is an instructive example of the interplay of theory and experiment. The application of equations (1), (3) (or more specifically (6), (3)) to a particular steady flow requires knowledge of the appropriate boundary conditions. Ignorance of the conditions at the solid–fluid interface delayed for some decades the establishment of the proper connexion between the general theoretical studies of Navier and his successors and the experimental work of Hagen and Poiseuille. In 1845 Stokes showed that a "no-slip" condition at the tube wall gave the Poiseuille flow as the appropriate solution of (1), (3) (or (6), (3)). He, however, treated the "no-slip" hypothesis as one of several possibilities, and was unaware of the work of Hagen and Poiseuille. It was left to the physiologist Jacobson (1860) to make the necessary connexion. He perceived that equation (7), derived by Neumann through a calculation similar to that of Stokes, was identical with Poiseuille's experimental law, and that this identity confirmed the "no-slip" hypothesis.

Darcy's Law

From his experiments on water flow through filter beds, Darcy (1856) proposed the law

$$Q = kA(h + L)/L$$

with Q the discharge rate through the filter, A its area, L its thickness, h the water depth over the filter, and k "un coefficient dépendant de la nature du sable". It is convenient here to rewrite this in the form

$$V = p\bar{U} = -\frac{K}{\nu}\nabla\bar{\Phi} \qquad (8)$$

V is the *macroscopic* vector flow velocity; p is the porosity (fractional pore volume) of the medium; $\bar{U}$ is the vector flow velocity U (cf. equations (1) and (6)) averaged over a fluid volume large compared with that of individual pores; $\bar{\Phi}$ is an average of the potential Φ (cf. equations (1) and (6)) over the same volume. K, the permeability, is a characteristic of the geometry of the medium and has the dimensions $(\text{length})^2$. K is a scalar for an isotropic medium and a second order tensor for anisotropic media.†

In general, the details of the internal geometry of a porous medium are random and unknown. The Navier-Stokes equation, nevertheless, leads to a definite assertion about flow through the medium: namely that, provided the inertia terms are negligible (and they demonstrably are, in a vast array of applications), the flow is everywhere directly proportional to the applied potential difference. A statistical requirement then completes the theoretical basis of Darcy's Law: the medium must be "sufficiently homogeneous" on the scale of the averaging volume (the "Darcy scale") for the quantities $\bar{U}$ and $\bar{\Phi}$ to exist (cf. Philip, 1968a).

Recognition of the connexion between Darcy's Law and the Navier-Stokes equation developed surprisingly late. The first correct discussion of the deviations from Darcy's Law at Reynolds numbers of order 1 to 10, due to the inertia terms, was apparently that of the Swedish engineer, Lindquist (1933). As recently as ten years ago it was necessary to complain (Philip, 1958a) that the most recent textbooks still subscribed to a wholly erroneous explanation involving turbulence.

General understanding of the mechanics of fluid flow in porous media has,

---

† An "operational" view of K may interest fluid-mechanicians. Integration of (6) over the averaging volume and division by (8) gives

$$\frac{K}{p} = -\frac{\bar{U}}{\overline{\nabla^2 U}}$$

which may be interpreted as minus a reciprocal U-weighted mean Laplacian.

perhaps, been impeded by the formal resemblance between Poiseuille's Law
(7) and Darcy's Law (8). Equation (7) refers to an exactly linear flow in a
special and precise geometry, whereas equation (8) applies to a conditionally
linear (Stokes) flow in a generally unknown geometry exhibiting certain
statistical regularities; but both state that a macroscopic flow velocity is
proportional to a macroscopic pressure gradient. This superficial similarity
has led many people to carry over into their mental picture of flow and transport in porous media notions that really apply only to Poiseuille flow (or to
exactly linear flows in the generalized cylinder).

We may get a first intimation of the difference in character between tube
flow and medium flow by considering the fate of a small parcel of fluid moving
through each system. In the tube the parcel possesses a constant linear velocity
throughout, while in the medium it is subject to accelerations which continuously change both the magnitude and direction of its velocity. This vital
difference finds quantitative expression in the 1,000 to 1 ratio of the critical
Reynolds numbers for failure of linearity of the two systems (Muskat, 1937;
Goldstein, 1938). In the following section we discuss a particular Stokes flow
which illustrates further aspects of the character of flow in porous media on
the microscopic scale.

DIVERGENT-CONVERGENT FLOW IN PORES

In many media we may identify the individual pores as the volumes contained
between consecutive constrictions in the flow path; the distance between
constrictions (i.e. the pore length) is commonly of the same magnitude as the
transverse dimensions of the pore. Fluid flow in such media is characterized
by successive sharp divergences and convergences on the scale of the individual
pore.

A simple but informative model of divergent-convergent flows of this
character is provided by the Stokes flow in a plane region bounded by a
circular wall from a point source in the wall to a point sink which is diametrically opposite.

We take the "pore" radius as the unit of length and (r, θ) as polar coordinates
with origin at the "pore" centre. Then, for a flux of magnitude 2 from a source
at $(1, \pi)$ to a sink at $(1, 0)$, the appropriate solution of equations (6) and (3) is

$$\Psi = \frac{2}{\pi}\left[\frac{(1 - r^4)r\sin\theta}{1 - 2r^2\cos 2\theta + r^4} + \tan^{-1}\frac{2r\sin\theta}{1 - r^2}\right] \tag{9}$$

Ψ is the stream function defined by

$$u = \partial\Psi/\partial y, \qquad v = -\partial\Psi/\partial x$$

with (u,v) the components of flow velocity in the directions of rectangular Cartesian coordinates (x, y), x being taken parallel to $\theta = 0$. Lord Rayleigh (1893) first obtained (9). He did not, however, explore the physical implications beyond some remarks on Ψ.

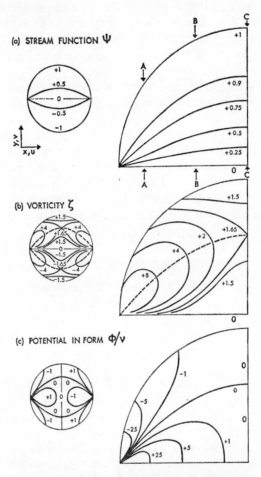

Fig. 1. Plane Stokes flow across a circular pore from a point source in the wall to a diametrically opposed point sink. (*a*) The stream function Ψ. Curves of constant Ψ are streamlines. Flow is left to right. (*b*) The vorticity ζ. (*c*) The potential in the form Φ/ν. The quarter-circles show detail. The small full circles show symmetries and antisymmetries for whole pore. Sections AA, BB, CC indicate locations of velocity profiles in Fig. 2.

Fig. 1*a* shows the streamlines, which are lines of constant Ψ. Fig. 1*b* depicts the distribution of the vorticity ζ, defined by

$$\zeta = \partial v/\partial x - \partial u/\partial y = -\nabla^2 \Psi$$

In the present context, ζ is closely related to the shearing stress along the streamline. Fig. 1*c* shows the distribution of potential in the form Φ/ν. The datum of Φ is chosen such that its mean value in the pore is zero. Fig. 2

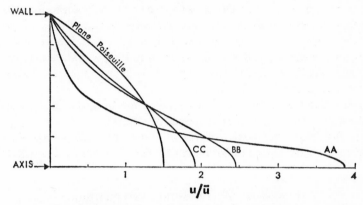

FIG. 2. Plane Stokes flow across a circular pore from a point source in the wall to a diametrically opposed point sink. Velocity profiles in the form $u/\bar{u}$. u is the component of velocity in the source–sink direction; $\bar{u}$ is the mean value of u over the cross-section. Letters on each profile identify appropriate section on Fig. 1(*a*). Profile for plane Poiseuille flow shown for comparison.

compares the shape of various profiles of u across the pore with the Poiseuille parabolic velocity distribution.†

This example affords a vivid picture of the character of divergent-convergent flow in the individual pore. We notice in particular:

(*i*) The maximum vorticity and shearing stress occur away from the pore wall (in contrast to Poiseuille flow where these quantities are maximal at the wall).

† It follows from (9) that

$$\zeta = \frac{16}{\pi} \frac{r \sin \theta[1 + 2r^2 - r^4(2\cos 2\theta + 1)]}{[1 - 2r^2\cos 2\theta + r^4]^2}$$

$$\frac{\Phi}{\nu} = -\frac{16}{\pi} \frac{r \cos \theta[1 - 2r^2 + r^4(2\cos 2\theta - 1)]}{[1 - 2r^2\cos 2\theta + r^4]^2}$$

$$u = \frac{2}{\pi} \frac{(1 - r^2)[3 + r^2(1 - 6\cos 2\theta) + r^4(1 - 2\cos 2\theta + 2\cos 4\theta) + r^6]}{[1 - 2r^2\cos 2\theta + r^4]^2}$$

These results were used to construct Figs. 1*b*, 1*c* and 2.

2*

(*ii*) There is no one-to-one relation between potential gradient and flow velocity: the potential gradient is, in fact, *reversed* in the outer region of the pore.

(*iii*) The velocity profiles deviate strongly from the Poiseuille parabolic profile (and exhibit points of inflexion related to the maxima of ζ and shearing stress away from the wall).

It must be recognized that the somewhat startling nature of Figs. 1*b* and *c* arises, in part, from the singularities associated with the point source and sink. It appears, however, that a more realistic representation of the entrance and exit flows would leave us with the same qualitative picture *in the broader parts of the pore*: velocity profiles with points of inflexion, and, associated with these, maxima of vorticity and shearing stress away from the walls and reversal of potential gradients near the walls.

It is clear that the notion that viscous flow in porous media takes place down a gradient of potential must be abandoned *on the microscopic scale.*† Thermo-dynamically based treatments of viscous flow and transport processes in porous media thus require rather more care than they sometimes receive.

TRANSPORT BY CONVECTION AND DIFFUSION

The transport by convection and diffusion of a solute (or of a dynamically neutral suspension or component of a gas mixture) is described by the equation

$$\frac{\partial\theta}{\partial t} + U\cdot\nabla\theta = D\nabla^2\theta \tag{10}$$

θ is the concentration of the transported material and D is the molecular (or Brownian) diffusivity, which, for simplicity, we take to be independent of θ.‡

The interactions between convection (which enters (10) through the term $U\cdot\nabla\theta$) and diffusion (the term $D\nabla^2\theta$) are complicated and subtle. Their significance for transport processes in pores and porous media have not yet, I think, been explored fully. Here we shall consider certain simple systems which offer some insights into the general character of convection-diffusion interactions.

† This is, of course, implicit in equation (6).

‡ The similarity of form of equations (1) and (10) will be noted. The Navier-Stokes equation can be interpreted as describing the convection and diffusion of three scalar components of momentum concentration. The term $-\nabla\Phi$ of (1) is analogous to the source strength term which appears in a slight generalization of (10).

Dispersion by convection and diffusion during Poiseuille flow

Fig. 3*a* shows schematically, for steady Poiseuille flow in a circular tube, the progressive displacement, relative to their centre of gravity, of marked fluid particles initially in a plane normal to the tube axis. This is simply an expression of the parabolic velocity profile. If convection alone were to

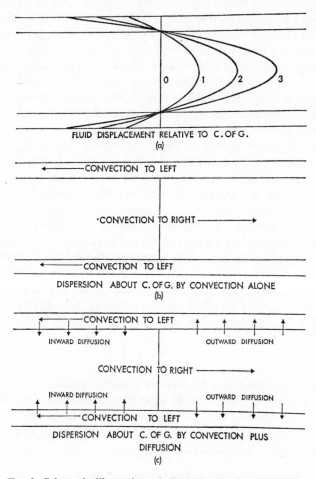

FIG. 3. Schematic illustration of dispersion by convection plus diffusion during Poiseuille flow in a circular tube. (*a*) The displacement, relative to their centre of gravity, of fluid particles initially in plane 0. 1, 2, 3 denote their positions after successive time-intervals. (*b*) The pattern of dispersion about the centre of gravity by convection alone. (*c*) The pattern of dispersion about centre of gravity by convection plus diffusion.

operate (i.e. in the absence of diffusion) the dispersion about the centre of gravity would consist of transport downstream in the central core and of transport upstream in the outer zone adjoining the wall (see Fig. 3b). Evidently the longitudinal spread of the dispersion would, in this case, be proportional to the time since the initial state.

Molecular diffusion modifies the longitudinal dispersion process profoundly. Fig. 3c gives a simplified picture of this. The convective motion sets up radial concentration gradients in the tube which, in a gross sense, produce diffusive transport *outward* downstream of the centre of gravity and *inward* transport in the upstream region. In both regions diffusion tends to move material into parts of the cross-section where the convective motion is directed back towards the centre of gravity. It is evident that, in this system, *molecular diffusion inhibits longitudinal dispersion*; and we shall expect that the larger the diffusivity, the less the dispersion. Of course, we shall expect also that the dispersion will be very much greater than it would be through molecular diffusion alone (i.e. if the convection produced by the radial variation of velocity in the tube were not taken into account).

Experiment and detailed analysis bear out these expectations. Although Westhaver (1947) previously obtained similar results in connexion with an electrochemical problem, Sir Geoffrey Taylor (1953, 1954) seems to have been the first to appreciate the significance of this process. He concluded that, for large enough times after its release, the longitudinal dispersal of a slug of marked fluid about its centre of gravity (as indicated by mean concentration in the cross-section) is describable as diffusion in the longitudinal direction† with diffusivity $\varkappa = a^2 \bar{U}^2/48D$. Here $\bar{U}$ is the mean flow velocity. Aris (1956) developed the more precise result

$$\varkappa = D + \frac{a^2 \bar{U}^2}{48D} \tag{11}$$

Carrier (1956) and Philip (1963) showed that the "diffusion" representation of this dispersion process is exactly equivalent to retaining only the leading term of an eigenfunction expansion of the appropriate solution of (10); and that (11) is valid only for aperiodic systems. For periodic systems $\varkappa$ is, in general, a complex function of frequency.

Dispersion by convection and diffusion in porous media

The analogous process of transport in porous media is similarly dominated by interaction between convection along the streamlines and diffusion across

---

† This result implies that the spread is proportional to (time)$^{1/2}$. Cf. dispersion by convection alone, with the spread proportional to time.

them; but there are important differences in detail, two of which we notice here:

(*i*) The dispersive spread *by convection alone* increases asymptotically as (time)$^{1/2}$ in the random geometry of a porous medium. In tubes the spread is directly proportional to time, as we have remarked above.

(*ii*) Diffusion transverse to the streamlines is not canalized in porous media by continuous walls, as it is in tubes. The intensity of longitudinal dispersal is consequently reduced.

Development of an adequate quantitative theory of transport of solutes in porous media remains, in my opinion, a challenging problem for fluid-mechanicians. Many attempts have been made to set up the needed theory, not all of them well-founded physically. The studies of the problem by Professor Saffman (1959, 1960) are noteworthy, and his current assessment of the field will be of interest.

It appears, both from the character of the physical processes and from the growing body of experimental data, that dispersion during Darcy flow in porous media is (at least asymptotically) describable on the Darcy scale as diffusion with the apparent diffusivity a tensor† function of the Péclet number Vl/D (l, a characteristic pore dimension). The effect is by no means trivial, in that the apparent diffusivities are typically observed to exceed D by as much as a thousandfold.

Reversible and irreversible components of transport

I cannot leave the topic of convection-diffusion interaction without referring to two "unmixing demonstrations", made by the petroleum engineer Heller (1960, 1961), which give a vivid picture of the reversible and irreversible components of transport by convection and diffusion.

The first is illustrated by Fig. 4. The experiment is performed in an apparatus made up of two concentric cylinders, the outer one fixed and the inner free to rotate, with water filling the annular space between them. A radial plane of the water is marked with dye. The inner cylinder is then turned slowly clockwise for 24 revolutions. The dye appears to be mixed evenly through the water. The inner cylinder is then slowly rotated anti-clockwise for 24 revolutions, so that the net convective movement is returned to exactly zero. The dye then appears to have become unmixed, the dispersion being restricted to a small sector of the annulus. Examination under a microscope, at the end of the clockwise rotations, reveals that the dye is, in fact, concentrated in a

† It will be understood that longitudinal and transverse dispersion may be quite different in magnitude.

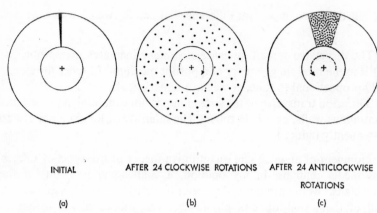

INITIAL   AFTER 24 CLOCKWISE ROTATIONS   AFTER 24 ANTICLOCKWISE

ROTATIONS

(a)   (b)   (c)

FIG. 4. Schematic illustration of Heller's unmixing demonstration for circular
Couette flow. See text for details.

24-turn spiral running from the inner to the outer cylinder; so that what seems
macroscopically to be irreversible mixing turns out to be largely the reversible
outcome of complicated convective transport. Finally, we note that the
circumferential dispersion at the instant when the net convection is returned
to zero is very much greater than it would have been in the same time-period
with the system left at rest.

We have thus the following schema:

$$\text{Convection alone} \;\rightarrow\; \text{Reversible transport, } X_r$$
$$\text{Diffusion alone} \;\rightarrow\; \text{Irreversible transport, } X_i$$
$$\text{Convection + diffusion} \;\rightarrow\; \text{Reversible transport + irreversible}$$
$$\text{transport, } X_r + X_i^*$$

In general, X_i^* differs from X_i, depending not only on diffusion, but also on
the convection history.

Heller's second unmixing demonstration (Fig. 5) illustrates this schema for
porous medium flow. Heller constructed a medium of a transparent mineral
and used as fluid a transparent liquid with the same refractive index. The
experiment consists of injecting a small quantity of dye at a point in the medium.
A slow flow to the right is then induced. The dye is seen to disperse into a
growing ellipsoidal cloud moving with the flow. After a suitable time-interval
the flow is reversed and the net convection slowly returned to zero. During the
return flow the dye moves back to the left and grows smaller, though, of course,
it does not shrink to the dimensions of the initial marker. At the end of the
experiment the cloud of dye is centred on the point of injection: it is much
larger than it would have been if produced by diffusion alone in the same

time-interval, and it is distorted from the (roughly) spherical shape it would have assumed in the absence of convection.

These considerations have consequences for transport of solutes or gases by periodic or pulsating flow systems in pores and porous media which are possibly of importance in physiology. A periodic flow system with zero *net* convection may produce dispersion very greatly in excess of that due to diffusion alone. Interest in processes of this type has developed recently

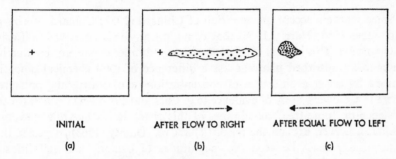

INITIAL   AFTER FLOW TO RIGHT   AFTER EQUAL FLOW TO LEFT

(a)   (b)   (c)

FIG. 5. Schematic illustration of Heller's unmixing demonstration for porous medium flow. See text for details.

amongst soil physicists; a preliminary study of transport during sinusoidal flow in circular tubes has been made by Farrell and Larsen (1968).

In the space remaining, I consider very briefly some aspects of physiological flow and transport which are connected (though perhaps somewhat loosely) with the processes discussed above, and with each other.

THE MECHANICS OF OSMOTIC TRANSFER

The passage of water through semi-permeable, membrane-like barriers is of great interest in physiology. Two kinds of experiments have been commonly made: flow experiments with an osmotically induced potential difference (e.g. Lucké, Hartline and McCutcheon, 1931; Collander and Bärland, 1933; Ordin and Bonner, 1956; Sidel and Solomon, 1957), and self-diffusion experiments using isotopically labelled water (e.g. Hevesy, Hofer and Krogh, 1935; Buffel, 1952; Ordin and Bonner, 1956; Paganelli and Solomon, 1957; Nevis, 1958). The interpretation of these experiments, in so far as they shed light on the flow mechanism and on membrane structure, seems to have been a matter of some confusion and disagreement.

Certain conceptual difficulties have arisen in connexion with the following facts which emerge from these, and related, experiments:

(*i*) A hydrostatic pressure difference and an equal osmotic pressure difference produce the same flow through a semi-permeable membrane† (e.g. Mauro, 1957; Robbins and Mauro, 1960).

(ii) The flow produced by a difference in total chemical potential (or activity) of osmotic or mechanical origin may differ from (and can be much greater than) the self-diffusive transfer produced by an equal potential difference arising from an isotopic concentration difference (e.g. Prescott and Zeuthen, 1953; Durbin, Frank and Solomon, 1956).

Some workers accept the assertion of Chinard (1952; Chinard, Vosburgh and Enns, 1955; Harris, 1956) that osmotic transfer is necessarily diffusive in character. This view is consistent with membranes capable of conducting water in an adsorbed phase across a difference of total chemical potential (caused by either a difference of concentration or of hydrostatic pressure). There is a growing body of evidence (e.g. Cass and Finkelstein, 1967) for the existence of "pore-free" membranes of this character. Chinard's viewpoint cannot, however, explain the result (ii) above. Dainty (1963) suggested that some discrepancies between the magnitudes of osmotic and self-diffusive transfer have arisen from "unstirred layers" (i.e. significant diffusive resistances outside the membrane). The discrepancies appear to be too large and too widespread, however, for them to be all explained in this way.

On the other hand, the result (ii) is consistent with the view (Kuhn, 1951; Ussing, 1952; Koefoed-Johnsen and Ussing, 1953; Pappenheimer, 1953; Renkin, 1954; Garby, 1955; Durbin, Frank and Solomon, 1956; Philip, 1958b; Ray, 1960; Solomon, 1960; Landis and Pappenheimer, 1963) that osmotic transfer can take the form of a pressure-induced "bulk flow" (i.e. viscous flow of liquid water, with some reservations for very narrow pores). This viewpoint seems to be generally defensible, though I believe that some of its exponents have not been justified in their quantitative use of naive and unsatisfactory models of flow and transport.

A question which has puzzled many people is how the concentration difference across a semi-permeable membrane could induce bulk flow, when there is no measurable pressure difference across it. The following explanation is essentially that of Mauro (1960), who acknowledged his debt to Schlögl (1955).

The total chemical potential across a semi-permeable membrane separating pure water and a solution (at the same hydrostatic pressure) must vary continuously across the membrane (Fig. 6). At each point in the system the total potential will be made up of a contribution due to the water concentration and a contribution due to the hydrostatic pressure. Water is effectively

† As well as being an experimental result, this is, of course, thermodynamically necessary.

incompressible, so that the contributions are independent of each other. Now, if the mechanism of semi-permeability is the total exclusion of solute from the pores of the membrane, then they can contain water only; so that the required decrease in total potential along a pore is realized through a pressure decrease. It follows that a pressure difference is sustained by the interface, at the pore exit, between the pure water phase and the solution phase. This appears to be essentially similar to other interfacial pressure differences, so that a kinetic explanation offers no serious conceptual difficulties.

The attempt by Ray (1960) 'to' develop this 'picture 'in more explicit detail seems open to several basic objections. He replaces the interface by an exit region of length equal to the pore radius, and sets up flow equations for both the exit region and the remainder of the pore. His equation for the exit region allows for diffusive transfer of water but ignores the (negative) hydrodynamic

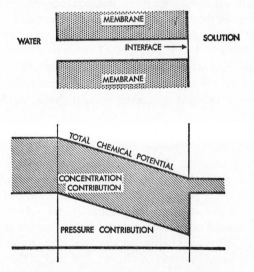

FIG. 6. Schematic illustration of osmotic transfer.

Upper figure shows a pore of a semi-permeable membrane interposed between pure water and an aqueous solution of a solute which is excluded from the membrane. There is no hydrostatic pressure difference across the membrane.

Lower figure shows, for this system, the profiles of total chemical potential and of the concentration and pressure contributions to this potential.

contribution to flow due to the very steep reverse pressure gradient. When this is included in the obvious way, the "hydrodynamic" terms turn out to be eliminable between the two flow equations, and one is left with purely diffusive transfer. This paradox seems to be an artifact of replacing the interface (which is properly treated as singular in macroscopic models of this type) by a specific model of transport over a finite region. I draw attention to these difficulties because the notion of osmotic transfer as a joint diffusion-viscous flow process, as developed in some important reviews (Dainty, 1963; Landis and Pappenheimer, 1963), involves Ray's proposal.

THE INFERENCE OF PORE PROPERTIES FROM FLOW AND TRANSPORT STUDIES

Modern studies of the structure of water (e.g. Lennard-Jones and Pople, 1951; Pople, 1951; Barker, 1963; Whalley, 1967) tend to favour the "uniformist" view that liquid water contains no special ice-like regions or long-range force fields. It would seem, in consequence, that water of normal properties (at least in the absence of very large molecules in solution) would exist in pores of widths as small as (say) tens of molecular diameters, and should move essentially by viscous flow of the type discussed in the earlier parts of this paper. As molecular numbers in the flow cross-section decrease, the continuum description of the process must become less precise; but it seems reasonable to suppose that, even then, it should retain some validity in a statistical sense.

I have devoted most of this paper to the discussion of viscous flow in pores and porous media, and to transport by viscous flow plus molecular diffusion in such systems. I have felt that it is useful for physiologists to appreciate that viscous flow is not necessarily Poiseuille flow, and that transport can be very much more complicated than a simple superposition of a mass flow term and a diffusion term. Unfortunately, the various approaches by the "bulk flow" school of physiologists to the estimation of pore geometry by flow and transport studies (which we shall not enumerate) do seem to have used unjustifiably simple models of viscous flow and of flow-diffusion interactions. It is doubtful if much reliance can be put on quantitative conclusions about pore dimensions made in this way.

THERMODYNAMICS AND THE TREATMENT OF TRANSFER IN HETEROGENEOUS SYSTEMS

I conclude with a brief remark on the formal problem of the macroscopic analysis of transfer in heterogeneous systems made up of a diversity of structures, with the transfer mechanism possibly differing in different parts of the system. This has, perhaps, been taken furthest in plant physiology, where the whole complex of water movement through the soil, the plant, and the atmosphere has been treated as transfer down a gradient of total potential of water in a thermodynamic continuum (Gradmann, 1928; van den Honert, 1948; Philip, 1957, 1966). The formalism is capable of incorporating into the one model the processes of viscous flow and vapour diffusion under capillarity and gravity in the soil, viscous flow in conducting organs and osmotic transfer across membranes in the plant, vapour (molecular) diffusion in the substomatal cavities, and both molecular and turbulent diffusion in the atmosphere.

In regions containing semi-permeable barriers, the appropriate total potential is made up of both a pressure component which is mechanical in character ("turgor pressure" and "tissue tension" in plant physiology; "interstitial" and "tissue pressure" in animal physiology) and a concentration component which is osmotic in character. (There may also be a gravitational component, which need not detain us here.) Animal physiologists call this "Starling's hypothesis" (Starling, 1896); plant physiologists refer to the "Höfler diagram" (Höfler, 1920), a graphical representation of the variation of the total potential, and its components, with cell volume or water content.

So far as transfer through tissue is concerned, a formalism first developed specifically in an analysis of the propagation of osmotic and turgor change through cell aggregations (Philip, 1958b) appears relevant. We give here, in very condensed form, a slight generalization of this approach. If both mechanical and osmotic components of $\overline{\Phi}$ (the total potential, averaged over a suitable volume in deference to our recognition of the failure of simple flow-potential gradient relations on the microscopic scale) are known, unique functions of the volumetric moisture content, ϑ, and the hydraulic conductivity of the tissue, k (possibly also a function of ϑ) is also known, the flow process can be shown to obey a concentration-dependent diffusion equation in material coordinate space. (By this we mean that the coordinates are fixed relative to the solid constituents of the tissue.) In one dimension the equation is of the form

$$\frac{\partial \vartheta}{\partial t} = \frac{\partial}{\partial m}\left[D \frac{\partial \vartheta}{\partial m}\right] \tag{12}$$

m is the material coordinate defined by the equation

$$m = \int^{x}(1 - \vartheta)\, dx$$

and the diffusivity D is the function of ϑ given by

$$D = (1 - \vartheta)^{3}\, k\, d\overline{\Phi}/d\vartheta \tag{13}$$

(See Philip, 1968b and Smiles and Rosenthal, 1968.) Methods of solving equations of the form (12) have been developed in some detail for soil systems (Philip, 1968a). Although processes of this type in three dimensions involve some unresolved difficulties, the approach may have relevance to the study of transient flow problems such as those occurring in the experiments of Guyton (1963; 1965; Guyton, Scheel and Murphree, 1966; Guyton et al., 1966).

SUMMARY

The mechanics of the viscous flow of Newtonian fluids through pores and porous media is reviewed. The relation between the general Navier-Stokes formulation and the empirical "laws" of Poiseuille and Darcy are developed. Whereas Poiseuille's Law represents an exactly linear solution of the Navier-Stokes equation, the much more general Darcy's Law is an expression of (i) linearity of the Navier-Stokes equation at small Reynolds number, and (ii) statistical homogeneity of the medium. It should be recognized that Darcy's Law connects a flow velocity averaged "on the Darcy scale" (i.e. over a volume large compared with that of the individual pore) with the gradient of a potential averaged on the same scale. Darcy's Law says nothing about potentials and velocities on the microscopic scale; and, in fact, *on this scale* the notion that viscous flow in porous media takes place down a gradient of potential is demonstrably wrong.

Complicated and subtle interactions of convection and diffusion may operate during solute transport by viscous flow in porous media. The reversible and irreversible aspects of transport are illustrated by two "unmixing demonstrations" due to Heller.

Some related physiological topics are discussed:

(i) The hydrodynamic explanation of osmotic transfer is presented; the basic difficulties of a too specific model due to Ray are indicated.

(ii) It is suggested that physiological estimates of pore geometry using oversimplified models of flow and transport may be in some doubt.

(iii) There are prospects of developing a diffusion formulation of the transient behaviour which follows a pressure change in tissue.

REFERENCES

ARIS, R. (1956). *Proc. R. Soc. A*, **235**, 67–77.
BARKER, J. A. (1963). *A. Rev. phys. Chem.*, **14**, 229–250.
BUFFEL, K. (1952). *Meded. K. vlaam. Acad. Wetenschap., België*, **14**, No. 7.
CARRIER, G. F. (1956). *Q. appl. Math.*, **14**, 108–112.
CASS, A., and FINKELSTEIN, A. (1967). *J. gen. Physiol.*, **50**, 1765–1784.

CHINARD, F. P. (1952). *Am. J. Physiol.*, **171**, 578–586.

CHINARD, F. P., VOSBURGH, G. J., and ENNS, T. (1955). *Am. J. Physiol.*, **183**, 221–234.

COLLANDER, R., and BÄRLAND, H. (1933). *Acta bot. fenn.*, **11**, 1–114.

DAINTY, J. (1963). *Adv. bot. Res.*, **1**, 279–326.

DARCY, H. P. G. (1856). *Les Fontaines publiques de la Ville de Dijon.* Paris: Victor Dalmont.

DURBIN, R. P., FRANK, H., and SOLOMON, A. K. (1956). *J. gen. Physiol.*, **39**, 535–551.

FARRELL, D. A., and LARSEN, W. E. (1968). *Proc. 6th int. Congr. Soil Sci.*, Adelaide, **1**, 173–184.

GARBY, L. (1955). *Acta physiol. scand.*, **35**, 88–92.

GOLDSTEIN, S. (ed.) (1938). *Modern Developments in Fluid Mechanics*, vol. 1, p. 319. Oxford: Clarendon Press.

GRADMANN, H. (1928). *Jb. wiss. Bot.*, **69**, 1–100.

GUYTON, A. C. (1963). *Circulation Res.*, **12**, 399–414.

GUYTON, A. C. (1965). *Circulation Res.*, **16**, 452–460.

GUYTON, A. C., PRATHER, J., SCHEEL, K., and McGEHEE, J. (1966). *Circulation Res.*, **19**, 1022–1030.

GUYTON, A. C., SCHEEL, K., and MURPHREE, D. (1966). *Circulation Res.*, **19**, 412–419.

HAGEN, G. (1839). *Poggendorfs Annln Phys.*, **46**, 423–442.

HARRIS, E. J. (1956). *Transport and Accumulation in Biological Systems*, p. 38. London: Butterworths.

HELLER, J. P. (1960). *Am. J. Phys.*, **28**, 348–353.

HELLER, J. P. (1961). Personal communication.

HEVESY, G., HOFER, E., and KROGH, A. (1935). *Skand. Arch. Physiol.*, **72**, 199–214.

HÖFLER, K. (1920). *Ber. dt. bot. Ges.*, **38**, 288–298.

HONERT, T. H. VAN DEN (1948). *Discuss. Faraday Soc.*, **3**, 146–153.

JACOBSON, H. (1860). *Arch. Anat. Physiol.*, 80–112.

KOEFOED-JOHNSEN, V., and USSING, H. H. (1953). *Acta physiol. scand.*, **28**, 60–76.

KOVÁSZNAY, L. S. G. (1948). *Proc. Camb. phil. Soc. math. phys. Sci.*, **44**, 58–62.

KUHN, W. (1951). *Z. Elektrochem.*, **55**, 207–217.

LANDIS, E. M., and PAPPENHEIMER, J. R. (1963). In *Handbook of Physiology, Section 2: Circulation*, vol. II, pp. 961–1033, ed. Hamilton, W. F. and Dow, P. Washington, D.C.: American Physiological Society.

LENNARD-JONES, J. E., and POPLE, J. A. (1951). *Proc. R. Soc. A*, **205**, 155–162.

LINDQUIST, E. (1933). *Proc. 1er. Congr. grands Barrages*, Stockholm, **5**, 81–101.

LUCKÉ, B., HARTLINE, H. K., and McCUTCHEON, M. (1931). *J. gen. Physiol.*, **14**, 405–419.

MAURO, A. (1957). *Science*, **126**, 252–253.

MAURO, A. (1960). *Circulation*, **21**, 845–854.

MUSKAT, M. (1937). *The Flow of Homogeneous Fluids Through Porous Media*, p. 56. New York: McGraw-Hill.

NAVIER, C. L. M. H. (1823). *Mém. Acad. r. Sci. Lett. Belg.*, **6**, 389–416.

NEVIS, A. H. (1958). *J. gen. Physiol.*, **41**, 927–958.

NEWTON, I. (1687). *Philosophiae naturalis Principia mathematica*, p. 373. London: Royal Society.

ONIONS, C. T. (Ed.) (1959). *The Shorter Oxford English Dictionary*, 3rd. edn., p. 1225, Oxford: Clarendon Press.

ORDIN, L., and BONNER, J. (1956). *Pl. Physiol.*, **31**, 53–57.

PAGANELLI, C. V., and SOLOMON, A. K. (1957). *J. gen. Physiol.*, **41**, 259–277.
PAPPENHEIMER, J. R. (1953). *Physiol. Rev.*, **33**, 387–423.
PHILIP, J. R. (1957). *Proc. 3rd int. Congr. Irrig. Drainage*, 8.125–8.154.
PHILIP, J. R. (1958a). *Highway Res. Board, Wash., Special Report* **40**, 147–163.
PHILIP, J. R. (1958b). *Pl. Physiol.*, **33**, 271–274.
PHILIP, J. R. (1963). *Aust. J. Phys.*, **16**, 287–299, 300–310.
PHILIP, J. R. (1966). *A. Rev. Pl. Physiol.*, **17**, 245–268.
PHILIP, J. R. (1968a). *Adv. Hydroscience*, **5**, 215–296.
PHILIP, J. R. (1968b). *Aust. J. Soil Res.*, **6**, 249–267.
POISEUILLE, J. L. M. (1840). *C. r. hebd. Séanc. Acad. Sci., Paris*, **11**, 961–967, 1041–
    1048; **12**, 112–115.
POISSON, S. D. (1831). *J. Éc. polytech.*, **13**, 139–166.
POPLE, J. A. (1951). *Proc. R. Soc. A*, **205**, 163–178.
PRESCOTT, D. M., and ZEUTHEN, E. (1953). *Acta physiol. scand.*, **28**, 77–94.
RAY, P. M. (1960). *Pl. Physiol.*, **35**, 783–795.
RAYLEIGH, Lord (1893). *Phil. Mag.*, Ser. 5, **36**, 354–372.
RENKIN, E. M. (1954). *J. gen. Physiol.*, **38**, 225–243.
ROBBINS, E., and MAURO, A. (1960). *J. gen. Physiol.*, **43**, 523–532.
SAFFMAN, P. G. (1959). *J. Fluid Mech.*, **6**, 321–349.
SAFFMAN, P. G. (1960). *J. Fluid Mech.*, **7**, 194–208.
SAFFMAN, P. G. (1967). *J. Fluid Mech.*, **28**, 826–828.
SAINT-VENANT, B. DE (1843). *C. r. hebd. Séanc. Acad. Sci., Paris*, **17**, 1240–1242.
SCHLÖGL, R. (1955). *Z. phys. Chem.*, **3**, 73–102.
SIDEL, W. V., and SOLOMON, A. K. (1957). *J. gen. Physiol.*, **41**, 243–257.
SMILES, D. E., and ROSENTHAL, M. J. (1968). *Aust. J. Soil Res.*, **6**, 237–248.
SOLOMON, A. K. (1960). *J. gen. Physiol.*, **43**, Suppl., 1–15.
STARLING, E. H. (1896). *J. Physiol., Lond.*, **24**, 317–330.
STOKES, C. G. (1845). *Trans. Camb. phil. Soc.*, **8**, 287–305.
TAYLOR, G. I. (1923). *Phil. Mag.*, Ser. 6, **46**, 671–674.
TAYLOR, G. I. (1953). *Proc. R. Soc. A*, **219**, 186–203.
TAYLOR, G. I. (1954). *Proc. R. Soc. A*, **225**, 473–477.
USSING, H. H. (1952). *Adv. Enzymol.*, **13**, 21–65.
WESTHAVER, J. W. (1947). *J. Res. natn. Bur. Stand., Wash.*, **38**, 169–183.
WHALLEY, E. (1967). *A. Rev. phys. Chem.*, **18**, 205–232.

DISCUSSION

Saffman: One should perhaps issue a warning that a two-dimensional model is not a good approximation for treating diffusion in porous media. In two-dimensional flow, constraints in the streamlines are imposed by continuity; these are not present in three dimensions, where streamlines can twist round one another and so accentuate the diffusion and the spread.

Philip: In a three-dimensional medium made up of an array of obstacles which are not touching, the order of the stream-tubes is preserved in an appropriate topological sense. If, however, the obstacles are multiply-connected (or consist of one highly multiply-connected object!), the possibility of disorder must be admitted. It is a nice, but I think unresolved, question whether the disorder in real porous media which arises from three-dimensionality, *per se*, is a major factor.

Muir: The concept of airflow reversibility seems to me to be the key to understanding what happens when aerosols are breathed into the lung; Dr. Altshuler was the first to show this (Altshuler, B., Yarmus, L., Palmes, E. D., and Nelson, N. [1959]. *J. appl. Physiol.*, **14**, 321–327). Despite the fact that each inhaled volume of air is divided up some millions of times on its passage into the lung until there can be only one particle in each airway, the particles come together again during the reverse process of exhalation.

Saffman: I am surprised by this observation, because reversibility usually occurs only when the Reynolds numbers are extremely small, so that inertial effects are negligible. I was under the impression that Reynolds numbers are quite large, at least in the upper branches of the lungs, so the reversibility you mention seems surprising.

Muir: The Reynolds numbers are exceedingly low in the depths of the lungs. I agree that in the upper airway this is not so. Where branching occurs and where one might expect non-reversibility, the Reynolds number has become so low that reversibility occurs. (See p. 214 for table of Reynolds numbers in airways.)

Davies: The explanation of this reversibility in the lung is that if you consider the intake of one breath, you start to generate a paraboloid which divides at the main bronchi and continues to bifurcate thousands of times; by the time the breath is completed the wall of the paraboloid in the upper airways is so close to the wall of the airway that hardly any air is left adjacent to the wall from the previous breath. What happens in the large airways, where the Reynolds number is high, is thus quite immaterial; however, when levels below the intrasegmental bronchi are reached, the Reynolds number is low and the flow is viscous. The envelope of the inhaled air is then axial and a long way away from the walls of the airways. The lack of mixing between the central air and the peripheral air must be quite remarkable because it is possible to recover so completely an aerosol, provided that it has the right particle size—about $0 \cdot 5 \, \mu$m.

Altshuler: In my paper (pp. 215–231) I shall show that there is quite a bit of axial dispersion of aerosol in the lungs even though a very large part of it is recovered in the expired air. How much of this is caused by irreversibility of flow—that is, convective mixing—has not been determined, but I expect it to play a major role.

Caro: Professor Guyton showed an enormous increase of conductivity when tissue pressure, measured from an implanted capsule, exceeded atmospheric pressure. I believe he also showed that tissue compliance was restored to its control low value if the limb was again dehydrated. I should like to know if the conductivity between the two capsules was also reversible—that is, if it also was restored to its previous value by such removal of excess tissue fluid? This seems to me important because it could be that tissue spaces had been torn. Apparently there was the creation of larger channels for flow in the sense that conductivity had increased.

Guyton: We have not looked for such reversibility. However, we changed the pressure at most 1 or 2 mm. Hg at a time so that the tearing force would have been extremely small. Yet, at the critical pressure point where we crossed from subatmospheric to atmospheric pressure, the conductivity increased four to five orders of magnitude. This indicated that the opening of channels was caused by pressure in the tissue overcoming the occluding force of atmospheric pressure.

Mead: In this connexion, you have the opportunity to examine the adhesive forces between cells in the subcutaneous tissues. I also wonder whether you examined the extent of the volume–pressure hysteresis in tissues, and whether you studied the morphology of these tears and separations? Quick-freezing methods would be illuminating here.

Guyton: We have studied tissue hysteresis. For example, we determined pressure–volume curves (Guyton, A. C. [1965]. *Circulation Res.*, **16**, 452–460), going up the curve either in 45 minutes or in as long as 12 hours. If we go up the curve over a period of hours rather than in less than one hour, the lower parts of the curves are almost identical, but the upper part is displaced downwards because of slow stress-relaxation of the tissue spaces.

We have not made the histological study you suggest. There would be the problem of measuring in two dimensions what are actually three-dimensional spaces.

Caro: Could you comment, Dr. Philip, on the changes in this porous medium which Professor Guyton may be inducing?

Philip: It seems to me that if a tissue contains fibrous walls separating cells, and the tissue distends as a whole, much freer pathways for flow will open up along these fibrous passages. In this case it wouldn't seem essential to postulate a gel state for the tissue water. The hydraulic conductivity would then be a function of the water content of the tissue. A relation of this type applies to water movement in unsaturated porous media, and leads to a diffusion formalism describing transient flow processes in such media. As I mentioned in my paper, the approach has been extended recently to media which swell and shrink.

Guyton: We invoked the existence of a gel in the interstitial spaces mainly because the chemists find the gel! Also, even when the interstitial fluid pressure is negative, diffusion studies show that there is still 12 to 17 per cent of water in the interstitial spaces, and we suppose that if there is so much fluid in the tissue spaces it ought to flow quite freely unless something prevents it. Therefore we need to invoke something that holds the fluid in an immobile state.

Philip: May it not be simply a matter of mechanical rearrangement of fibrous material?

Guyton: This would be easy to believe if there were not so much water in the interstitial spaces.

Renkin: In ordinary circumstances, in this poorly conductive gel there is a continuous flow of lymph. This does not seem to fit with your idea of very restricted conductivity in the tissue spaces.

Guyton: When we implant two capsules an inch apart and have a pressure gradient of 1 mm. Hg between them, we observe movement of about 1 mm.^{3} of fluid from one capsule to the other in ten minutes. This is in the same order of magnitude as movement of lymphatic fluid. There is some movement of fluid, but it does seem to be restricted. What is striking is the enormous increase of conductivity when interstitial fluid pressure becomes positive.

Philip: From the point of view of normal physiology there should be great interest in these low tissue conductivities. They seemingly represent the normal state of affairs, while the spectacular high conductivities are a manifestation of a pathological, oedematous, condition.

Burton: Dr. Philip has illustrated that microscopic complexities may lead to macroscopic relative simplicity, and that it is important to specify which level one is working on. A minor illustration of this is the millipore filter which is extensively used and yet remains something of a mystery, because the filters are said to consist of rectilinear cylindrical pores, of diameter a fraction of a micrometre. I have not been able to get an electron microscopist to show me what is inside them because the materials apparently dissolve in the usual fixatives, but certainly under a high-power light microscope one sees an irregular felt-work with strands of beads of material going in all directions, layer on layer. Yet the mercury intrusion method of measuring critical pore size shows that the filter behaves as if made up of pores of the size stated by the manufacturers. It seems curious that the irregular fibrous structure that we see can behave like a set of regular geometrical pores.

Renkin: J. C. Bugher ([1953]. *J. gen. Physiol.*, **36**, 431–448) made surface replica electron micrographs of collodion membranes prepared and calibrated by a standard procedure for use as ultra filters to determine virus particle size. As Professor Burton describes for the millipore filters, these collodion filters have an irregular meshwork structure in which the spacings are very close to what was calculated by dynamic methods (water content and hydraulic conductivity), and correspond to the limiting dimensions of filterable viruses.

Philip: The measured "air entry value" in soil physics is analogous to the mercury entry pressure in the system mentioned by Professor Burton. This type of measurement gives a reasonably reproducible figure for a typical porous medium; but it measures no more than the way the advance of an interface is governed by what I suppose to be the effective neck radius of the largest pores. In soil physics the fact of this reproducibility has never been held to imply that the geometry of the medium is simple. Much more elaborate methods are used to estimate the detailed internal geometry of the medium and to relate it to hydraulic conductivity; and even these are not wholly convincing.

SECTION II
MASS TRANSPORT IN BLOOD VESSELS

EXCHANGE OF SUBSTANCES THROUGH CAPILLARY WALLS

EUGENE M. RENKIN

Department of Physiology and Pharmacology, Duke University,
Durham, North Carolina

INTERCHANGE of materials by the circulatory system depends on two processes: (1) circulation of blood through the capillary beds of all tissues and organs and (2) transport of various components of the blood through the capillary walls. Both processes are examples of "transport in porous media", though at different scales of porosity, and the interaction between them is the determining factor in overall blood–tissue transport.

Net transport across capillary walls can arise from driving forces of two kinds: (1) differences in hydrostatic or effective osmotic pressure of the fluids on either side and (2) differences in concentration of permeating solutes on either side. Kedem and Katchalsky (1961) derived a generalized transport equation encompassing both of them, and used it to analyse interactions between osmosis and diffusion in biological membranes. However, transcapillary ultrafiltration in response to hydrostatic and osmotic forces is the principal mechanism for control of plasma and interstitial fluid volumes, while transcapillary diffusion of specific substances along their individual concentration gradients is the mechanism by which tissue metabolism is sustained. Thus in terms of their physiological functions and controls, it is convenient to consider them separately.

The basis for control of ultrafiltration transport is the balance between capillary hydrostatic pressure and plasma protein osmotic pressure. Starling (1896) proposed that if the capillaries were freely permeable to the water and crystalloids of plasma and impermeable to plasma colloids, fluid balance (i.e., no net fluid movement) would be achieved when the difference in hydrostatic pressure across the capillary wall was equal to the difference between plasma and interstitial fluid colloid osmotic pressures. Inequality results in net translocation or ultrafiltration of fluid. Direct experimental proof of Starling's hypothesis was obtained by Landis (1927) for capillaries of the frog's mesentery and by Pappenheimer and Soto-Rivera (1948) for capillaries of mammalian muscle. Besides confirming the conditions for fluid balance, they showed that the rate of transcapillary ultrafiltration (F) was proportional to the difference between the opposing forces

$$F = K_F[(P_C - P_T) - (\Pi_p - \Pi_T)] \tag{1}$$

where $P_{C,\,T}$ represent hydrostatic pressure in capillary and interstitial fluid, respectively, and $\Pi_{p,\,T}$ the respective colloid osmotic pressures. The proportionality coefficient or capillary filtration coefficient, K_F, is the product of the effective capillary surface area in a given mass of tissue and the permeability per unit surface area of the capillary wall to filtered fluid.

Two terms in equation (1) are responsible for the most important influence of capillary circulation on ultrafiltration transport: P_C and K_F. A gradient of hydrostatic pressure along the capillary bed is necessary to maintain blood flow, and the shape of this gradient depends on geometrical or hydrodynamic factors. Fig. 1 is a model of the microvascular bed in the form of two hydro-

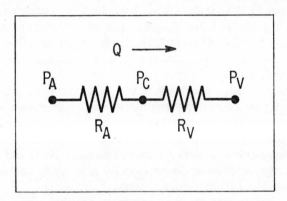

FIG. 1. Diagram of the capillary circulation to illustrate pre- and postcapillary hydrodynamic resistances (R_A and R_V, respectively) and their influence on capillary hydrostatic pressure (P_C). See text.

dynamic resistances in series, precapillary resistance R_A and postcapillary resistance R_V. P_C represents hydrostatic pressure at the functional midpoint of the capillary bed, and P_A and P_V arterial and venous pressure, respectively. Q represents blood flow. The pressure drop across the whole bed,

$$P_A - P_V = Q(R_A + R_V) \tag{2}$$

and across the postcapillary part,

$$P_C - P_V = Q(R_V) \tag{3}$$

From these it follows (Q dropping out) that

$$\frac{P_C - P_V}{P_A - P_V} = \frac{R_V}{R_A + R_V} \tag{4}$$

or
$$P_C = \frac{R_V}{R_A + R_V} (P_A - P_V) + P_V \tag{5}$$

In most vascular beds, the greater part of the resistance is on the precapillary side. If $P_A = 100$ mm. Hg and $P_V = 0$ and assuming that P_C must be 20 mm. Hg to balance P_T and $(\Pi_p - \Pi_T)$,

$$\frac{R_V}{R_A + R_V} = \frac{20 - 0}{100 - 0} = \frac{1}{4 + 1}$$

Vasomotor mechanisms can alter this ratio, thereby producing shifts in fluid balance. Such changes have been studied by Mellander (1960), Folkow and others (Folkow, Mellander and Öberg, 1961; Folkow, Lundgren and Wallentin, 1963; Öberg, 1964; Mellander and Öberg, 1967; Öberg and Rosell, 1968). In general vasoconstriction lowers P_C and tends to move fluid from interstitium to blood whereas vasodilatation tends to raise P_C and tends to move fluid from blood to interstitium.

The capillary filtration coefficient is also subject to control by vasomotor mechanisms, by the precapillary sphincters which determine the fraction of capillaries open at any time and thus the effective capillary surface (Krogh, 1929; Zweifach and Metz, 1955). The studies of Cobbold and co-workers (1963); Kjellmer (1964) and Lewis and Mellander (1962) and others have shown that large increases or decreases in K_F accompany vasomotor adjustments, presumably without change in permeability *per se*.

Tissue hydrostatic pressure is an important variable in the ultrafiltration equation (equation 1), but it is difficult to specify what its determining factors are. To a large extent, it must depend on the balance between fluid and protein leakage from the capillaries into the interstitial space, and removal and return by the lymphatics. Measurements by Guyton and his co-workers (Guyton, 1963, 1965) of sub-atmospheric tissue pressures in implanted plastic spheres indicate that the difference in effective protein osmotic pressure across the capillary wall must exceed the hydrostatic pressure difference.

Effective osmotic pressure difference between plasma and interstitial fluid depends not only on their concentrations of proteins and other colloidal material, but on the impermeability of the capillary wall to these substances. Even in skeletal muscle, the capillaries are not completely impermeable to plasma proteins, since they appear in lymph (Yoffey and Courtice, 1956;

Mayerson *et al.*, 1960). In capillaries of mammalian skeletal muscle, however, Pappenheimer and Soto-Rivera (1948) have shown that the effective osmotic pressure is about 95 per cent of the total osmotic pressure. Various sorts of injury may reduce this (see Landis and Pappenheimer, 1963), though the mechanisms are not clear. Apparently, normal permeability of the capillary wall depends on an interaction between the endothelium and plasma proteins. Pappenheimer and W. B. Kinter (unpublished observations; see Landis and Pappenheimer, 1963) found that clinical dextran, which was capable of maintaining colloid osmotic pressure in the perfused cat's hind leg preparation in the presence of plasma proteins, exerted little osmotic effect in its absence. The capillary filtration coefficient was also increased greatly if the plasma protein was diluted to less than 10 per cent of its normal value (to less than 0·6 g./100 ml.). It was restored to normal by replacing the plasma, or by purified serum albumin or purified haemoglobin (Pappenheimer and Renkin, unpublished observations). The extent to which permeability is controlled physiologically is unknown.

Transient contributions to effective osmotic pressure difference across capillaries may arise from concentration differences of permeating solutes, if they diffuse more slowly than water (Pappenheimer, Renkin and Borrero, 1951). This mechanism has been proposed to account for at least part of the large translocation of fluid observed after burn injury (Arturson and Mellander, 1964).

There remains to consider the direct influence of capillary blood flow on ultrafiltration. This is not explicit in equation (1), but acts through increase of Π_p by concentration of the plasma protein in proportion to the fraction of plasma volume lost. At ordinary blood flows, the filtration fraction is too small to make this effect important, but at low flows for the capillary bed as a whole, or in individual capillaries with flows much less than the average for the bed, some impairment of filtration may result. Assuming Π_p to be a linear function of protein concentration, we may modify equation (1) as follows

$$F = K_F \left(P_C - P_{Ci} \left\{ \frac{1 - f/2}{1 - f} \right\} \right) \tag{6}$$

where P_{Ci} represents the mean capillary hydrostatic pressure required for fluid balance, and f is the filtration fraction, F divided by the plasma flow. The $f/2$ in the numerator arises from the assumption that loss by ultrafiltration along the capillary is linear, and thus at the mid-point, the protein osmotic pressure has risen half-way to the venous level. Fig. 2 is a graph of this function. As long as plasma flow (Q) is more than 200–250 times greater than the capillary filtration coefficient (K_F) there is little effect of flow on filtration. In mammalian skeletal muscle at rest, $K_F = 0 \cdot 01$ ml./min. $\times$ 100 g., and Q is about $5 \cdot 0$ ml./min. $\times$ 100 g. The ratio Q/K_F is 500, which appears safely above this limit. However, in a non-uniformly perfused vascular bed, there may be some capillaries in which ultrafiltration transport is limited by blood flow.

Diffusion of specific solutes across capillary walls takes place according to individual concentration gradients, set up by their consumption or production

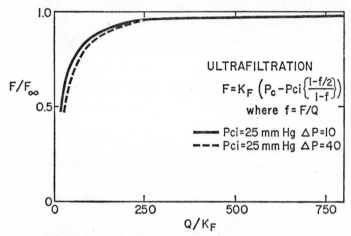

FIG. 2. Influence of capillary blood flow on ultrafiltration transport. F = filtration rate at actual flow Q, F_∞ = filtration rate at infinite flow, $\Delta P = P_c - P_{ci}$.

in the tissues. At any point along a capillary, the relation between a solute flux (M) and its concentration difference (Δc) across the capillary wall may be represented by Fick's Diffusion Law for a thin membrane

$$M = -PS\Delta c \tag{7}$$

where P represents capillary permeability to a particular solute per unit surface area and S is effective capillary surface. In capillaries of the central nervous system, there is evidence of chemically specific transport mechanisms (Crone, 1965; Cunha-Vaz and Maurice, 1967), but in peripheral capillaries, transport appears to be entirely passive. Permeability is high to small solutes, and falls with increasing molecular weight, to apparent impermeability at 20–40,000 (Pappenheimer, Renkin and Borrero, 1951; Landis and Pappenheimer, 1963). Above this level a trace amount of permeability exists (Yoffey and Courtice, 1956; Mayerson et al., 1960). It is not clear whether this "leakage" of protein represents passive diffusion or active transport by cytoplasmic vesicles (Bruns and Palade, 1968; Karnovsky, 1967).

At the smaller end of the molecular size spectrum, lipid solubility is an important factor influencing permeability. Lipid-soluble substances penetrate more readily than lipid-insoluble substances of comparable molecular weight (Renkin, 1952). For the small molecular species, lipid-soluble and insoluble, which constitute the substrates and products of cell metabolism, rates of transcapillary diffusion are so rapid that capillary blood flow becomes an important limitation to transport.

The influence of capillary blood flow on diffusion from blood to the tissues can be illustrated by a relatively simple capillary model consisting of a single capillary surrounded by a homogeneous pool of tissue fluid (Kety, 1951; Renkin, 1959) (Fig. 3). This model does not take into account diffusion

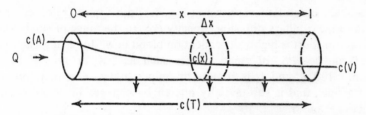

FIG. 3. Diagram to illustrate the effect of capillary blood flow on diffusion transport. $c(A)$ = arterial, $c(V)$ = venous, $c(T)$ = tissue solute concentration; $c(x)$ = concentration in capillary segment Δx. See text for explanation. (From Renkin, 1968 with permission.)

gradients and permeability barriers outside the capillary, or non-uniformity of permeability and blood flow within the capillaries. More complicated models which deal with these matters have been developed (see, for example, Blum, 1960; Martin de Julian and Yudilevich, 1964; Zierler, 1965).

Fig. 3 is a drawing of the simplified capillary model. Blood flows into its arterial end at rate Q and concentration $c(A)$ of a specific solute. As the blood moves along the capillary, the solute diffuses into the tissue, and its concentration within the capillary $c(x)$ falls progressively. At any point along the capillary the rate of diffusion is proportional to the concentration difference between $c(x)$ and $c(T)$ in the tissue. By integration of Fick's Law over the length of the capillary, an expression for the concentration of the solute in the emerging venous blood, $c(V)$ is obtained:

$$\frac{c(V) - c(T)}{c(A) - c(T)} = e^{-PS/Q} \tag{8}$$

3

The symbol e is the base of natural logarithms. An equilibration fraction E may be defined as follows

$$E = \frac{c(A) - c(V)}{c(A) - c(T)} = 1 - e^{-PS/Q} \tag{9}$$

Capillary clearance C may be defined (by analogy with renal clearance) as the imaginary volume of blood which is fully equilibrated with tissue in a given time with respect to a specific solute (Kety, 1951):

$$C = QE = Q(1 - e^{-PS/Q}) \tag{10}$$

The exponent PS represents the capillary diffusion capacity for a specific solute—that is, the maximum clearance attainable at infinite Q. At all real blood flows, C must be less than PS.

A graph of the relation predicted by equation 10 between capillary clearance and capillary blood flow is shown in Fig. 4. Both C and Q are represented relative to the capillary diffusion capacity PS. In the range of values shown, diffusion transport is highly dependent on blood flow. In resting mammalian skeletal muscle, PS for small solutes such as ^{42}K or urea is about 5 ml./min. $\times$ 100 g., and Q is about 5 ml./min. $\times$ 100 g. C is therefore about 0·63 maximal, and is substantially altered by changes in either Q or the product of P and S.

In other organs, a similar relation between Q and PS for ^{86}Rb or ^{42}K has been found. In intestine, Dresel, Folkow and Wallentin (1966) found $PS(Rb)$

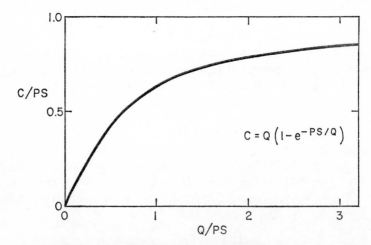

FIG. 4. Influence of capillary blood flow on diffusion transport. C = capillary clearance, Q = capillary blood flow.

to be 30–40 ml./min. × 100 g., and blood flow 30–60 ml./min. × 100 g. In the heart, PS(Rb) is about 80 ml./min. × 100 g., and blood flow 70–120 ml./min. × 100 g. (Winbury and Gabel, 1967; see also Renkin, 1967).

Control of capillary blood flow by arteriolar smooth muscle is well known. Experimental studies of transcapillary diffusion show that PS is subject to physiological control as well (Renkin and Rosell, 1962a, b, c; Renkin, Hudlická and Sheehan, 1966). Fig. 5 shows experimental data obtained in two perfused

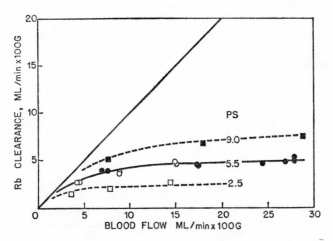

FIG. 5. Capillary clearance of ^{86}Rb in isolated, blood-perfused gracilis muscle of dog.

    ○, ● Controls, experiments 1 and 2, respectively.
    □ Maximum sympathetic vasoconstriction (experiment 1).
    ■ Maximum vasodilatation by motor nerve stimulation
    (experiment 2).

Data from Renkin and Rosell, 1962a; Renkin, Hudlická and Sheehan, 1966. (Reproduced from Renkin, 1967, by permission of the publisher.)

dog gracilis muscles, with ^{86}Rb as a tracer. The circles represent values of clearance at various blood flow rates produced by varying the perfusion pressure. For both preparations, they conform to prediction for a PS value of 5·5 ml./min. × 100 g. In the experiment represented by open symbols, the sympathetic vasoconstrictor nerves were stimulated electrically. This reduced clearance at every perfusion rate; PS was cut to less than half its control value. In other experiments, PS was reduced to as little as one-fourth of the control value. In the experiment designated by filled symbols, the motor nerve to the gracilis muscle was stimulated, producing muscular contractions. This increased clearance at every flow, and nearly doubled PS. The total range of variation of PS in experiments similar to these is about 8-fold from full vaso-constriction to vasodilatation.

The simplest explanation of the changes in PS is the same as for the changes in K_F described previously: changes in effective capillary surface due to the opening and closing of precapillary sphincters. If this is the mechanism, we should expect changes in PS and K_F to be parallel and similar in magnitude. This is the case in some conditions but not in others. Table I enumerates

TABLE I

COMPARISON OF CHANGES IN CAPILLARY FILTRATION COEFFICIENT (K_F) AND CAPILLARY DIFFUSION CAPACITY (PS) WITH VASOMOTION IN MAMMALIAN SKELETAL MUSCLE

Vasomotor mechanism	K_F	PS	Reference
Sympathetic adrenergic vasoconstriction	Decrease, then return to control	Sustained decrease	1, 2
Sympathetic cholinergic vasodilatation	No change	No change	3, 4
Metabolic vasodilatation			
muscular contraction	Increase	Increase	5, 6
reactive hyperaemia	Increase	Increase	7, 6
Intra-arterial vasodilator drugs	Increase	No change or decrease	8, 9
Decreased blood flow	Increase	No change or decrease	1, 6, 10
Increased transmural pressure	Decrease	Decrease	11, 12

References: 1. Cobbold *et al.* (1963); 2. Renkin and Rosell (1962*a*); 3. Folkow, Mellander and Öberg (1961); 4. Renkin and Rosell (1962*b*); 5. Kjellmer (1964); 6. Renkin, Hudlická and Sheehan (1966); 7. Lewis and Mellander (1962); 8. Kjellmer and Odelram (1965); 9. Renkin, Sheehan and Hudlická, unpublished observations; 10. Renkin (1959); 11. Mellander, Öberg and Odelram (1964); 12. Renkin and S. Gray, unpublished observations.

instances in which changes in these quantities can be compared. Values for PS were taken from published and unpublished work from my own laboratory and for K_F from the experiments of Folkow, Mellander and their associates. Since the measurements of ultrafiltration and diffusion were made in different preparations, caution must be used in comparing them. In the case of sym-pathetic vasoconstriction, measurements of PS(Rb) and K_F were made simultaneously in segments of cat's intestine by Dresel, Folkow and Wallentin (1966). Both coefficients were reduced during the period of maintained vasoconstriction, and returned to control levels when stimulation ceased, or when autoregulatory escape occurred. The return to control K_F during sympathetic stimulation in the normally circulated skeletal muscles studied by Cobbold and co-workers (1963) occurred while vasoconstriction was still maintained. The failure of PS to follow the same course may be due to a diminished autoregulatory reactivity of the precapillary sphincters in the muscles perfused at constant flow by Renkin and Rosell (1962*a*). This may also account for part of the difference in response to decreased blood flow. However, the entirely different response to a number of intra-arterial vaso-dilator agents cannot be explained by this mechanism.

Even when the changes in PS and K_F have the same direction, their magnitude is not always the same. In metabolic vasodilatation, the maximum increase in K_F is 3–4-fold (Kjellmer, 1964) and in PS(Rb), 2–2·5-fold (Renkin, Hudlická and Sheehan, 1966), but these were not in the same preparations. In their simultaneous measurement on cat's intestine, Dresel, Folkow and Wallentin (1966) reported that the change in K_F produced during sympathetic vaso-constriction was always greater than that in PS. In general, the range over which K_F can vary is slightly but distinctly greater than that for PS(Rb or K).

These discrepancies probably reflect the oversimplification of the capillary model explicit in the derivation for PS, and implicit in its comparison with K_F. The capillaries are not a uniform array. Their anatomical configuration suggests a wide range of path length of exchange vessels from arteriole to venule, with wide divergence of individual flow rates relative to surface area (Zweifach and Metz, 1955; Weideman, 1963; see also Renkin, 1964). Further-more, in the course of a single capillary path, there may be differences of structure and permeability (Landis and Pappenheimer, 1963; Majno, 1965; Wiederhielm, 1966). Although it has been generally assumed that ultra-filtration permeability and diffusion permeability depend on the same ultra-structural features of the capillary wall (Pappenheimer, Renkin and Borrero, 1951; Landis and Pappenheimer, 1963), this is not an absolute certainty. Intaglietta and Zweifach (1966) have studied the distribution of transmural pressures and ultrafiltration flows in the capillary network of rat mesentery and found that it is not balanced, but that the number of capillaries with outward filtration greatly exceeds those with inward filtration. No comparable analysis has been made for capillary diffusion.

It is possible in an exchange vessel network with local differences in ultra-filtration and diffusion permeabilities that a suitable arrangement of smooth muscle elements might provide for separate control of ultrafiltration and diffusion transport. No such mechanism is presently known, but it might be worth looking for. It seems closer to our current understanding of trans-capillary exchange to attribute the discrepancies observed in these two forms of transport to the effects of non-uniform distribution of capillary blood flow in relation to capillary surface and permeability.

Diffusion transport of solutes of low molecular weight is highly sensitive to capillary blood flow within its normal range (equation 10, Fig. 4). The relation is non-linear: an increase in flow of a given magnitude produces a smaller change in capillary clearance than a decrease in flow of the same magnitude.

Thus any deviation from a uniform distribution of flow relative to PS must reduce transcapillary diffusion, and lower the PS measured experimentally (Renkin, 1964). Ultrafiltration transport is also sensitive to blood flow (equation 6, Fig. 2), but the principal effect is in a range of flows considerably below the mean capillary flow in mammalian skeletal muscle. Consequently only marked reduction in mean flow will lower the ultrafiltration rate at a given driving force, and only very severe non-uniformity of flow rates within a network of many capillaries will lower the K_F measured experimentally.

In a real capillary network, then, two mechanisms may be concerned in the regulation of exchange of materials: (1) an all-or-none action of the precapillary sphincters, opening or closing individual capillary pathways, and (2) graded activity of terminal arterioles and precapillary sphincters which controls the distribution of flow among pathways. The all-or-none mechanism would alter filtration and diffusion coefficients proportionately; the graded mechanism would change PS more than K_F.

Non-uniformity of capillary blood flow in relation to capillary surface can also account for the fall in effective PS produced by intra-arterial infusion of vasodilator drugs. Intra-arterial distribution of such drugs must result in a highly non-uniform pattern of vasodilatation, which may be great enough to overcome the effect of the greater number of open capillaries. Increased flow in the first channels reached by the drug brings more drug to them, and diverts drug from other channels. Of all the vasodilator substances my colleagues and I have tried (including acetylcholine, ATP, nitroglycerine, papaverine and chloral hydrate) only one group is able to increase PS. These are the beta-adrenergic vasodilators—isoprenaline (isoproterenol) or adrenaline after alpha adrenergic blockade (Sheehan and Renkin, 1965). It is possible that this is indicative of an indirect vasodilator action of these substances, as proposed by Lundholm (1956). The action of beta adrenergic vasodilators on ultrafiltration transport in skeletal muscle has not been reported.

Another form of non-uniformity of capillary circulation which has been proposed as a mechanism for controlling transport is parallel division of the microcirculatory A–V paths into exchange or nutritional capillaries, and non-nutritional channels or shunts (Barlow, Haigh and Walder, 1961; Ballard, Fielding and Hyman, 1964; Friedman, 1968). It seems unlikely that this mechanism can be responsible for control of transport in skeletal muscle, though it may function in other tissues. In skeletal muscle A–V equilibration fractions (E) of very highly diffusible substances such as water (tritium labelled) and phenazone (antipyrine) may approach $1\cdot00$, while simultaneously measured E for more slowly diffusing substances such as urea or ^{86}Rb are much lower and vary for each substance according to its diffusibility

(Renkin, 1959, 1968; Yudilevich and Martin de Julian, 1965). Inefficiency of transport in short arterio-venous pathways is due not to an anatomical distinction of such paths, but to the high ratio Q/PS.

In a capillary network with A–V pathways of many lengths, if we assume all to have the same diameter and permeability per unit surface area, both PS and hydrodynamic resistance must increase linearly with length. According to Poiseuille's Law, however, blood flow will be in inverse relation to length. Such a bed represents the worst of all possible distributions. One of the functions of the terminal arterioles and precapillary sphincters must be to diminish this maldistribution by selectively increasing resistance in the shorter paths (Renkin, 1964). A relatively uniform pattern of distribution is probably maintained by a feedback link to tissue metabolism through the vasodilator action of certain metabolic products. In accordance with this hypothesis, optimal vasodilatation in terms of diffusion transport occurs at somewhat less than maximum vasodilatation. Vasodilatation beyond this optimum is associated with a fall in PS, though K_F continues to rise (Renkin, Hudlická and Sheehan, 1966; Kjellmer, 1964). This phenomenon may be an important limiting factor in local circulatory adjustment to exercise, and may contribute to the ineffectiveness of vasodilator drug therapy in peripheral vascular insufficiency. Perhaps the best "vasodilator" drug would not be a vasodilator itself, but would act to increase the sensitivity of arteriolar smooth muscle to normally produced metabolic vasodilators.

Another deficiency of the simplified capillary model used to analyse diffusion exchange is its failure to take into account diffusion barriers outside the capillary. This deficiency is shown by the large difference between the capillary diffusion coefficients based on transient osmotic measurements, which presumably reflect gradients only across the capillary wall, and the measurements based on the equilibration-flow relation (equation 10). The latter are very much smaller. For example PS(urea) in mammalian skeletal muscle calculated from $A/\Delta x$ (urea) measured by Pappenheimer, Renkin and Borrero (1951) comes to about 60 ml./min. × 100 g. The PS value directly measured is $5 \cdot 5$ (Renkin, 1967; see also Landis and Pappenheimer, 1963). Part of this difference may be attributed to the reduction in diffusion efficiency through non-uniformity of the capillary circulation. However, restriction of cell membranes to entry of urea and other substances is probably also important. Dr. Robert Sheehan, working in my laboratory, has succeeded in showing that cell membrane resistance to diffusion of K or Rb can account for one-fourth to one-half the total resistance represented by PS (Renkin and Sheehan, in preparation). The role of both cell membranes and interstitial substance in the control of transport between blood and tissue needs to be studied more extensively. It appears, however, that the dominating factor in the control of transport is the peripheral vasomotor apparatus, which controls capillary blood flow, hydrostatic pressure, surface area and distribution of blood flow with respect to surface area. The extent to which changes in permeability may also be involved is not clear, but it is probably far from unimportant.

SUMMARY

Transport across capillary walls by ultrafiltration and diffusion depends not only on capillary permeability but also on capillary haemodynamics, and is therefore subject to control through vasomotor mechanisms, both intrinsic metabolic and extrinsic nervous mechanisms. Control of ultrafiltration transport is brought about by changes in the ratio of postcapillary to total vascular resistance, and by changes in the number of open capillaries. Control of diffusion transport is brought about by changes in the number of open capillaries and by changes in local distribution of capillary blood flow relative to capillary surface and permeability. The role of changes in permeability in control of transport is not known.

Acknowledgement

This work was supported by National Institutes of Health Grant No. HE10936 and National Science Foundation Grant No. GB-5063X.

REFERENCES

ARTURSON, G., and MELLANDER, S. (1964). *Acta physiol. scand.*, **62**, 457–463.
BALLARD, K. W., FIELDING, P. A., and HYMAN, C. (1964). *J. Physiol., Lond.*, **173**, 178–189.
BARLOW, T. E., HAIGH, A. L., and WALDER, D. N. (1961). *Clin. Sci.*, **20**, 367–385.
BLUM, J. J. (1960). *Am. J. Physiol.*, **198**, 991–998.
BRUNS, R. R., and PALADE, G. E. (1968). *J. Cell Biol.*, **37**, 277–299.
COBBOLD, A., FOLKOW, B., KJELLMER, I., and MELLANDER, S. (1963). *Acta physiol. scand.*, **57**, 180–192.
CRONE, C. (1965). *Acta physiol. scand.*, **64**, 407–417.
CUNHA-VAZ, J. G., and MAURICE, D. M. (1967). *J. Physiol., Lond.*, **191**, 467–486.
DRESEL, P., FOLKOW, B., and WALLENTIN, I. (1966). *Acta physiol. scand.*, **67**, 173–184.
FOLKOW, B., LUNDGREN, O., and WALLENTIN, I. (1963). *Acta physiol. scand.*, **57**, 270–283.
FOLKOW, B., MELLANDER, S., and ÖBERG, B. (1961). *Acta physiol. scand.*, **53**, 7–22.
FRIEDMAN, J. J. (1968). *Am. J. Physiol.*, **214**, 488–493.
GUYTON, A. C. (1963). *Circulation Res.*, **12**, 399–414.
GUYTON, A. C. (1965). *Circulation Res.*, **16**, 452–460.
INTAGLIETTA, M., and ZWEIFACH, B. W. (1966). *Circulation Res.*, **19**, 199–205.

KARNOVSKY, M. J. (1967). *J. Cell Biol.*, **35**, 213–236.

KEDEM, O., and KATCHALSKY, A. (1961). *J. gen. Physiol.*, **45**, 143–179.

KETY, S. S. (1951). *Pharmac. Rev.*, **3**, 1–41.

KJELLMER, I. (1964). *Acta physiol. scand.*, **62**, 18–30.

KJELLMER, I., and ODELRAM, H. (1965). *Acta physiol. scand.*, **63**, 94–102.

KROGH, A. (1929). *The Anatomy and Physiology of Capillaries*, rev. edn. New Haven: Yale University Press.

LANDIS, E. M. (1927). *Am. J. Physiol.*, **82**, 217–238.

LANDIS, E. M., and PAPPENHEIMER, J. R. (1963). In *Handbook of Physiology, Section 2: Circulation*, vol. II, pp. 961–1033, ed. Hamilton, W. F., and Dow, P. Washington, D.C.: American Physiological Society.

LEWIS, D. H., and MELLANDER, S. (1962). *Acta physiol. scand.*, **56**, 162–188.

LUNDHOLM, L. (1956). *Acta physiol. scand.*, **39**, Suppl. 133, 1–52.

MAJNO, G. (1965). In *Handbook of Physiology, Section 2: Circulation*, vol. III, pp. 2293–2375, ed. Hamilton, W. F., and Dow, P. Washington, D.C.: American Physiological Society.

MARTIN DE JULIAN, P., and YUDILEVICH, D. (1964). *Am. J. Physiol.*, **207**, 162–168.

MAYERSON, H. S., WOLFRAM, C. G., SHIRLEY, H. H., and WASSERMAN, K. (1960). *Am. J. Physiol.*, **198**, 155–160.

MELLANDER, S. (1960). *Acta physiol. scand.*, **50**, Suppl. 176, 1–86.

MELLANDER, S., and ÖBERG, B. (1967). *Acta physiol. scand.*, **71**, 37–46.

MELLANDER, S., ÖBERG, B., and ODELRAM, H. (1964). *Acta physiol. scand.*, **61**, 34–48.

ÖBERG, B. (1964). *Acta physiol. scand.*, **62**, Suppl. 229, 1–98.

ÖBERG, B., and ROSELL, S. (1968). *Acta physiol. scand.*, **71**, 47–56.

PAPPENHEIMER, J. R., RENKIN, E. M., and BORRERO, L. M. (1951). *Am. J. Physiol.*, **167**, 13–46.

PAPPENHEIMER, J. R., and SOTO-RIVERA, A. (1948). *Am. J. Physiol.*, **152**, 471–491.

RENKIN, E. M. (1952). *Am. J. Physiol.*, **168**, 538–545.

RENKIN, E. M. (1959). *Am. J. Physiol.*, **197**, 1205–1210.

RENKIN, E. M. (1964). In *Effects of Anesthetics on the Circulation*, pp. 171–181, ed. Price, M. L., and Cohen, P. J. Springfield, Ill.: Thomas.

RENKIN, E. M. (1967). In *Coronary Circulation and Energetics of the Myocardium*, pp. 18–30, ed. Marchetti, G., and Taccardi, B. Basel and New York: Karger.

RENKIN, E. M. (1968). *J. gen. Physiol.*, **52**, 96s–108s.

RENKIN, E. M., HUDLICKÁ, O., and SHEEHAN, R. M. (1966). *Am. J. Physiol.*, **211**, 87–98.

RENKIN, E. M., and ROSELL, S. (1962a). *Acta physiol. scand.*, **54**, 223–240.

RENKIN, E. M., and ROSELL, S. (1962b). *Acta physiol. scand.*, **54**, 241–251.

RENKIN, E. M., and ROSELL, S. (1962c). *Acta physiol. scand.*, **54**, 381–384.

SHEEHAN, R. M., and RENKIN, E. M. (1965). *Pharmacologist*, **7**, 178 (abstract).

STARLING, E. H. (1896). *J. Physiol., Lond.*, **19**, 312–326.

WEIDEMAN, M. P. (1963). In *Handbook of Physiology, Section 2: Circulation*, vol. II, pp. 891–933, ed. Hamilton, W. F., and Dow, P. Washington, D.C.: American Physiological Society.

WIEDERHIELM, C. A. (1966). *Fedn Proc. Fedn Am. Socs exp. Biol.*, **25**, 1789–1798.

WINBURY, M. M., and GABEL, L. P. (1967). *Am. J. Physiol.*, **212**, 1062–1066.

YOFFEY, J. M., and COURTICE, F. C. (1956). *Lymphatics, Lymph and Lymphoid Tissue*, 2nd edn. Cambridge, Mass.: Harvard University Press.

3*

YUDILEVICH, D., and MARTIN DE JULIAN, P. (1965). *Am. J. Physiol.*, **208**, 959–967.
ZIERLER, K. L. (1965). *Fedn Proc. Fedn Am. Socs exp. Biol.*, **24**, 1085–1091.
ZWEIFACH, B. W., and METZ, D. B. (1955). *Angiology*, **6**, 282–290.

DISCUSSION

Saffman: In the calculation of the diffusion of solutes from capillaries into the tissues do you assume that the concentration of solutes is uniform across the capillary? If so I would be rather suspicious of the result, because I would not think that was a good assumption.

Renkin: It is possible that there are gradients in solute concentrations from the centre to the periphery of the capillary, but if resistance at the capillary wall is large, as is implied by permeability–surface area products of the order of 5 or 10 ml./min. × 100 g., it is unlikely that these gradients will be great. F. Pollock and J. J. Blum ([1966]. *Biophys. J.*, **6**, 19–28) have shown that for the normal range of capillary parameters (radius, length, blood flow, permeability, diffusion coefficient) the influence of radial gradients within the capillaries is negligible. Gradients outside the capillary are a much more severe problem.

Davies: I agree with this for the low rates of blood flow, but you have shown that diffusion transport is very dependent on the rate of flow and one would expect a more considerable gradient inside the capillary at the higher rates of flow.

Renkin: The main factor in the flow dependence is the longitudinal concentration gradient. According to Pollock and Blum, radial gradients contribute to flow dependence only at flow rates far beyond the highest ever reached in skeletal muscle under physiological conditions. The highest physiological flows obtain during maximum metabolic vasodilatation. I. Kjellmer ([1964]. *Acta physiol. scand.*, **62**, 18–30) found that in these conditions, the capillary ultrafiltration coefficient was increased 3 to 3·5 times above the control value. However, the diffusion coefficient for Rb goes up only 2 to 2·5 times (Renkin, E. M., Hudlická, O., and Sheehan, R. M. [1966]. *Am. J. Physiol.*, **211**, 87–98). It may be that the discrepancy is due to radial diffusion gradients within the capillaries, but this is not the only possible explanation.

Caro: Can one ignore the presence of red cells in the model, in considering the question of gradients of solute concentration across the capillary?

Renkin: I like to imagine that the red cells help to stir up the fluid phase and therefore diminish the gradients!

Burton: When we think of the filtration coefficient increasing with the area of the capillary wall, we have to remember that pores in the capillary, which are normally estimated as about 70 Å (7 nm.) diameter, will enlarge relatively more than the surface area does when the wall is stretched mechanically in vaso-dilatation. The increase in pore area for isotropic membranes was calculated for me by a colleague (Dr. D. R. Miller, Dept. of Applied Mathematics, University of Western Ontario), and the increase does not depend upon the individual elastic constants of the wall, but only on Poisson's ratio of stretch and contraction in directions at right angles. Unfortunately he is unable as yet to produce a solution if the membrane is anisotropic. However, one can verify this empirically by stretching bits of rubber and cloth; the hole is stretched much more than the membrane itself. You can demonstrate this quite well on a buttonhole!

Renkin: A buttonhole is probably a very good model of a capillary pore, because the pore is between two endothelial cells and if the capillary is stretched longitudinally the pore may be pulled open widely. However, it seems un-likely under physiological conditions that stretch of the pores is a major factor controlling capillary transport capacity. Baez and his associates (Baez, S., Lamport, H., and Baez, A. [1960]. In *Flow Properties of Blood and other Biological Systems*, pp. 122–135, ed. Copley, A. L., and Stainsby, G. Oxford: Pergamon Press) have shown that capillaries of the rat mesoappendix, once they are opened, do not change much in diameter with further increase in pressure. Capillaries appear to have a pressure–diameter curve like that of veins: once opened they seem to be only slightly distensible.

Taylor: Professor Burton's colleague seems to have solved the wrong problem, because if the capillary diameters do not change very much with increasing pressure one cannot expect much change in pore size. The converse does apply to arterioles.

Renkin: Professor Burton's point is relevant to another matter. If venous pressure is raised abnormally high—to 50 or 60 mm. Hg—protein loss from the capillaries is increased considerably. Mayerson and his colleagues (Shirley, H. H., Wolfram, C. G., Wasserman, K., and Mayerson, H. S. [1957]. *Am. J. Physiol.*, **190**, 189–193) have attributed this loss to widening of capillary pores—they called it the "stretched-pore phenomenon". The magnitude of pressure required to induce protein leakage might be a source of valuable information about the forces determining the shape and dimensions of the pores in capillary walls.

Floyer: We have attempted to study changes in the size of capillary pores using a Guyton capsule implanted into the subcutaneous tissue of a rat and measuring the albumin/gamma globulin ratio in the capsule fluid and in plasma. We assume that the A/γG ratio in the capsule fluid is affected by the rate of flow of fluid from the capillaries into the capsule and by the size of the pores in the capillary wall. If the mass flow rate remains constant, the ratio (capsule A/capsule γG)/(plasma A/plasma γG) will give an indication of the selective permeability of the capillary membrane. In an experiment on a group of rats, we measured selective capillary permeability before and after increasing the blood volume (with haematocrit constant) by regular infusions of a mixture of blood and dextran. In the hypervolaemic rats, the decreased A/γG ratio in the capsule fluid suggested that the pores had been stretched and had allowed more of the larger molecule to enter the extra-vascular fluid.

THE MECHANICS OF THE RED CELL IN RELATION TO ITS CARRIER FUNCTION

ALAN C. BURTON

*Department of Biophysics, University of Western Ontario,
London, Ontario*

IN preparing this contribution I have found great difficulty in choosing among a variety of points relevant to the subject of the symposium that have resulted from research in our laboratory over the past seven years, without the paper becoming very tedious, certainly indigestible, and almost unintelligible. I shall therefore use the device of asking you to form a Celestial Sub-committee on the design of "carriers" to transport haemoglobin in the blood stream from lung capillaries to tissue capillaries, and to consider the points that would be discussed by such a Celestial Sub-committee. This device protects me from accusations of teleology; we can be as teleological as we like (and most of us find it essential in our research thinking) without the necessity of speaking of optimal arrangements arrived at by random variation, combined with testing for survival in an evolutionary process.

The specific mission of the Sub-committee is to decide on the best type of "vehicle" to transport haemoglobin, and it will lead us to see the importance of mechanics and geometry in the "design" of such vehicles. The background to my discussion is a number of researches made in our laboratory by graduate students and colleagues in the past six or seven years. I have been fortunate to have had such original and productive collaborators as R. Haynes, Peter Rand, J. Prothero, Roderic Phibbs, Peter Canham and B. Shrivastav, many of whom are now known for their independent work elsewhere. Without their work I would have nothing worth saying.

Perhaps this relief from specialized factual papers, and the flight of imagination, may serve to link together usefully the contributions that precede and follow mine.

The tentative agenda for the first meeting of SCOTCH is given below.

*Celestial Sub-Committee on Carriers for
Transport of Haemoglobin (SCOTCH)*

AGENDA

(1) Should haemoglobin be transported in solution or in "packets" (red cells)?

67

(2) The best size of terminal blood vessels.
(3) The best size of the "packets".
(4) The mechanical properties of membranes for enclosing haemoglobin.
(5) The best shape of the "packets".
(6) The best concentration of the "packets" (haematocrit).
(7) Planned obsolescence and replacement (lifespan of red cells).

Vive Charles Darwin!

   This agenda did not satisfy the biophysicist on the committee, who thought that the physical forces maintaining the equilibrium of the proposed "red cells" of various shapes and sizes should be considered. The chairman ruled that there would not be time to discuss this if important practical decisions were to be reached, but promised consideration of the basic physics at a later meeting.
   The first item was included because a chemist on the committee was not convinced that a solution of haemoglobin in the plasma would not serve just as well as packaging the haemoglobin in red cells. He had heard that a physiologist (Amberson *et al.*, 1933) had shown many years ago that dogs could live and function satisfactorily for some time when all their blood was

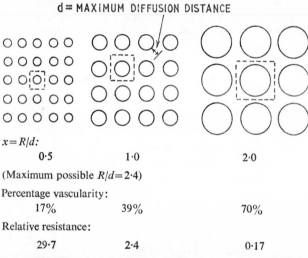

$d =$ MAXIMUM DIFFUSION DISTANCE

$x = R/d$:

| 0·5 | 1·0 | 2·0 |

(Maximum possible $R/d = 2·4$)

Percentage vascularity:

| 17% | 39% | 70% |

Relative resistance:

| 29·7 | 2·4 | 0·17 |

FIG. 1. This illustrates how the condition of maximum diffusion distance d could be satisfied with capillaries in parallel of different diameters, and how the opposing factors of excessive vascularity for large capillaries and high resistance to flow for small capillaries combine to produce an optimal diameter. $R =$ radius.

exchanged for a haemoglobin-glucose-Ringer solution. The other items seem to be logical for a committee charged with doing the job with the greatest economy and efficiency (as the acronym SCOTCH suggests). Discussion of each point follows.

(1) SHOULD HAEMOGLOBIN BE IN SOLUTION OR CONTAINED IN PACKETS?

The obvious reason why haemoglobin must be transported inside "bags" whose membranes are selectively permeable to water, ions and sugars but will not pass larger molecules is that the size of the haemoglobin molecule (about 60 Å diameter) is such that it passes (though not very readily) the glomerular membrane of the kidney (if there is haemolysis in the blood, haemoglobin appears in the urine). An additional advantage of packaging haemoglobin in red cells is that at the same concentration of haemoglobin free in the plasma, the viscosity of the blood flowing through the resistance vessels would be much greater than it is. (This is discussed under item 3.) In the terminal vessels of small diameter the effective viscosity of blood (cells and plasma) actually approaches that of plasma alone, by the curious rheology of flow of cells in very small tubes (the Fahreous-Lindquist effect).

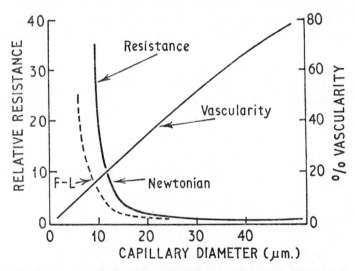

FIG. 2. The opposing factors of excessive vascularity and of increased resistance to flow suggest an optimal capillary diameter of 5–10 μm. (assuming a maximum diffusion distance of 10 μm.). The broken line represents the modification of the resistance curve by the Fahreous-Lindquist effect.

(2) HOW LARGE SHOULD THE SMALLEST BLOOD VESSELS BE?

This should be determined by the need for easy diffusion of gases and nutrients to the tissue cells. It had been laid down by a previous committee that no cell in metabolically active tissue should be more than roughly 10 μm. from the nearest blood vessel (capillary). Figs. 1 and 2 show how the committee decided between having a large number of very small capillaries in parallel, or a smaller number of larger vessels in parallel, either of which could satisfy the condition of a maximum distance for diffusion. An obvious disadvantage of choosing larger vessels is shown: a high proportion of the total tissue space will be occupied merely by vessels. However, as vessels become smaller and smaller the resistance to flow through the terminal vascular bed rises quite abruptly to very high values (the abruptness reflects the modified fourth power law of Poiseuille), so we cannot go very far in making the capillaries small. Two considerations, however, indicate that we might go further in reducing the size of capillaries than the resistance curve of Fig. 2 indicates.

The first is that the major part of the total resistance to flow is not in the capillaries (about 25 per cent) but in the arterioles (about 60 per cent). The second is that, as discussed in the next section, by choosing the size of the red cells appropriately we can effectively lower the viscosity in the capillaries far below that in the large vessels. In view of these considerations the decision of the committee to have most capillaries of diameter less than 10 μm. (the lung capillaries are exceptionally larger), seems logical. Of course the chosen maximum distance for diffusion must depend on the level of need of cells—that is, on their metabolic rate—and the ease of diffusion in the intervening tissue. This distance could be greater for metabolically inactive tissue, and at lower tissue temperatures. The decision of the committee to have a capillary diameter range of 5–10 μm. seems logical.

(3) HOW LARGE SHOULD THE CARRIERS (RED CELLS) BE?

Having settled the size of the smallest vessels, we are in a position to discuss the optimal size of the red cells. They must be small enough in diameter to pass the capillaries. However, they may be a little larger if the red cell is deformable enough to pass through the capillaries in a sausage shape. In fact, as Prothero and Burton (1962a) showed with millipore filters some years ago, Rand and Burton (1964) with micropipettes, and most recently Canham and Burton (1968) from studies of the population of red cells in blood samples, red cells of maximum diameter 8 μm. can pass through cylindrical channels down to 3·7 μm. in diameter, without trapping or haemolysis. Capillaries are usually 5–10 μm. in diameter, while the red cells have a maximum diameter of 8 μm. Prothero and Burton (1962b) also showed by modelling theory, and by experiments with micropipettes, that the passage of single red cells, separated by trapped plasma, in tandem down capillaries (bolus flow) uses so little energy that the effective viscosity approaches that of plasma, rather than of blood flowing in tubes larger than 1 mm. in bore. This is the classical Fahreous-Lindquist effect, namely that the relative viscosity of blood measured in glass capillary tubes decreases greatly when the diameter of the tubes is less than about 0·3 mm. This explains the original finding of Whitaker and Winton (1933) that the relative viscosity in the hind limbs of cats is much less than that expected from tests of relative viscosity in large-bore viscometers. The best reviews of the rival theories explaining this are still those of Haynes (1960, 1962). Fig. 3 summarizes this point. H. L. Goldsmith, with Professor Mason, has been making fascinating observations on the dynamics of blood cells and of plastic spheres moving through micropipettes only a little larger than the particles. No doubt Professor Lighthill and Professor Mason will mention these experiments.

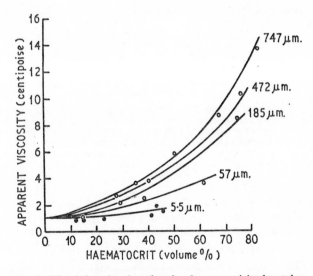

FIG. 3. Blood viscosity plotted against haematocrit in glass tubes of various diameters. The data for 5·5 μm. tubes is from the work of J. Prothero with micropipettes, added to a graph already published (Haynes and Burton, 1959). For very small tubes the effective viscosity approaches that of plasma, even at high haematocrits.

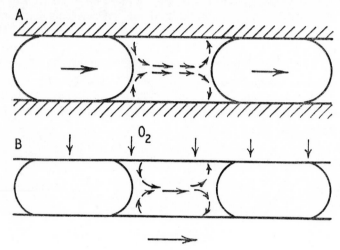

We demonstrated that there is an extra dividend in bolus flow, where the cells fill the lumen of the capillary, separated by trapped plasma. Prothero and Burton (1962c) showed that in the segments of plasma between the cell boluses there has to be a "circus" or "fountain" motion (Fig. 4) which greatly facilitates the equilibration of the plasma with substances or gases being exchanged through the capillary walls. In addition, no capillary is a smooth uniform tube and the contents of the deformed red cells travelling through are thoroughly churned up in passage. (This churning takes place even in large vessels.) Thus the seemingly paradoxical decision of the committee to

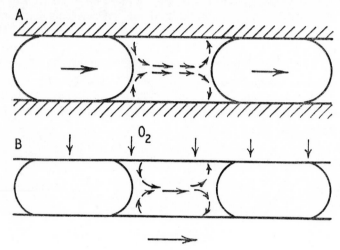

FIG. 4. Diagram of bolus flow. Plasma on the axis of the tube moves forward twice as fast as the cells, catches up the cell ahead, moves to the sides and waits for the cell behind to catch up. This circus or fountain motion is repeated at least ten times in the length of a capillary, and aids in equilibration. A shows the motion with respect to a stationary observer, B for an observer moving with the red cells. (From Burton, 1965.)

have red cells with a maximum diameter of about 8 μm., even though many capillaries are much smaller than this, was fully justified.

I was intrigued to discover from a recent article (Jensen and Ellis, 1967) on the transportation of substances by pipe-lines that this group of engineers has at last discovered the Fahreous-Lindquist effect (or the sigma effect of Dixon and Scott Blair, 1950) that those in our field have known so long. Solid substances such as ore or coal could be carried in the form of a "slurry" of powder in water, in small lumps, in large lumps, or in special capsules. To quote the article: "Experiments showed that the most favorable [least energy required for a given flow] cylindrical or spherical capsules were those large enough to fill 90 to 95 per cent of the pipe diameter . . . The driving of a slurry calls for a greater consumption of pumping power".

(4) AND (5) THE MECHANICAL PROPERTIES OF THE RED CELL MEMBRANE, AND THE SHAPE OF RED CELLS

The astonishing work of Rand on micromanipulation of single red cells, in which he sucks portions of the membrane into micropipettes down to fractions of a micrometre in diameter, has provided direct information on the stiffness of the red cell membrane—Young's Modulus, the viscoelastic properties—and on its resistance to haemolysis. Rand's work also gives plausible but indirect evidence of a uniform tension (probably an interfacial tension) in the membrane and, strangely enough, of a positive rather than a negative pressure (only about 3 mm. water, but very significant) inside the cell. Details of this work can be found in Rand and Burton (1964); what is relevant here are the conclusions.

The membrane of the red cell is easily "bent"—that is, it has a very low modulus of bending—but the membrane exhibits a high Young's Modulus of elasticity when the area is increased. A very small increase in area, which Rand estimated to be less than 10 per cent but Seeman (1967) finds to be at most only 4 per cent, results in the development of a high tension, rigidity of the cell, and reversible haemolysis. Since the membrane can flow—that is, it is viscoelastic—it might withstand more stretch than this if the deformation were very slow.

The red cell must in its life in the circulation tolerate a high degree of deformation, not only when it is in the capillaries, but also in the crowded, jostling blood stream of larger vessels such as the arteries and veins. This intolerance of the membrane to stretch makes it mandatory, therefore, that the cells are *non-spherical* (Burton, 1966), since for a given volume a sphere has less surface area than any other shape into which it might be deformed. *A spherical red cell, such as can be produced in hypotonic osmotic swelling, cannot tolerate any degree of deformation, however small.* The tolerance to deformation of each red cell in a population of red cells of blood samples has been related by Canham (Canham and Burton, 1968) to its volume and area (and an index called the sphericity index, $4 \cdot 8 \times \text{volume}^{2/3}/\text{area}$; this index is $1 \cdot 0$ for a sphere and zero for an infinitely thin disc). Moreover, we had demonstrated that haemolysis resulted from an increase of membrane area alone (by sucking the membrane into a sufficiently narrow micropipette) without any swelling, so this inability to withstand stretch is basic to the problem of survival of the red cell in the circulation. The electron micrographic work of Seeman (1967) has made it quite certain that haemoglobin leaves the normal red cell only when the membrane is stretched.

The actual biconcave discoid shape of the red cell is sufficiently non-spherical to allow a great deal of deformation, even to the extent of enabling the cell to pass through tubes $3 \cdot 7$ μm. in diameter.

The biconcave shape of the normal red cell has often been said to allow gases to diffuse most rapidly to the haemoglobin in the centre of the cell. This argument is quite unrealistic on two grounds. First, a thinner disc would theoretically allow an even greater speed of diffusion, so other considerations must be important. Secondly, equilibration does not have to depend on diffusion, since there is mixing of the contents of the cell as it moves. Canham (private communication) in our laboratory has just completed some computer calculations on the total bending energy of the membrane of a red cell, if it could take the many shapes that are possible even when both area and volume are kept constant. The theoretical shapes for minimum total bending energy, calculated for the different volumes associated with a constant area, agree very well with those observed in osmotic swelling by Rand and Burton (1963).

(6) HOW MANY PACKETS OF HAEMOGLOBIN PER UNIT VOLUME OF BLOOD?

Once one has settled the size and shape of the carriers of haemoglobin, the question arises of the optimal haematocrit; that is, the number of packets that could be carried in the blood before disadvantages arise. It is important to realize that a haematocrit of 50 per cent with red cells of the biconcave discoidal shape of the human red cell represents an extremely crowded suspension. In fact, a haematocrit of more than 65 per cent is certainly impossible, from purely geometrical considerations, without deforming the cells. (Spheres, of course, can be more tightly packed than this.) A picture of the actual conditions of blood flowing in an artery was provided by the photographs made by Phibbs in our laboratory (see Phibbs and Burton, 1968). He froze the blood flowing in the femoral artery of rabbits very rapidly (in $0 \cdot 1$ sec.) and by slow freeze-substitution produced histological slides of thin sections (Fig. 5). The impression of crowding is very strong. Many cells at different levels fill the apparent gaps in the thin slice. Moreover, the haematocrit was only 36 per cent. (The obvious orientation of the cells does not concern us here.) Clearly, haematocrits higher than those found in most mammalian species would mean that the blood was rheologically more like a solid than a liquid, resulting in a very great increase in effective viscosity.

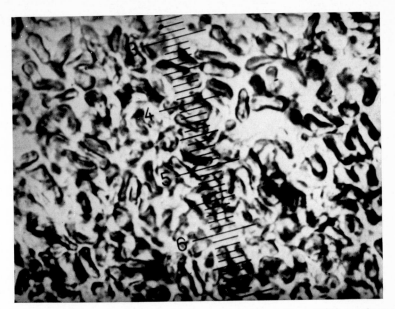

FIG. 5. Photomicrograph of blood quick-frozen during flow in the rabbit femoral artery, followed by slow-freeze substitution.
    The figure illustrates how crowded and exposed to deformation are the red cells flowing in an artery, even at a haematocrit of only 34 per cent. The section is about 5 μm. thick; smallest scale division, 2 μm. (From the work of R. Phibbs.)

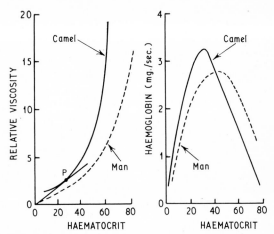

FIG. 6. For maximum efficiency in transport, the maximum weight of haemoglobin per sec. should be obtained for the same driving pressure. This is proportional to the ratio haemato-crit/viscosity. The curves on the right are data of blood flow through glass tubes from the work of Stone, Thompson and Schmidt-Nielson (1968) simplified from one of their graphs. The usual haematocrit of the camel is 27 per cent, and of man, 47 per cent. The maximum haematocrit value is the point, P, of contact of the tangent from the origin to the curve of viscosity against haematocrit.

[To face page 74

An interesting paper by Stone, Thompson and Schmidt-Nielsen (1968) has recently appeared on the very different normal haematocrits found in different species of mammals (camel, 27 per cent; goat, 33 per cent; sheep, 32 per cent; dog, 46 per cent; man, 47 per cent). Stone and his co-workers point out that for maximum efficiency in oxygen transport the haematocrit value should give the maximum rate of flow of haemoglobin (mg./sec.), rather than of the whole blood (ml./sec.). If we assume that the concentration of haemoglobin in the cells is constant in different species, then since the volume flow under a constant arterial pressure varies inversely with the viscosity, the rate of flow of haemoglobin is proportional to haematocrit/viscosity, and for maximum efficiency this ratio should have a maximum value (Fig. 6). The numerator of the ratio can be increased by increasing the haematocrit, but as is well known, viscosity increases markedly with increase of haematocrit; thus a maximum value for flow of haemoglobin occurs at a particular haematocrit value. Since the increase of viscosity with haematocrit differs in different species, presumably because of variation in the size and shape of the red cells, the optimal haematocrit so calculated will also vary. The calculated optimal value for each species was found to be very close to the normal haematocrit for that species. (This consideration of optima was mentioned by Guyton in his book [see Guyton, 1961]; I do not know whether it was original with him or not.) My own contribution is limited to pointing out that the point of contact of a tangent from the origin to the curve of relative viscosity against haematocrit indicates the optimal haematocrit.

I found this matter a delightful example of adaptation for best physiological function. Perhaps if the number of species were increased exceptions might be found, but I am sure we could think of special reasons for such exceptions! One weakness of the logic must be pointed out. Stone, Thompson and Schmidt-Nielsen (1968) measured the flow of haemoglobin through glass tubes of quite large bore with the same pressure gradient for all species, but the relevant comparison would be of flows through tubes of smaller bore, comparable to the resistance vessels. While the increase of viscosity with haematocrit would be much less, I have no doubt that the maximum ratio of haematocrit to viscosity would occur at about the same optimal haematocrit.

(7) PLANNED OBSOLESCENCE: THE LIFESPAN OF RED CELLS

The recent work of my colleague Peter Canham has revealed the importance of geometry in determining the lifespan of normal red cells. Any committee of biologists would know that the carriers for haemoglobin that it has designed in the way suggested cannot last for the life-time of the animal, so that arrangements for the selective removal of old cells (presumably in the spleen) and for either a continuous renewal or supply (from the bone marrow) must be made. The lifespan of human red cells is from 100 to 140 days, which means that about 0·8 per cent of the cells are removed and replaced by new ones every 24 hours. This mechanism for "turnover" is also essential in order that it can be accelerated, by feedback mechanisms, to deal with emergency losses of red cells, as in haemorrhage. How is this selective removal of old cells to be accomplished?

Our approach seemed at first sight rather unlikely to supply the answer. There is a great variety of sizes and shapes of red cells in a sample of normal blood. We made enlarged prints of individual cells hanging on edge beneath a coverslip and supplied data on the profile of the hanging cells to a computer, which gave us the area, volume and diameter of each cell, and histograms of the distribution of these. It also gave correlation plots between the various parameters—for example, area against volume. The distributions of any one parameter, such as area or volume, were remarkably Gaussian and told us nothing new. However, the plots of interrelation between the parameters showed that they did not vary independently.

For example, while cells of less than average volume have a wide range of sphericity, from markedly spherocytic to very thin, those of more than average volume are nearly all thinner than normal. We were able to track down a hidden geometrical restriction in the data. The computer calculated for us, from the area and volume of individual cells, the smallest diameter of a cylindrical channel through which a particular cell could pass without having to increase its area (which would result in trapping and haemolysis). This minimum cylindrical diameter was remarkably similar for all the cells in the population, and from subject to subject. In eight normal subjects 95 per cent of the cells had geometry such that they could just pass a cylindrical channel of from 3·5 to 3·8 μm. diameter (mean 3·66 ± 0·037 s.e.m.). This was not just the usual cut-off at the tail of a normal distribution. The geometrical theory predicted accurately that there should be a straight-line boundary in the plot of area against volume, beyond which no points representing cells occur. Other postulated restrictions, such as the passage of red cells through orifices (stomata) in membranes, or between two parallel membranous sheets, did not predict nearly as good fits to the data.

In splenectomized subjects this boundary was transgressed; after the spleen had been removed, many cells were circulating in the blood stream that would be unable to pass channels of 3·7 μm. in diameter. We are, therefore, convinced that the Celestial Sub-committee met the problem of the removal of old cells by arranging that in their passage through the spleen, red cells sooner or later take some route through cylindrical channels of about $3 \cdot 7$ μm. diameter. There may be overwhelmingly more probability that, in a single circuit, a given cell will not encounter these channels, but pass instead by many parallel routes with larger vessels. Yet mathematically it is easy to show that in the many circuits made by each cell in 24 hours, the probability of encountering these critically narrow channels is quite high (see Appendix, p. 79). Cells with inappropriate area and volume will be trapped, and probably haemolysed chemically (or perhaps osmotically) after trapping. The critical channels need not be cylindrical tubes. They might be quasi-cylindrical channels between columns of cells packed into sinusoids.

The missing link in the chain of logic is why it is that as red cells grow older, they fail to pass the geometrical test as they did when they were younger. Studies of distribution of the geometry of old and young cells (they may be separated by centrifugation, since older cells have a higher density) show that with age the cells present in a sample are more spherocytic for the same volume; this is consistent with the idea that the area of membrane is unchanging, and that with age the cell tends to increase in volume. A taking in of water would be expected if the metabolic pump of the membrane decreased in activity with age. (The concentration of enzymes and lipids in red cells is known to decrease with age.)

At risk of confusing you, I must report that both the area and volume of old cells are slightly but significantly *less* than for young cells, though the minimum cylindrical diameter is not different, which at first sight seems to contradict what I am suggesting. This is not so, for in flowing blood we examine what is left after the cells which have increased in volume have been removed by the spleen. Perhaps the most convincing demonstration of this geometrical theory of ageing is that from the measured distribution of the area, volume and sphericity of old and young cells, Canham could compute osmotic fragility curves (Fig. 7), and his predicted curves agree closely with the well-known finding (Prankerd, 1958) that there is a slight shift in the sigmoidal curve of osmotic fragility for old red cells. The osmotic fragility curve is a very sensitive index of change in the geometry of red cells. As little as a 5 per cent increase in volume of all the cells in the population would cause a crisis in the circulation, similar to that seen in hereditary spherocytosis.

Mr. Alfred Jay, working with great skill and patience in our laboratory, can now measure the electrical potential inside single red cells (average $8 \cdot 0$ mv, $\pm 0 \cdot 2$ s.e.m., negative inside). We are hoping that use of this tool may show us a decline in voltage with age, as an indication of the suggested metabolic decline.

The mechanics of the membrane and the geometry of individual red cells are, therefore, of great importance in the functioning and life of erythrocytes. In every respect the "design" of the carriers of haemoglobin seems to show optimal arrangements for their vital function. To the biophysicist there is the remaining fascinating problem of how the normal shape of red cells, and the variety of shapes they can assume in altered environments (such as crenation, cup shapes, osmotic swelling up to a sphere; the effects of surfactants, pH, electric fields) can represent a physical equilibrium of the membrane in

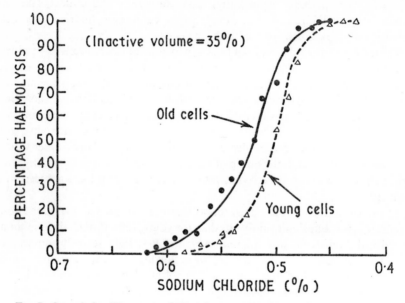

FIG. 7. Osmotic fragility curves of old and young red cells, computed entirely from the distribution of geometrical parameters in samples of old and young cells separated by centrifugation. The basic assumption is that haemolysis occurs when the cell is swollen to a sphere. (From Canham, 1967.)

terms of the forces acting upon it. We feel that in the past five years we have made progress towards the solution of this problem, which however it is inappropriate to discuss here.

As so often when we learn more of the details of living things, in the study of the biophysics of the red cell we encounter many examples of optimal "design" for physiological function. The great usefulness of thinking in terms of optima is that when we encounter some feature that does not appear to be well adapted to function, we can be sure that some important factor of physiology is operating of which we are unaware. Discrepancies of this sort are the most promising starting points for new research.

SUMMARY

Erythrocytes present many examples of optimal "design" as carriers of haemoglobin from lung capillaries to peripheral capillaries; the design is here discussed by a fictitious committee. Haemoglobin cannot be dissolved in plasma because the viscosity would be excessive and it would leak from the kidney; it must be enclosed in "packets". The best size of these depends on the size of capillaries, which is itself determined by the maximum diffusion distance allowable. A capillary diameter of 5–10 μm. is the best compromise between excessive vascularity (larger capillaries) and excessive resistance to flow (smaller capillaries). The packets should have diameters similar to this, because of the facilitated equilibration of gases in "bolus flow", and the remarkable lowering of effective viscosity (Fahreous-Lindquist effect). The best haematocrit value is also discussed. The shape of red cells depends on the mechanical properties of the membrane, which may easily be bent but not stretched without becoming rigid or haemolysing. Non-sphericity is essential. Statistical study of the geometry of populations of blood cells indicates that limiting cylindrical channels of diameter 3·7 μm., probably in the spleen, filter out cells of inappropriate geometry (old cells). The lifespan of red cells can be explained on this basis.

APPENDIX

THE PROBABILITY OF CAPTURE IN THE SPLEEN OF RED CELLS OF UNSUITABLE GEOMETRY (OLD CELLS)

Let the probability of capture in the critical (3·7 μm. diameter) channels of the spleen in a single circulation of blood be p. This would correspond to the proportion of all the parallel routes available for passage that were of this size at some place.

Then the probability that a given cell survives a single passage will be $(1-p)$. This a $priori$ probability is independent of the number of times the cell has circulated. Therefore, the probability of $surviving$ two successive passages is $(1-p)^2$, and of surviving n passages is

$$P = (1-p)^n \tag{1}$$

The probability that a cell is $captured$ in n passages is

$$P^1 = 1 - (1-p)^n \tag{2}$$

Taking natural logarithms of (1), and using the well-known series for $\ln(1 - x)$, when $x \ll 1$

$$\ln P = n\ln(1 - p) \simeq -np \tag{3}$$

Let us calculate how many passages, N, on the average, are required before the chances of capture are even or better than even, i.e. before $P^1 \geqslant 1/2$, and therefore $P \leqslant 1/2$. Since $\ln 1/2 = -0\cdot69$, (3) gives

$$-0\cdot69 = np$$

$$N = \frac{0\cdot69}{p} \tag{4}$$

Circulation times vary from as little as 10 seconds for the coronary circuit to several minutes for longer routes. Let us assume that the mean circulation time is of the order of 60 seconds. The probability of capture by the restricting vessels in the spleen in a single complete circulation will depend on what proportion of the cardiac output goes through the spleen (e.g. 2 per cent) and on what proportion of the routes through the spleen are restrictive (e.g. 5 per cent). If p be taken as $1/1,000$, equation 4 gives $N = 700$; that is, after 700 circulations (11 to 12 hours) a cell with inappropriate geometry would probably be trapped by the critical vessels in the spleen. In two days the probability of capture has become 94 per cent.

As long as the time for the probability of capture to become high is only a few days, it would play little part in the mean lifespan of red cells (120 days), but merely widen the range of the lifespan (100 to 140 days). The mean lifespan is determined, not by this probability, but by how long it takes the ageing process to make the cell geometrically susceptible to trapping. The normal distribution of geometrical parameters in the new red cells will also contribute to the range of lifespan.

The point of this order-of-magnitude calculation is to show that specific restricting channels in the spleen (e.g. cylindrical channels of $3\cdot7$ μm. diameter) need form only a very small fraction of the possible routes of the circulation through the spleen, and yet may effectively filter the blood free of "senescent" cells.

REFERENCES

Amberson, W. R., Flexner, J., Pankratz, D. R., Steggerda, F. R., and Mulder, A. G. (1933). *Am. J. Physiol.*, **105**, 2 (Abstract).

Burton, A. C. (1965). *Physiology and Biophysics of the Circulation.* Chicago: Year Book Medical Publishers.

Burton, A. C. (1966). *Fedn Proc. Fedn Am. Socs exp. Biol.*, **25**, 1753–1760.
Canham, P. B. (1967). Ph.D. Thesis, University of Western Ontario.
Canham, P. B., and Burton, A. C. (1968). *Circulation Res.*, **22**, 405–422.
Dixon, F. J., and Scott Blair, G. W. (1950). *J. appl. Phys.*, **11**, 574.
Guyton, A. C. (1961). *Textbook of Medical Physiology*, 2nd edn, p. 546. Philadelphia and London: Saunders.
Haynes, R. H. (1960). *Am. J. Physiol.*, **198**, 1193–1200.
Haynes, R. H. (1962). *Biophys. J.*, **2**, 95–103.
Haynes, R. H., and Burton, A. C. (1959). *Am. J. Physiol.*, **187**, 943–950.
Jensen, E. J., and Ellis, H. S. (1967). *Scient. Am.*, 62–72. See also (1963). *Ind. Engng Chem.*, **55**, no. 8, 18–26 and **55**, no. 9, 29–34.
Phibbs, R. H., and Burton, A. C. (1968). In *Proc. 1st int. Conf. Hemorheology*, pp. 617–632, ed. Copley, A. L. Oxford: Pergamon Press.
Prankerd, T. A. J. (1958). *J. Physiol., Lond.*, **143**, 325–331.
Prothero, J., and Burton, A. C. (1962a). *Biophys. J.*, **2**, 213–222.
Prothero, J., and Burton, A. C. (1962b). *Biophys. J.*, **2**, 199–212.
Prothero, J., and Burton, A. C. (1962c). *Biophys. J.*, **1**, 565–579.
Rand, R. P., and Burton, A. C. (1963). *J. cell. comp. Physiol.*, **61**, 245–253.
Rand, R. P., and Burton, A. C. (1964). *Biophys. J.*, **4**, 115–135.
Seeman, P. (1967). *J. Cell Biol.*, **32**, 55–70.
Stone, H. D., Thompson, H. K. Jr., and Schmidt-Nielson, K. (1968). *Am. J. Physiol.*, **214**, 913–919.
Whitaker, S. R. F., and Winton, F. R. (1933). *J. Physiol., Lond.*, **78**, 339–369.

DISCUSSION

Taylor: One other point in favour of carrying haemoglobin in packets relates to osmotic pressure. The osmotic pressure of haemoglobin at 15 gm. per cent is about 80 mm. Hg. To maintain the Starling equilibrium with haemoglobin in solution would need a much higher mean blood pressure, so this is another reason why packets are necessary.

Farhi: Another argument in favour of carrying haemoglobin inside cells pertains to exchange across the capillary walls. A haemoglobin solution would leave a sizeable unstirred boundary layer on the capillary wall, impeding diffusion, while each red cell that passes "scrapes" the walls clean.

Burton: The theory of the origin of the remarkably low effective viscosity of whole blood is still controversial. There are two rival theories of how the Fahreous-Lindquist effect operates in vessels less than 0·5 mm. in bore; one is that there is a cell-free layer of plasma against the wall; the other is based on the fact that the problem has a "graininess"; you must not in Poiseuille's Law "*integrate*" (but rather "summate") because there are only five blood cells across a diameter. Thus you get what is called the sigma effect. Both explanations are plausible at normal haematocrits, but R. H. Haynes ([1962].

Biophys. J., **2**, 95–103) has shown that both theories become implausible at extreme haematocrits. The true theory may be a mixture of these two aspects. Certainly Phibbs has shown by freezing the blood in the rabbit femoral artery (diameter 1 mm.) that the plasma layer is only a statistical occurrence and its mean thickness is not more than 1 or 2 μm. We have no other direct evidence of what happens at high haemocrits (up to 50 per cent). (See Phibbs, R. H., and Burton, A. C. [1968]. In *Proc. 1st int. Congr. Hemorheology*, pp. 617–632, ed. Copley, A. L. Oxford: Pergamon Press.)

Lighthill: What was the velocity in your experiment on the very low effective viscosity of blood in very narrow tubes?

Burton: In spite of ingenious methods for measuring very slow flows, the least flow we achieved was about a hundred times the normal rate of flow in capillaries (1 mm.^{3} in 7 hours).

We discussed earlier the possible stretching of capillary walls (p. 64). However it is probable that capillaries do not distend very much when pressure is increased. We measured microscopically the distension of frog capillaries and found that they are like rigid tubes when pressure is increased mechanically (Nichol, J., Jerrard, W., Claxton, E. B., and Burton, A. C. [1957]. *Am. J. Physiol.*, **164**, 330–344). If histamine is injected they dilate, but one can put 300 mm. Hg of pressure on capillaries and fail to measure an increase in diameter. This is because they are so small, in accordance with Laplace's Law which predicts that the tension in the wall is the product of transmural pressure and radius. On the other hand if the pressure is lowered the capillaries disappear altogether. But once they reach their normal size the distensibility curve is flat.

Caro: Has anyone any views on how capillaries are able to distend when for example vasodilator drugs are given, and yet a change of hydrostatic pressure will not distend them?

West: The pulmonary capillaries are apparently different; their mean diameter does increase when the pressure within them is raised (see my paper, pp. 256–272). Of course they are not surrounded by a mass of tissue as systemic capillaries are.

Burton: They are also much larger than systemic capillaries (10–20 μm. mean diameter as against 5–10 μm.). An important idea is that of Y. C. Fung ([1966]. *Fedn Proc. Fedn Am. Socs exp. Biol.*, **35**, 1761–1772), that one should not think of the rigidity of the systemic capillary in terms of the strength of its wall; rather the capillary is supported by the whole tissue, which is like a gel with holes bored through it.

Caro: Perhaps then histamine changes the properties of the surrounding material?

Burton: One can clearly change the properties of the basement membrane chemically, with pitressin for example. We were unable to measure the distension of frog capillaries *under pressure*, though we could measure distension under pressure in arterioles and venules quite easily by our method.

Taylor: This is supported by C. A. Wiederhielm's direct observations of capillary diameter and pressure. His observations and those of P. C. Johnson showed the very variable pressures in the microcirculation, depending on whether the precapillary sphincters are open or not (Johnson, P. C., and Wayland, H. [1967]. *Am. J. Physiol.,* **212,** 1405–1415). The idea of capillary pressure is indeed only a statistical mean. It can go up to 60 or 70 mm. Hg at the arterial end of a capillary or alternatively be very much lower than that if the precapillary sphincter is shut. The mean is presumably struck among the various capillaries themselves.

Renkin: The statistical mean pressure in a capillary network is important from the point of view of net ultrafiltration of fluid, since this is the value that must balance colloid osmotic forces, according to Starling's hypothesis. Local fluid movements in and out of capillaries with pressures above and below the mean must sum to this net movement. The locus of mean capillary pressure represents a functional mid-point of the capillary bed. Direct measurements of local ultrafiltration rates by M. Intaglietta and B. W. Zweifach ([1966]. *Circulation Res.,* **19,** 199–205) show that this point may lie downstream of the anatomical midpoint of the capillary network. Of a large number of capillaries measured, presumably uniformly distributed over the capillary network, 80 per cent showed outward fluid movement, 20 per cent inward. We know that normally most of the filtered fluid gets back into the circulation because lymph flow is much less than total ultrafiltration loss from the capillaries. The only possible conclusion is that much of the return of fluid is through the walls of vessels downstream of the capillaries—the small venules. Our notions of what constitutes an "exchange vessel" must be re-examined.

Burton: The method used here defeats the object, which was to discover the normal filtration. They blocked capillaries by the pressure of a glass rod and observed whether red cells moved towards or away from the block, but surely the rod causes pressure to rise upstream to where it joins a free flowing channel.

Renkin: On the far side of the blockade pressure would be expected to fall to that of the downstream free flowing channel; they found that on both sides of the block red cells moved towards the block. Physiologically the most questionable part of their experiment is that the mesentery was exposed and covered with a 1 or 2 per cent solution of gelatin. This changes the osmotic pressure of the fluid outside. It may have been the abnormal external environment that shifted the balance towards filtration through parts of the capillary where fluid normally goes back.

West: The permeability of vessels slightly larger than capillaries is an interesting problem. C. A. Wiederhielm ([1966]. *Fedn Proc. Fedn Am. Socs exp. Biol.,* **25,** 1789–1798) has some evidence that the small venules in the mesentery of the frog are very permeable to highly diffusible dyes. We would like to know the permeability of the somewhat larger vessels in the lung, say above 100 μm. in diameter, which have exceedingly thin walls. Is it possible that fluid moves out of these and contributes to the perivascular cuff of fluid which is seen when the lung has interstitial oedema? Certainly oedema formation in the excised lung is hastened by large inflations of the lung which do not increase the transmural pressure across the capillaries but do across the larger extra-alveolar vessels.

MOTION IN NARROW CAPILLARIES FROM THE STANDPOINT OF LUBRICATION THEORY

M. J. LIGHTHILL

Imperial College of Science and Technology, London

PRELIMINARY NOTES ON MOTIONS WITH NEGLIGIBLE INERTIA

I WANT to discuss motion in very narrow capillaries from the point of view of physics, and it follows that I shall be describing studies which in most respects are simply a continuation of Professor Burton's well-known researches on the mechanics of erythrocytes in capillaries (see for example Prothero and Burton, 1961, 1962a, 1962b; Rand and Burton, 1964; Burton, 1966). I shall be discussing the passage of red cells through narrow capillaries particularly from the standpoint of lubrication theory, with a view to estimating the thickness of any layer of plasma separating a cell from the endothelial wall, and determining how such a layer may contribute to mass transport and to resistance. The work is described in a tentative, preliminary fashion, on the lines of an earlier paper (Lighthill, 1968) and of some more recent work by my research associate J. M. Fitz-Gerald.

Lubrication theory is concerned with fluid motions in which there is a direct balance between pressure gradients and viscous forces, and inertia plays a totally insignificant role in the balance. Actually the small blood vessels in general are places where inertial effects are totally negligible in this way, because the Reynolds numbers R of motion in those vessels are very small; actually, less than 1. In all vessels with $R < 1$, which in practice means vessels with diameter less than about 100 μm., a fluid motion completely different in character from those inertia-influenced flows that are familiar to us in everyday experience is necessarily present.

Scientists in other disciplines than fluid mechanics often think of Reynolds number principally as an indicator of whether or not turbulence will be present, but it is of course important for a far wider range of purposes than that as an indicator of the type of fluid motion to be expected, and *within* the field of purely laminar flows its value continues to determine the relative significance of inertia and viscosity and, through that, the type of laminar motion that occurs. The total insignificance of inertia in vessels of diameter below

100 μm. follows from the circumstance that $R < 1$, and is supported further by the fact that Womersley's parameter α is considerably less than 1 (see, for example, McDonald, 1960).

The special type of flow expected when pressure gradients are directly balanced by viscous forces is one lacking all the characteristic and familiar effects produced by fluid inertia. One can forget Bernoulli's equation; there is no difference between static and dynamic pressures; there are no centrifugal forces; fluid can negotiate sharp bends without difficulty; no secondary flow is set up by the curvature of vessels, and generally motion is much less sensitive to vessel geometry. There is no tendency to flow separation, and indeed (as other contributors have mentioned) there is a sense in which motions at $R \ll 1$ are completely reversible.

The insensitivity to geometrical detail is further shown by the virtual disappearance of any "entry length". If fluid enters a tube at a marked angle to the axis, say, then the difference between the motion and a Poiseuille motion with the same total flow is reduced by an order of magnitude already (that is, by a factor of 10) in an axial distance of half a tube radius; an exceedingly quick adjustment to Poiseuille flow.†

Propagation of changes of pressure, which in the large arteries is a wave propagation, governed mainly by a balance between distensibility and inertia, is in the peripheral circulation governed entirely by a balance between distensibility and resistivity (that is, compliance and resistance). Changes of pressure are there subject to a purely diffusive spreading, exactly as if the blood vessels were wires along which thermal conduction was diffusing changes of temperature. There is, actually, a precise analogy between the diffusion of temperature changes, a diffusion governed by the ratio between thermal conductivity k and heat capacity per unit volume ρc_p, and the diffusion of pressure changes in the microcirculation.

Thus, we know that k is *heat* flow rate across unit area per unit gradient of *temperature*, while ρc_p is *heat* addition per unit volume for unit increase of *temperature*, their ratio being the diffusivity of temperature changes. If in the peripheral circulation we read "fluid volume" in these definitions for heat and "pressure" for temperature, we deduce the diffusivity D of pressure changes as the ratio of a fluid conductivity σ (*volume* flow rate across unit area per unit gradient of *pressure*, which on Poiseuille's Law would be $a^2/8\mu$ where a is tube radius and μ viscosity) to a distensibility K (*volume* addition per unit volume for unit increase of *pressure*).

---

† The Stokes stream function of such differences decays exponentially like $e^{-\alpha x/a} f(r/a)$ where x is axial distance, a is tube radius and α is the root of $J_0^2(\alpha) + J_1^2(\alpha) = (2/\alpha)J_0(\alpha)J_1(\alpha)$ with least positive real part, whose value may be proved to be $\alpha = 4 \cdot 5 \pm 1 \cdot 5i$.

I have mentioned this analogy for demonstrating that pressure changes will simply diffuse through the peripheral circulation with a diffusion coefficient $D = \sigma/K$ principally because that result is used in arguments to be presented by Dr. Caro (see pp. 153–168). It allows an estimate of the time delay taken for a signal to propagate a distance l as l^2/D, or, when diffusivity takes different values $D_1, D_2, \ldots$ in different parts $l_1, l_2, \ldots$ of the total path l, as a time delay $(\sum l_n D_n^{-1/2})^2$. If the fluid conductivity is written in terms of an "effective viscosity" as $a^2/8\mu$, this time delay may be written

$$[\sum (8\mu_n K_n)^{1/2} (l_n/a_n)]^2 \tag{1}$$

in terms of the distensibility K_n and effective viscosity μ_n and ratio of length to radius for the nth component of the total path.

I come next to how the total insignificance of inertia influences some aspects of motion of particles within the blood in the small vessels. A simple spherical particle, with radius b and density ρ, has any differences between its velocity and that of the fluid reduced by a factor of ten in a time $0 \cdot 5\rho b^2/\mu$; furthermore, in a shear flow such a particle is set rotating with an angular velocity equal to half the fluid vorticity in a time still shorter than this.[†] For non-spherical particles the time lags are still shorter, but when b has a typical value for an erythrocyte of 4 μm., even the upper limit $0 \cdot 5\rho b^2/\mu$ is only 2×10^{-6} seconds.

This negligible time lag within which the single erythrocyte in a fluid takes up the motion determined by the fluid's local velocity and vorticity is a further illustration of the insignificance of inertia; yet another is that, at these Reynolds numbers, the Magnus force on a body in a sheared stream is totally negligible. When blood flows in these narrow tubes, however, there is an effective radial force operating essentially through interactions of particles with each other and with the vessel walls. For example, the existence of a relatively cell-free layer of plasma immediately adjacent to a wall probably comes about partly as a result of what we may loosely call the pressure, within the ensemble of red cells, of collisions with the wall.

PRELIMINARY NOTES ON AXIAL CONCENTRATION

Let me follow this up a little farther. For shapes as irregular as those of erythrocytes it is easy to see how their flailing motions near a wall might be imagined to produce continual collisions whose pressure might force the

† Stokes's Law, valid at these low Reynolds numbers, gives for the difference velocity v the equation $\rho(\frac{4}{3}\pi b^3)dv/dt = -6\pi\mu bv$, from which the above time requirement is deduced; the analogous equation for the difference angular velocity Ω is $\rho(\frac{8}{15}\pi b^5)d\Omega/dt = -8\pi\mu b^3\Omega$, giving a time requirement smaller by a factor $0 \cdot 3$.

4

whole ensemble of red cells towards the interior. Even for such shapes, however, and certainly for particles of more spherical shape, the interactions probably do not involve physical collision. This already is a topic where lubrication theory is helpful, indicating that fluid pressure forces come into play in thin layers between surfaces in relative sliding motion to oppose collision. Such forces would probably constitute the individual components of the overall wall pressure on the ensemble of red cells.

Within the fluid a similar centripetal pressure force on the red cell ensemble may continue to act, because interactions between red cells, at given volume concentration, are greatest where they are spinning fastest, that is, where the fluid vorticity is greatest (near the wall). These forces of interaction between cells are also probably mainly generated in lubricating layers between spinning deformable cells. They give a distribution of internal pressure in the red cell ensemble[†] with a centripetal gradient that must help to maintain the well-known axial concentration with its various well-known consequences.

These include a net lowering of resistance in vessels of diameter between (say) 10 and 40 μm., arising from the fact that resistance is reduced by lowered viscosity near the wall more than it is increased by higher viscosity near the axis. This is expressed well by the formula

$$\sigma = (2a^2)^{-1} \int_0^a \mu^{-1} r^3 \, dr \qquad (2)$$

for conductivity of fluid in a tube where the viscosity μ varies with distance r from the axis. This formula shows that values of μ^{-1} near the wall are weighted by the large factor r^3 for large r. That formula corresponds to a distribution of velocity proportional to

$$\int_r^a \mu^{-1} r \, dr \qquad (3)$$

which varies most in the outer low-viscosity region.

Whitmore (1967) gave a useful discussion of this, and of how it affects variations in red cell *concentration* in different parts of the microcirculation. He came particularly near the subject of lubricating layers when he considered

† Here, the red cell ensemble is looked at from the point of view of the kinetic theory of gases, and its pressure from this point of view is the rate of transfer of momentum per unit area by interactions between the particles. Goldsmith and Mason (1964, p. 591) pointed out that although there is a measurable tendency for an individual deformable cell in Poiseuille flow to move towards the axis, essentially as a result of changes of shape under straining by the fluid shear, nevertheless at high volume concentrations this must be supplemented to an important extent by the effect of collisions taking place most frequently on the side of the cell farthest from the axis.

the very narrow vessels in which the cells form an axial train. To a rough approximation, the mean velocity of the cell-free plasma is half that of the axial train—that is, of the cells and of the discs of plasma swept along between the cells. (This is inferred from equation (3), where μ is the viscosity of plasma and $r\,dr$ weights the integral in proportion to the actual volume of fluid.) We can describe this as a leakback of plasma relative to the motion of the cells.

Now the volume flow of red cells as a proportion of total volume flow must have the same value essentially at all levels of vessel size through which the blood passes,[†] and this ratio for large vessels where red cells and plasma have essentially the same mean velocity is the haematocrit c_0. In very small vessels, if the axial train has radius r_c and velocity v_c and the mean volume concentration of red cells within the vessel is $\bar{c}$, this gives for the ratio of red cell flow to total flow

$$\frac{\bar{c}v_c}{(r_c^2/a^2)\,v_c + (1 - r_c^2/a^2)\tfrac{1}{2}v_c} = c_0 \tag{4}$$

Accordingly, the mean volume concentration of red cells is

$$\bar{c} = \tfrac{1}{2}(1 + r_c^2/a^2)\,c_0 \tag{5}$$

a value reduced below the haematocrit value c_0 characteristic of the larger vessels. On the other hand, the concentration c_t within the axial train itself is

$$c_t = \tfrac{1}{2}(1 + a^2/r_c^2)\,c_0 \tag{6}$$

(greater than (5) by the area ratio a^2/r_c^2), which exceeds the haematocrit value. Whitmore (1967) plotted these quantities against the ratio b/a of red cell radius to tube radius, assuming that the core radius r_c could be taken as approximately equal to b itself when this is near a; in this plot (Fig. 1), c_0 is taken as $0 \cdot 4$.

For rather smaller values of b/a, an admittedly cruder approximation of Whitmore's involves a cell-free region of thickness b, the cell radius, *and* the possibility of still ignoring variation of velocity in the core region where at least viscosity is much greater than the plasma viscosity; Whitmore pointed out that this crude approximation leads to identical results when b/a is rather less than $0 \cdot 5$ with r_c/a replaced by $1 - (b/a)$; see Fig. 1. No doubt the true curves are not so symmetrical, but possibly the prediction of a minimum mean concentration of red cells $\bar{c}$ in vessels of somewhere around twice a red cell diameter may have value.

† Strictly, this assumes that all the cells and all the plasma pass through vessels of all these size levels; to this assumption there can be exceptions in parts of the peripheral circulation that are significantly shunted by anastomoses (see, for example, Pappenheimer and Kinter, 1956).

Of course, the actual geometries of red cells in an axial train are quite variable, and for this reason the amount of leakback of plasma relative to the motion of cells must vary. Whitmore (1967) points out how this would produce variation in the amounts of plasma between successive cells, or in other words would lead to the "bunching" of cells that is frequently observed.

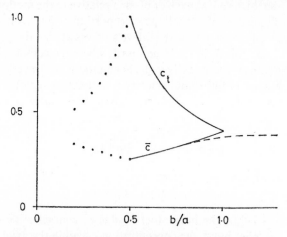

FIG. 1. Suggested type of variation of concentration of red cells of undeformed radius b in a capillary as a function of its radius a, when the haematocrit is 0·4 in large arteries. Here $\bar{c}$ is overall volume concentration of red cells in the capillary, and c_t a rough value of concentration within the core region (of radius r_c).
——— theory (Whitmore, 1967) for fairly large b/a using $r_c = b$; ······ rough approximation (Whitmore, 1967) for smaller b/a, using $r_c = a - b$; – – – – – extended theory (see p. 92) for b/a near to or exceeding 1.

The viscous properties of plasma itself have recently been studied particularly carefully by Gabe and Zatz (1969), whose detailed comparisons of phase as well as amplitude as a function of distance from the axis of an oscillating cylindrical viscometer show how accurately cell-free plasma behaves as a Newtonian viscous liquid. Its viscosity μ_p is about 0·015 poise. In the axial train regime conductivity according to equation (2) is about

$$\sigma = \frac{a^2}{8\mu_p}\left(1 - \frac{r_c^4}{a^4}\right) \tag{7}$$

so that the effective viscosity in those circumstances is

$$\mu_p\bigg/\left(1 - \frac{r_c^4}{a^4}\right) \tag{8}$$

which does not rise to be equal to a typical whole-blood viscosity of $0 \cdot 04$ poise until r_c/a is about $0 \cdot 89$.

It is in the region $b/a > 0 \cdot 9$, then, that we can look for resistances greater than would be given by Poiseuille's Law with an effective viscosity equal to a typical whole-blood value. But new features must in any case be present when b/a is near 1, or (as of course can occur) greater than 1. It is then essential to consider the rather special pressure distribution associated with the non-uniform thickness of the very thin lubricating layer round the cell rim, *and* the effects of deformations of red cells, *and* the interactions between these.

MOTION IN THE NARROWEST CAPILLARIES

It may be thought unnecessary to investigate circumstances in which capillary resistance may be enhanced, since it is known that the highest resistance in the peripheral circulation (the greatest pressure drop) is located (roughly speaking) in arterioles, whereas the pressure drop across capillaries is much less, in spite of their very small diameter, because there is such an enormous number of them in parallel. If, however, as I shall suggest, there is a tendency for capillary resistance to become substantially enhanced at low flow rates, this might be significant in certain contexts.†

One possible relevance of such a property is to the detailed mechanism by which the rate of perfusion of part of the peripheral vascular bed can be controlled, often within a factor of more than 10, by vasomotor muscular activity in the arterioles. I will emphasize again that for $R < 1$ there is no possibility of sphincters being able to operate a sluice-gate effect, involving separation behind the constriction. The pressure drop associated with that would be of purely inertial character. At $R < 1$ this is impossible, and vasomotor muscles can control the flow, at any rate if it is steady, only by changing the *resistance* of arterioles.

To be sure, the greatest resistance *is* in the vessels on which vasomotor control acts, but not all the resistance is there, and it is not easy to explain how changes in that resistance can produce the very big overall changes in flow that are observed. This is where some special non-linear property of capillary resistance, whereby it increased at low flow rates, might help to explain why vasomotor control is so effective.

† Such a prediction would not be in conflict with findings referred to by Professor Burton that very low resistances occur in narrow capillaries of $5 \cdot 5$ μm. diameter at velocities greater by orders of magnitude than those occurring in the actual circulation; it is argued below that resistance essentially varies with velocity, and may take substantially enhanced values at more normal, and especially at subnormal, velocities.

It seems desirable also to estimate what degree of leakback through the lubricating layer remains under tight-fit conditions—not simply for inferring how Whitmore's curve (Fig. 1) for mean red cell concentration $\bar{c}$ is extended into the region where b/a is near or above 1, but also for making predictions relevant to mass transfer. The diffusion coefficients D of dissolved gases in the blood are actually three orders of magnitude lower than the diffusivity of momentum μ/ρ, so that in capillaries convection and diffusion of dissolved gas are on a par (Ud/D is of order 1, as Prothero and Burton, 1961, 1962a have emphasized) even though Reynolds number $\rho Ud/\mu$, which indicates the relative importance of convection and diffusion of momentum, is so very small.

Prothero and Burton pointed out the possible convective role of a toroidal circulation in the "bolus" of plasma between two successive cells, and performed an excellent experiment using the correct value of Ud/D in which transport was shown to be approximately doubled because of convection in the bolus. The toroidal motions, however, may be enhanced by inertial effects tending to maintain the rotary motion at the Reynolds number of those experiments, which was around 10, and the toroidal motion may be less pronounced at very small Reynolds number. In those circumstances the flow associated with leakback (Fig. 2) may play the more prominent role in mass transport.

The mathematical models that I, and more recently Fitz-Gerald, have used to estimate the characteristics of the lubricating layer are quite complicated, and I do not propose to describe them in detail, but only to mention three perhaps essential features they possess. First, in the use of lubrication theory;

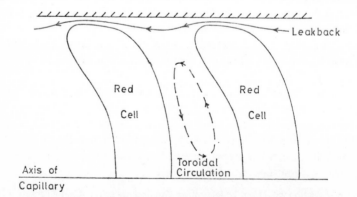

FIG. 2. Sketch of the toroidal flow of the plasma bolus between cells, and the flow associated with plasma leakback past cells, in very narrow capillaries. The predicted proximal "necking" of the gap between cell and tube wall is also sketched.

this relates the pressure distribution when viscous fluid is forced through a gap by the sliding of one surface over another to the details of the variation of gap thickness. Next, in the use of data on the distortion of red cells; consideration of their elastic properties provides a second link between distributions of rim pressure and of gap thickness. A third essential feature of the models is that the pressure difference between the two sides of a cell must be just sufficient to balance the viscous resistance to its motion due to the thin plasma layer.

A general feature of the mathematical models is their critical dependence on a parameter relating what we may call red cell "constrictability" to characteristic viscous stresses. I use constrictability as a sort of opposite to Burton's word "distensibility" that I used earlier for tubes. The constrictability k means a relative change of dimension per unit additional pressure applied in the lubricating layer. It has the dimensions mb^{-1} and from the work of Rand and Burton (1964) and of Fung (1966) I estimate it as between 1 and 2 in those units. The key parameter relating constrictability to viscous stresses is

$$A = k(\mu_p U/a) \tag{9}$$

where U is the red cell velocity and a the tube radius.

For typical values $U = 0 \cdot 1$–2 mm./sec. and $a = 3$–4 μm., the parameter A is around 10^{-3}. The mathematical models indicate under these circumstances something like a 7 per cent leakback of plasma relative to the red cells (in tubes somewhat less in diameter than the undistorted cells). This means that mean plasma velocity is 93 per cent of mean erythrocyte velocity, and film thickness is about $0 \cdot 07a$ (say, between $0 \cdot 2$ and $0 \cdot 3$ μm.). On this assumption the reduced mean concentration of red cells in capillaries would even out at about $0 \cdot 95c_0$ (see broken line on Fig. 1). There is a rather more critical dependence of resistance on the particular model used, but the more sophisticated models show it to be at least twice what would be calculated from Poiseuille's Law using the viscosity of whole blood.

The distribution of lubricating-layer thickness h is influenced by the need to build up a pressure maximum such as will sufficiently squash the cell. Sliding at velocity U without leakback sets up a negative pressure gradient proportional to $-\mu_p U/h^2$. This can help pressure fall away on the distal side of its maximum but cannot allow it to rise up to a maximum on the proximal side. However, a leakback flow Q through a gap of small thickness h and width $2\pi a$ demands a positive pressure gradient proportional to $+ \mu_p Q/ah^3$, by the appropriate form of Poiseuille's Law. The combination of the positive gradient proportional to h^{-3} and negative gradient proportional to h^{-2} permits passage of the pressure through a maximum, provided that the film thickness h has the right distribution.

Film thicknesses are required that are least on the proximal side of the pressure maximum, where the models indicate a pronounced "necking" of the gap (Fig. 2). The arguments also explain why for fixed properties of the cell the film thickness h has to vary roughly as the square root of the velocity U, so as to maintain about the same contribution $\mu_p U/h^2$ to pressure gradient. The calculations indicate, in fact, that leakback varies approximately as the square root of the velocity parameter A, and that the same is true of ratios of a typical film thickness to the tube radius.

Also, the pressure difference required to push the cell depends on viscous stresses like $\mu_p U/h$, where h is proportional to $\sqrt{U}$, so we have the unusual

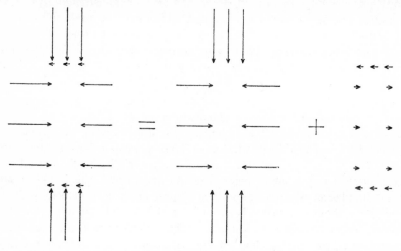

FIG. 3. Illustrating the idea that the total system of stresses acting on a red cell is equivalent to the sum of a system of "squashing" stresses (in which equal and opposite proximal and distal pressures are accompanied by larger circumferential pressures) and of a system of "bowing" stresses shown at right (in which circumferential shear stress is balanced by two equal forces, distributed respectively over the cell's proximal and distal faces).

phenomenon of fluid flow at velocity U appearing to require a pressure difference proportional to $\sqrt{U}$. The ratio of resistance predicted to resistance given by Poiseuille's Law then varies as $1/\sqrt{A}$, so that figures of at least 2 for this ratio mentioned earlier for $A = 10^{-3}$ become much larger at low values of the parameter A. This is the non-linear kind of resistance, increasing at low flow velocities, that I suggested earlier. Furthermore, at these lower values of A, the film thicknesses are predicted to fall considerably below the values of $0 \cdot 2$–$0 \cdot 3$ μm. already quoted. Those are circumstances when a lubrication engineer might expect failure of hydrodynamic lubrication, and the kind of abrupt rise in resistance that he calls "seizing up".

It is possible that complete seizing up would be prevented by the presence of the kind of mucopolysaccharide layer of thickness a few hundredths of a micrometre that Luft (1966) has inferred from his observations. Such a layer, both far thinner *and* more viscous than the lubricating layers of plasma postulated here, would create an upper limit to resistance, but that upper limit would be at least an order of magnitude above the values that I have suggested as normal. Thus a big rise in resistance at low flow rates would still be predicted.

The mathematical models that we first used were axisymmetric, so that we were trying to estimate approximately the mutual dependence of various parameters of the motion by averaging all properties round the circumference. More recent studies using a non-axisymmetric model have given this crude approach support, by indicating that the hydrodynamic distributions of pressure may compress the cell most where the layer is thinnest and therefore tend to increase the axisymmetric character of the layer. Another recent development is to decompose the stress system deforming the cell into two systems (Fig. 3), namely the effect of excess circumferential pressures squashing the cell directly, and that of the circumferential shear stress balanced by pressure difference tending to make the cell bow-shaped.

I shall mention only one more refinement of the model that is now in progress. Fitz-Gerald is considering the effect on the lubricating layer of loss of plasma through those crevices in the capillary endothelial wall which Professor Guyton (1966) estimated may accept perhaps 1 per cent of capillary flow near the proximal end of a capillary. It was thought that this loss of fluid might be influential when possibilities of seizing-up had to be considered, but the preliminary indications from this study are that these losses do not significantly disturb the fundamental balance between compliance and viscosity, which I have made the main theme of this contribution.

Acknowledgement

It is a pleasure to acknowledge many helpful discussions with Dr. Colin Caro on the subject of this paper.

REFERENCES

BURTON, A. C. (1966). *Fedn Proc. Fedn Am. Socs exp. Biol.*, **25**, 1753.
FUNG, Y. C. (1966). *Fedn Proc. Fedn Am. Socs exp. Biol.*, **25**, 1761.
GABE, I. T., and ZATZ, L. (1969). In preparation.
GOLDSMITH, H. L., and MASON, S. G. (1964). *Proc. R. Soc. A*, **282**, 569.
GUYTON, A. C. (1966). *Textbook of Medical Physiology*, 3rd edn. London: Saunders.
LIGHTHILL, M. J. (1968). *J. Fluid Mech.*, **34**, 113.
LUFT, J. H. (1966). *Fedn Proc. Fedn Am. Socs exp. Biol.*, **25**, 1773.
    4*

McDONALD, D. A. (1960). *Blood Flow in Arteries.* London: Arnold.
PAPPENHEIMER, J. R., and KINTER, W. B. (1956). *Am. J. Physiol.*, **185**, 377.
PROTHERO, J., and BURTON, A. C. (1961). *Biophys. J.*, **1**, 565.
PROTHERO, J., and BURTON, A. C. (1962a). *Biophys. J.*, **2**, 199.
PROTHERO, J., and BURTON, A. C. (1962b). *Biophys. J.*, **2**, 213.
RAND, R. P., and BURTON, A. C. (1964). *Biophys. J.*, **4**, 115.
WHITMORE, R. L. (1967). *J. appl. Physiol.*, **22**, 767.

DISCUSSION

Saffman: May I make two comments? On your assumption of axisymmetry, there is experimental evidence by D. C. Christopherson and D. Dowson ([1959]. *Proc. R. Soc. A*, **251**, 550) using solid spheres that motion is not axisymmetric. Secondly, F. P. Bretherton ([1961]. *J. Fluid Mech.*, **10**, 166) has considered air bubbles rising through tubes, which is a similar type of problem to the red cell, and found that seizing up could occur when a certain parameter of the problem was less than some critical value.

Lighthill: We were much influenced by Christopherson and Dowson's paper because it is one of the few in which lubrication theory has been used and the criterion applied of a pressure difference on the two sides which has to balance the viscous resistance in order to determine the rate of leakback. We concluded that their sort of asymmetry would not apply to erythrocytes because it depended very much on the fact that they used spheres which would rotate, and the spinning was causing the asymmetry. We came to the conclusion that irregular shapes like erythrocytes would not spin as they go down the tube, which would remove that source of asymmetry. Certainly our calculations seem to indicate that there is an automatic tendency to go nearer to symmetry than you start with in the unstressed state. I would like to look up the paper on bubbles.

Mason: May we have more details of your model? Does it apply to a single isolated cell or do you consider a train of cells, as in a rouleau? And are you considering a rigid body?

Lighthill: We think of the erythrocyte as existing in a train of cells but the mathematics is mainly confined to a single lubricating layer. We tried one or two different models of the elasticity and they all seem to depend on a parameter which is some ratio of compliance forces to viscous forces; but we are not yet satisfied with our model. We have tended to use simple Hookian models of various types, but we have included models influenced by Professor Burton's studies of the cell wall as a membrane under tension.

The tube is rigid. We first worked it out for a non-rigid tube but after combing the literature we decided that the elasticity of the tube ought to be neglected.

Mason: There is considerable difference between a rigid and a deformable particle in this context. An air bubble, as in Sir Geoffrey Taylor's ([1961]. *J. Fluid Mech.*, **10**, 161) experiments, is automatically self-centring, and I imagine that you assume your model behaves similarly. On the other hand, rigid particles such as discs do not centre themselves automatically, as we have shown experimentally. Instead they tend to rattle down the tube rotating very erratically. The self-centring mechanism in your model arises from the apparent deformability of the particles.

Lighthill: The theory certainly indicates that it comes from the deformability, but as I say, most experiments which have shown this rattling have not been on bodies as extremely different from a spherical shape as are red cells, so there is a possible difference. Certainly spheres are not self-centring but I am not sure whether experiments on markedly different shapes have been done. And even supposing that a single cell was flapping about a lot, there would be definite constraints on a train of cells that should make them less likely to flap about.

Mason: The deformability is important in another context, in that the pressure difference across your model red cell produces a re-entrant cavity, as first shown by P. I. Branemark and J. Lindstrom ([1963]. *Biorheology*, **1**, 139). This also occurs with liquid drops and gas bubbles (Goldsmith, H. L., and Mason, S. G. [1963]. *J. Colloid Sci.*, **18**, 237). A theoretical analysis of this phenomenon would be interesting.

Lighthill: The re-entrant cavity *is* predicted by the latest model, referred to in the written version of my paper (see Fig. 3, p. 94).

Burton: Professor Lighthill, have you had cases where the time of transit through the tube of the plasma is *less* than the time of transit of the cells? Dr. A. C. Groom ([1968]. In *Proc. 1st int. Conf. Hemorheology*, pp. 643–653, ed. Copley, A. L. Oxford: Pergamon Press) has labelled plasma and cells with different radioactive isotopic markers and so been able to measure simultaneously the time of transit of both plasma and cells through isolated organs (skeletal muscle). While at relatively low haematocrits (below 70 per cent) the expected result is found—the red cells come through faster—at high (more than 70 per cent) haematocrits this reverses, and plasma comes through faster than red cells. When cells are touching each other, as in sedimenting red cells in a tube, one could imagine that the plasma could move more easily through the matrix of cells than the cell matrix could move.

Lighthill: The leakback of plasma gets less at the lower flow rates, but we have no evidence of a "leak forward"; in fact we feel that the more the cells get squashed in the tube, the more the two velocities should approach equality. If there is such an effect as you describe it might arise in the slightly bigger tubes and not in these very narrow ones.

Burton: It may be that what Groom is measuring is related to the larger tubes rather than to the very small ones in the vascular bed. He is studying a whole organ so he is measuring across a whole vascular bed. But the net result is that at high haematocrits the plasma is coming through faster than the red cells, not the opposite which is invariably found at low haematocrits.

Lighthill: Does all the plasma or just a tail out in front come through faster? Is the actual mean flow faster?

Burton: The velocity is faster over the whole curve.

Mead: Professor Lighthill, how do you measure the compliance of the red cell? Is the pipette method directly applicable?

Lighthill: That is one method. We obtain orders of magnitude only. A result we found very useful is that on osmotically produced changes in red cell geometry, as we feel that osmotic forces would produce something similar to the corresponding mechanical pressure difference. We were able to see how sphericity changes were associated with changes of radii, and then Professor Burton's work and Fung's on possible membrane tensions using a Laplace Law gave us something that agreed with the more direct estimates from the pipette measurements.

Burton: We have a fair idea of the force it takes to bend the red cell—expressed in ergs/cm.[2]—and to stretch the membrane, that is, Young's Modulus for the red cell membrane. By integrating the bending moments over the whole shape (see my paper, p. 74) Peter Canham finds that the normal shape of the red cell represents a minimum total bending energy. The red cell has to have a certain fixed volume and area but that allows an infinite number of shapes, and the computer calculation shows that the minimum total bending energy will be when it is the shape it actually is. With the same area and a larger volume, as in a cell in osmotic swelling, the shape for minimum bending energy is different and corresponds to the actual shape of swollen cells. This is very satisfactory.

Lighthill: It will be interesting to correspond with you and perhaps make use of this programme. We would ideally like a separate estimate of the constrictability by each of the two systems of forces in Fig. 3 of my paper (p. 94).

Mead: What is the unstressed shape of a red cell?

Burton: I am quite sure that it has a *uniform* cell membrane, because when a red cell is swelled to a sphere it is a perfect sphere—a real object of admiration! Peter Rand and I once made rubber models cast into the shape of red cells, and if we blew them up by positive pressure inside they were never accurately spherical. So the membrane itself must be the same everywhere, at the rim as at the dimple, and therefore some unknown force holds it in its shape. It saves some total bending energy by being the shape it is rather than being spherical.

Philip: Professor Burton, your calculations on bending energy carry an implication of the actual model of deformation of the membrane itself. Are you treating the red cell as simply being a perfectly elastic membrane?

Burton: The red cell is bounded by a uniform cell membrane with a uniform bending moment but the cell membrane is not stretched until the red cell is spherical.

Philip: If you are making calculations on what you call bending energy, work must be being done against some mechanical resistance to bending.

Altshuler: Bending implies a shell, not a membrane; by definition a membrane means no bending. The term "membrane" refers to surface forces.

Burton: "Membrane" is the term used by physiologists for what you call a "shell"; the red cell is not a membrane in the mechanical sense.

Philip: The question is whether the red cell is behaving as a thin elastic plate in the mechanical sense. If energy is stored in the bending, then the cell must be behaving as an elastic object.

Davies: With a shell of uniform thickness with curvatures in different directions there must be differences in the tensions or structural–mechanical properties of the shell, in order to maintain these opposed curvatures by surface tension.

Burton: If the red cell were like a soap film with energy required to bend it, it could not have the shape it has. There is therefore a missing force which we think is an attraction between the opposing membranes of the disc, which may be exactly similar to the attraction between the membranes of two adjacent red cells in a rouleau, which we know depends on long-chain (protein) molecules being in the medium (rouleaux do not form in saline solution). So we infer that long-chain molecules are present across the red cell, and by polarized light studies we have shown that something is indeed lined up across the middle of the cell.

Philip: Professor Lighthill's calculations must depend rather critically on his model of deformation of the red cell, and I hate to see him do a lot of work until this aspect has been clarified.

Lighthill: That is true, but we have used rather simple models first. I think we have shown that it does not matter tremendously what we assume provided the red cell is constrictable, because there is a gross change from normal hydrodynamics: there is a pressure difference which may vary like the square root of velocity. This is the simple *qualitative* point we are bringing to the notice of physiologists. We are asking whether it is conceivable that a rise in capillary resistance occurs at low flow rates.

Philip: What I have in mind particularly is that your results must be very sensitive to the details of the shape of the cell.

Lighthill: We do not have confidence in the exact numbers that come out of our calculations.

Cumming: Professor Lighthill, is your analysis applicable with equal validity to the pulmonary circulation?

Lighthill: I cannot see why it should be different.

Cumming: If that is so, do I understand that the resistance in the capillary would be higher than you would compute were simple Poiseuille forces applicable, and therefore the pressure drop over the capillary bed itself will be greater?

Lighthill: We think this would be particularly true at the lower flow velocities, of the order of tens rather than hundreds of micrometres a second.

Cumming: In that case perhaps I can give you some data. We have studied the pulmonary circulation by making a cast and then measuring the length and diameter of all the constituent vessels. Some 12,767 branches were considered and from the measurements the flow down each branch was found, total flow being 5 litres per minute. If we consider the flow of a Newtonian fluid in this structure the pressure drop across it can be computed. It turns out that if one assumes a value for viscosity of 3 centipoises, then the drop from the pulmonary artery to vessels of the order of 100 μm. is about 3 cm. of water. The evidence suggests also that at least a similar drop occurs in vessels from 100 to 20 μm. (though we have not measured this directly).

Thus the bulk of the pressure drop appears to occur before the capillaries, though this conclusion is based on the somewhat fallacious application of fully developed laminar flow in the system.

West: I wonder whether Professor Lighthill's analysis helps to explain the patchy flow and filling that we have observed in the pulmonary capillary circulation. It is possible to raise the pulmonary arterial pressure to 10 or 15 mm. Hg above alveolar pressure and still find no red blood cells in many of the capillary channels, and we do not understand why. Is it possible that because of some perturbation, the flow in some of the many communicating mesh-like channels becomes very low, and as a result the resistance to flow becomes very high and flow ceases? In other words, in a mesh-like system like the pulmonary circulation with its many parallel networks, flow might be inherently unstable.

Burton: This is an excellent point, the same sort of result as the surfactant story—that without lung surfactant there will be an instability of volume (atelectasis). If Professor Lighthill's calculation predicts resistance that increases when the flow is lower, rather than decreasing as in the ordinary case, it will lead to instability in vessels in parallel. It would be valuable if Professor Lighthill would analyse the situation for several vessels in parallel, following this law that resistance increases when flow decreases.

Caro: If I may return the discussion from pulmonary to systemic capillaries, vasomotion of precapillary sphincters might have an important effect if capillary resistance rises at low flow rates. Indeed red blood cells presumably come to rest in capillaries when the relevant precapillary sphincter closes (Wiederhielm, C. A. [1967]. *Fedn Proc. Fedn Am. Socs exp. Biol.,* **26,** 495) and their motion will have to be restarted when the sphincter opens.

Taylor: Flow seems to start again quite easily in the systemic circulation. One sees red cells jammed into a narrow vessel where a precapillary sphincter has closed or a bit of smooth muscle has contracted; when the sphincter re-opens or smooth muscle relaxes the train of cells starts moving again, and the sticking and slipping seems to be more in the nature of plugging, where the vessel is too narrow for the red cell to squeeze through.

West: It depends what you mean by "easily"; in the systemic circulation an enormous arterial pressure is available when the arteriolar sphincter opens up. In the pulmonary circulation by contrast the pressures are very low. Additionally, the mesh-like character of the pulmonary bed may mean that the pressure across a single capillary segment may be only a fraction of a centimetre of water.

Taylor: Even in the systemic circulation one sees regions in the capillaries with cross-connexions having a high pressure at both ends and a very small gradient. In those circumstances the red cells drift very slowly in one direction, come to rest and drift back again; you may see platelets in suspension which are obviously not sticking to anything and they too move around quite freely. The red cells do not seem to become adherent to the lining endothelium. White cells certainly do. I have seen white cells go one way while the platelets and red cells were flowing the other way; the white cells, which are actively motile, give the impression that they wet the endothelium and roll along its surface whereas red cells seem to be like mercury on glass and barely touch the endothelial lining.

Burton: May I turn again to the lung? The size of the smallest vessels in the pulmonary circulation is considerably greater than that of systemic capillaries. Very few capillaries in the lungs are smaller in diameter than red cells, whereas perhaps the majority of systemic capillaries are narrower than the diameter of the red cell.

West: It depends on the capillary pressure; it is true that for high pressures the capillaries easily accommodate the red cells (see Figs. 1A–D in my paper, p. 256) but at lower pressures the capillaries appear narrower than the red cell diameter.

Caro: So the lung capillaries are quite distensible?

West: It depends what you mean by distensibility. Certainly we believe that the mean diameter of the capillaries, measured across the septum, increases as capillary pressure is increased up to 50 cm. water. However this does not necessarily mean that the perimeter of the capillary stretches; the behaviour may be like that of a collapsed plastic bag which can be inflated up to a certain volume without stretching its walls.

Burton: Has anyone watched a white cell going through a capillary? There is one white cell for every 600 red cells. Does flow in that capillary stop while it crawls through, or is it driven through by pressure, or what?

Taylor: White cells get pushed along by the red cells. They can elongate enormously, and they go through capillaries like a plug, rather slowly with a lot of impatient red cells queuing up behind. The whole lot suddenly pops out at the other end of the capillary, almost audibly!

Lighthill: It seems to be generally agreed in the literature that the residence times of cells are lower than that of the plasma in the peripheral circulation, but I am not emphasizing this for the smallest vessels. I was only quoting Whitmore's argument that this effect would be most pronounced (more precisely, leakback would be greatest) for a vessel of twice the diameter of the red cell (Whitmore, R. L. [1967]. *Nature, Lond.*, **215**, 123–126).

Caro: Is there in fact a slowing up of cells when a white cell goes through a capillary?

Taylor: I think there is, but it is a rare event—one in many hundred.

Mead: In a parallel system of vessels, moreover, the probability of white cells occupying many parallel capillaries simultaneously is very low.

Cumming: If the effect of white cells on flow were important, in leukaemia where you may have not one white cell to 600 red cells but one white cell for every single red cell, one should see a disastrous effect on the circulation; and we see no such thing.

Renkin: White cells seem to hold up flow only in closed or narrowed pre-capillary sphincters in mammals. There is a momentary interruption of flow while the white cell oozes through the sphincter region but as soon as the white cell is free in the capillary, all the blood cells move rapidly on again. This produces momentary interruptions in flow but no great distortions (see Zweifach, B. W. [1957]. *Am. J. Med.*, **23**, 684–696). However, large aggregates of cells in capillaries and venules may be associated with low velocities of blood, and I wonder what Professor Lighthill would say about the movement of aggregates of red cells in capillaries as a source of resistance to blood flow.

Lighthill: This needs considering. I did quote the point about the variation of geometry of cells, which might be expected to produce a variation in leak-back, so that there might be a bunching of cells with rather small amounts of plasma between them.

Mead: If capillary resistance accounts for only a small fraction of the total resistance to flow in the circulation, perhaps 1 per cent, such variation would have a barely detectable influence on resistance.

Caro: A simple calculation, based on classical measurements of micro-vascular pressures, shows that the pressure drop down the capillary bed is roughly one quarter of the total. But this does not make sense in relation to exercise, because even if the arteriolar resistance then fell almost to nothing a substantial pressure drop would remain and not allow the great increase of flow that is seen for example in muscle. It would seem that there must then be a significant reduction of the pressure drop down the capillary and post-capillary vessels.

Renkin: In a muscle at rest, precapillary resistance has to be roughly four times postcapillary resistance in order to maintain fluid balance (Pappen-heimer, J. R., and Soto-Rivera, A. [1948]. *Am. J. Physiol.*, **152,** 471–491; Mellander, S. [1960]. *Acta physiol. scand.*, **50,** Suppl. 176, 1–86). Precapillary resistance extends from large arteries down to an imaginary mid-point of the capillaries, and postcapillary resistance from the capillary mid-point to the large veins. The greatest value that half the capillary resistance could have would be equal to the total postcapillary resistance, and it follows that all capillary resistance can be no more than two-fifths of total vascular resistance.

Lighthill: I said that capillary resistance is probably very much less than that, probably 20 per cent of the total, but even if vasodilatation removes all the arteriolar resistance, this would produce only a 5-fold increase in the rate of perfusion and I understand that flow may increase 10 or 15 times, so there is something to explain!

In this connexion, may I revert to Dr. Cumming's experimental data on the pressure drop in the pulmonary circulation (p. 100). It is central to my thesis that in the great bulk of the small vessels effective viscosity might be expected to be reduced to near plasma viscosity, for the reason Professor Burton mentioned, that what matters most is the viscosity of fluid near the wall. Hence it does not seem clear that you can get the whole pulmonary pressure drop without taking capillary resistance into account. You assumed that the viscosity of blood is 3 centipoise, about three times that of water, in comparing the calculated and observed pressure drops, but we are suggesting that the viscosity of whole blood has no real meaning in small vessels. In much of the microcirculation you are nearer the plasma viscosity.

Cumming: These calculations were made for the large vessels, not the microcirculation; we took vessels down to about 50 μm.—what one calls the arterioles.

West: Professor Renkin's comments on resistance apply of course to the systemic circulation and not to the pulmonary circulation. There is evidence that much of the resistance to blood flow in the pulmonary circulation is located in the capillaries, especially at low lung volumes (Fowler, K. T., West, J. B., and Pain, M. C. F. [1966]. *Resp. Physiol.*, **1**, 88–98).

THE FLOW BEHAVIOUR OF PARTICULATE SUSPENSIONS

S. G. MASON AND H. L. GOLDSMITH

Department of Chemistry, McGill University, and
University Medical Clinic, Montreal General Hospital, Montreal, Canada

THIS paper describes some flow properties of dispersions subjected to steady and oscillatory flow through rigid tubes in terms of the motions of the individual suspended particles and their effect on the surrounding liquid. This approach, in which the flow properties of the aggregate system are obtained from a knowledge of the detailed behaviour of the elements of which it is composed, is the method of microrheology. Here we are concerned with suspensions of rigid and deformable spheres, discs and rods in which the elementary volumes of Newtonian liquids each containing a particle are viewed under a microscope, first in isolation from each other and then in interaction, in dilute and concentrated suspensions up to 50 per cent by volume. The microrheology of such dispersions has been extensively studied in a variety of shear flows including Couette, Poiseuille and hyperbolic flow and fully described elsewhere (Goldsmith and Mason, 1967). The present discussion is confined to steady and oscillatory laminar flow in tubes because of its application to blood flow. Wherever possible, the observed particle motions have been interpreted in terms of rigorous hydrodynamic theory. The experiments with model spheres, discs and rods have laid the basis for an extension of the work to human red cell suspensions using similar techniques adapted to viewing microscopic particles (Goldsmith, 1967). It has emerged that many of the phenomena first described in model systems are also observed in erythrocyte suspensions.

Both investigations were carried out over a range of the tube Reynolds number $Re = R\bar{u}\rho/\eta$ (R being the tube radius, $\bar{u}$ the mean linear flow rate, ρ and η the respective fluid densities and viscosities) from 10^{-3} in the Stokes or creeping flow regime to values greater than 1 where inertia of the fluid becomes important in determining particle behaviour.

The phenomena described below were observed with model particles and red blood cells whose diameter was small compared to that of the tube ($< 0 \cdot 2$). The present *in vitro* results are therefore relevant only to blood vessels larger

105

than 50 μm. diameter. An investigation of the flow and deformation of large liquid bubbles in small tubes which has been used as a model for the passage of red blood cells through the capillaries of the microcirculation (Goldsmith, 1968) has been described elsewhere (Goldsmith and Mason, 1963) and will not be discussed here.

TECHNIQUES AND SUSPENSIONS

(a) Model studies

The particle movements in precision bore glass tubes having $R = 0 \cdot 10$ to $1 \cdot 00$ cm. were observed through a travelling microscope so that continuous viewing over 50–75 cm. travel was possible. The events were recorded with still and ciné cameras and subsequently analysed on a projection table.

Steady flow was provided by an infusion-withdrawal pump, oscillatory flow by a sinusoidally reciprocating pump and pulsatile flow by the two pumps in parallel (Takano, Goldsmith and Mason, 1968a).

Particles consisted of rigid polystyrene, lucite and polymethylmethacrylate spheres and discs (made by compressing the spheres between the heated plates of a press), nylon and dacron rods and filaments, and pulpwood fibres suspended in Newtonian oils whose viscosities ranged from $0 \cdot 1$ to 500 poise. Suspensions of deformable water or oil drops were made with ranges of viscosity ratios $\lambda =$ drop phase/suspending phase viscosity from 10^{-3} to 50 and of interfacial tensions γ from 2 to 40 dynes/cm.

The viewing of particles in concentrated suspensions was made possible by rendering them transparent, through the matching of the refractive indices of the disperse and suspending phases. A small fraction of particles with the same geometry and density but of different refractive index was then added to serve as visible tracers (Karnis, Goldsmith and Mason, 1966a).

(b) Blood

Freshly drawn, heparinized human blood obtained by venipuncture from healthy persons, in which red cells were resuspended in the plasma to give volume concentrations of less than 2 per cent, was used to study single particle motions. At low flow rates both single cells and straight chain (rod-like) and branched aggregates or rouleaux could be seen (Fig. 1). Their behaviour was observed in glass or polypropylene tubes of radius from 25 to 100 μm. In this

FIG. 1. Photomicrographs of rouleaux of human erythrocytes showing two separate aggregates in the upper portion and a network of rouleaux in the lower part. The tendency to form rouleaux in whole blood is in part responsible for the suspension's non-Newtonian behaviour; i.e. as the blood is sheared, the network of rouleaux progressively breaks down and the measured viscosity decreases. (After Goldsmith and Mason, 1967.)

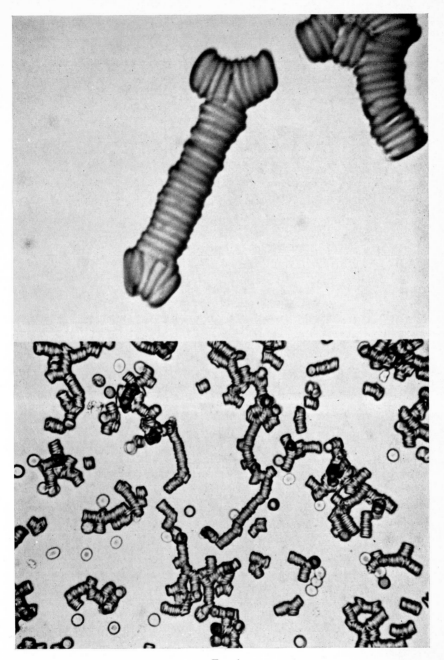

Fig. 1

[To face page 106

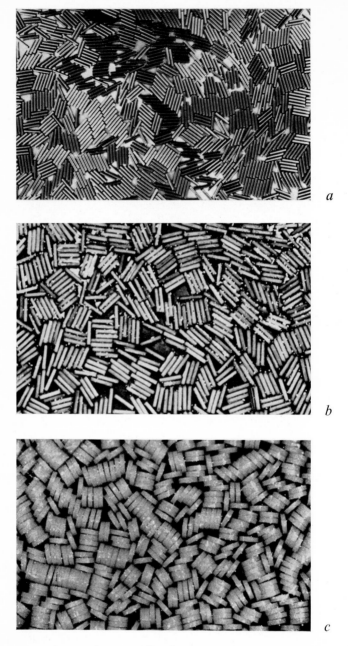

a

b

c

Fig. 2

case, the cells were kept in the field of view by moving the tube and attached infusion pump with the aid of a mechanically driven microscope stage (Goldsmith, 1967).

The occurrence of rouleaux in mammalian blood, first investigated in modern times by Fahraeus (1929), is of more general interest as an example of ordered arrays of particles having uniform geometry. Other examples are mosaics produced in towing rafts of pulpwood logs or in a vibrating monolayer of cylinders, as shown in Fig. 2a, b. As first demonstrated by Norris (1869), rouleaux of rigid discs are formed when these float with their faces vertical at an aqueous surface (Fig. 2c).

Transparent concentrated suspensions of blood were made by reconstituting red cell ghosts in biconcave form in plasma and adding a small fraction of the original red blood cells (Goldsmith, 1967).

POISEUILLE AND LAMINAR OSCILLATORY TUBE FLOW

The Poiseuille or laminar viscous flow of a Newtonian liquid in a rigid circular tube, as seen in the median or diametrical plane, is shown in Fig. 3. The fluid velocity $u(r)$ in the X- or axial direction increases parabolically from zero at the wall, with decreasing radial distance r, to a maximum at the centre, according to

$$u(r) = \frac{k}{2}(R^2 - r^2) \qquad (1)$$

where

$$k = \frac{dP}{dx} \cdot \frac{1}{2\eta} = \frac{4Q}{\pi R^4} \qquad (2)$$

Q being the volume flow rate and P the pressure. The velocity gradient or shear rate, G, increases linearly with r:

$$G = kr$$

In laminar oscillatory flow having a sinusoidal pressure gradient

---

Fig. 2. Mosaic of ordered structures of model particles produced by vibrating them in a monolayer (Shah, 1967).
(a) Steel rods resting on a solid surface.
(b) Wooden rods floating at a water surface.
(c) Polyethylene discs, poised to float vertically in an aqueous salt solution. The aggregates here resemble the rouleaux of red blood cells shown in Fig. 1.

$\partial P/\partial x = \varkappa \cos \omega t$ in the axial direction, the velocity distribution at time t is given by (Womersley, 1955; Takano, Goldsmith and Mason, 1967)

$$u(r, t) = \frac{\varkappa \eta M_0'}{\rho \omega} \sin (\omega t + \varepsilon_0) \qquad (3)$$

Here ω is the angular velocity of oscillation, ε_0 the phase angle which together with M_0' is a function of the radial distance and the dimensionless parameter

$$\alpha = R \left(\frac{\omega \rho}{\eta} \right)^{1/2} \qquad (4)$$

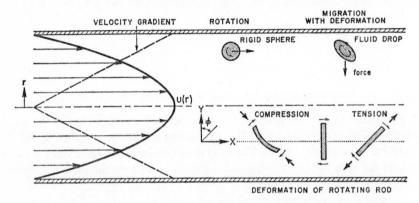

FIG. 3. Poiseuille flow of a viscous liquid as seen in the median or diametrical plane of a circular tube. The diagram shows the parabolic velocity distribution according to equation (1) and the velocity gradient, responsible for the fluid stresses which lead to the particle behaviour schematically portrayed. Thus a rigid sphere and flexible rod rotate; the fluid drop and the rod are subject to deforming stresses, compressive and tensile in alternate quadrants of the angle φ. The interaction of the ellipsoidal drop with the tube wall leads to axial migration.

and may be calculated from tables of Bessel functions (Womersley, 1955); $\varkappa$ is defined by

$$\varkappa = \frac{\Delta V \alpha^2 \omega}{2 \pi R^4 M_{10}'} \qquad (5)$$

ΔV being the volume displacement per half cycle, and values of M_{10}' have been tabulated (Womersley, 1955).

FIG. 4. Displacement profiles at 30° intervals over a half cycle of oscillation of a liquid in a tube, $\alpha = 7 \cdot 1$, obtained by following the motion of tracer spheres. The lines drawn are calculated from equation (6) using the experimental values of the volume displacement per half cycle—ΔV, ω and the phase angle ε_0. (After Shizgal, Goldsmith and Mason, 1965.)

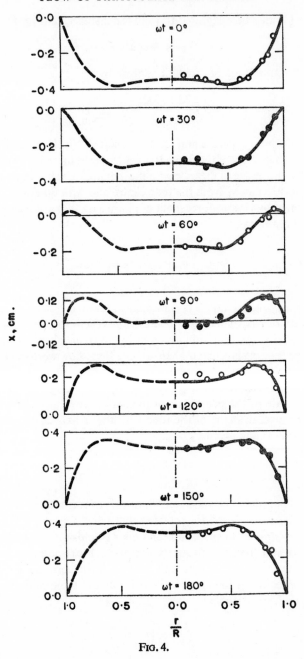

FIG. 4.

Equation (3) may be integrated to yield the displacement profiles

$$x(r, t) = A(r) \cos(\omega t + \varepsilon_0) \qquad (6)$$

where A is the amplitude of oscillation, given by

$$A(r) = \frac{2\varkappa \eta M_0'}{\rho \omega^2} = \frac{\Delta V M_0'}{\pi R^2 M_{10}'} \qquad (7)$$

Fig. 4 gives some experimental and calculated displacement profiles at $\alpha = 7 \cdot 1$ over a half cycle of the flow. It is evident that the velocity distributions are blunted in the centre of the tube with the maximum displacement amplitude at a radial position away from the tube centre and with fluid motion near the wall (dominated by viscous forces) out of phase with that at the centre (dominated by inertial forces).

SINGLE PARTICLE BEHAVIOUR

(a) Rotation

When the suspending liquid is subjected to laminar flow, the fluid stresses on the surface of suspended *rigid* bodies cause them to rotate as they travel down the tube (Fig. 3). The spin and rotation of rigid spheroids, either oblate (saucer-shaped) or prolate (cigar-shaped), in a shear flow were treated theoretically by Jeffery (1922), who found the motion of the particle axis of revolution to be somewhat like that of a precessing top. The angular velocity $d\varphi/dt$, φ being the angle of the projection of the axis of revolution of the spheroid in the XY or median plane of the tube with the Y-axis, as shown in Figs. 3 and 5b, is variable and given by

$$\frac{d\varphi}{dt} = \frac{G}{r_p^2 + 1} (r_p^2 \cos^2 \varphi + \sin^2 \varphi) \qquad (8)$$

where r_p is the particle axis ratio: length of axis of revolution/diametrical axis (<1 for oblate spheroids, >1 for prolate spheroids). Experiments have shown that the theory applies to small rods and discs (Goldsmith and Mason, 1967), and red cells and linear rouleaux (Goldsmith, 1967) at low shear rates in Poiseuille flow provided that r_p is replaced by r_e, an experimentally determined axis ratio representing the spheroid which has the same period of rotation, T, as the cylindrical particle

$$T = \frac{2\pi}{G} \left(r_e + \frac{1}{r_e} \right) \qquad (9)$$

For a rigid sphere, $r_e = r_p = 1$; the particle rotates with uniform angular velocity, which from equation (8) is $d\varphi/dt = G/2$ with a period of rotation $T = 4\pi/G$.

A consequence of the variable angular velocity of non-spherical particles

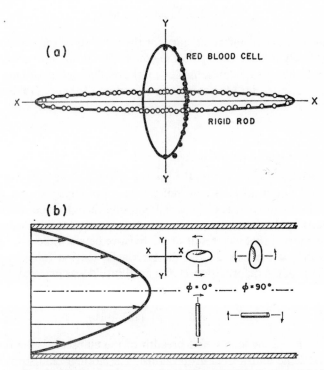

FIG. 5. (a) The square root of the differential distribution $p(\varphi)$ of the φ-orientation (plotted as the radius vector on a polar diagram) of the axis of revolution of a rod having $r = 14\cdot2$ (open circles) and a red blood cell having $r_e = 0\cdot40$ (closed circles). The lines were calculated from equation (10).

(b) The orientation of a rod and red blood cell in the median plane of the tube.

The plot shows that there is a much higher probability of finding the particles with their major axes aligned with the flow than across the flow.

is that the particles spend more time in each orbit aligned with the direction of flow ($\varphi = 0°$ for a disc or red cell, $\varphi = 90°$ for a rod or rouleau of more than five cells), a fact which measurement of the instantaneous orientation distribution of model particles (Anczurowski and Mason, 1967) and red cells

(Goldsmith, 1968) has confirmed. This is illustrated in Fig. 5a, a plot of the differential distribution function $p(\varphi)$, derived from equation (9), giving the relative probabilities of finding the particle axis of revolution at various values of the angle φ,

$$p(\varphi) = \frac{r_e}{2\pi(r_e^2\cos^2\varphi + \sin^2\varphi)} \qquad (10)$$

It is remarkable that Jeffery's theory for the rotation of spheroids which is strictly valid only in the creeping flow regime has been found to apply to rods and discs in oscillatory and pulsatile flows if the oscillating value of the velocity gradient G is inserted into the equations of motion (Takano, Goldsmith and Mason, 1967).

(b) Deformation and radial migration

The fluid stresses which act on the surface of rigid bodies causing them to rotate, act on liquid droplets deforming them into ellipsoids and on rods, filaments, fibres and rouleaux of red cells causing them to bend or buckle as they rotate (Fig. 3). The case of the liquid drop was considered by Taylor (1934) who showed that as a result of the balance between the viscous forces tending to distort the particle and the interfacial tension forces tending to keep it spherical, the deformation D into an ellipsoid was given by

$$D = \frac{L-B}{L+B} = \frac{Gb\eta}{\gamma} \cdot \frac{(19\lambda + 16)}{(16\lambda + 16)} \qquad (11)$$

Here, L and B are the length and breadth of the ellipsoid, γ the interfacial tension, and b the undistorted drop radius. The normal fluid stresses which are tensile and compressive in alternate quadrants of the angle φ (Fig. 3) orientate the drop with its major axis at an angle $45°$ to the flow, and the tangential stresses are transmitted into the interior of the drop, resulting in internal circulation patterns (Taylor, 1932).

As a result of the orientation and deformation of the drop and its interaction with the tube wall, the particle experiences a net inwardly directed force and migrates to the tube axis (Fig. 6) with a radial velocity which varies as Q^2, $(b/R)^4$, and the ratio, $r^2/(R-r)^2$; that is, it decreases rapidly with decreasing radial distance (Chaffey, Brenner and Mason, 1965; Karnis and Mason, 1967). This effect, which occurs in the viscous flow regime, is not observed with rigid particles (Goldsmith and Mason, 1962). Inward radial migration at low Reynolds numbers was also observed with human erythrocytes (Goldsmith,

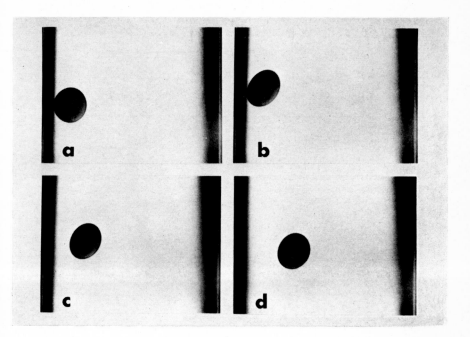

FIG. 6. Photomicrographs of the deformation and accompanying axial migration of an aqueous drop of 300 μm. radius suspended in silicone oil of 50 viscosity poise in a tube of $R = 0.4$ cm. (a) Drop at rest close to the tube wall. (b) to (d) Successive positions of drop, deformed into an ellipsoid, as liquid flows upward through the tube. The drop migrates away from the wall, the velocity gradient and the deformation decreasing with decreasing r. At (d) the drop has moved 18 cm. along the tube and migrated 0.13 cm. inward.

[To face page 112

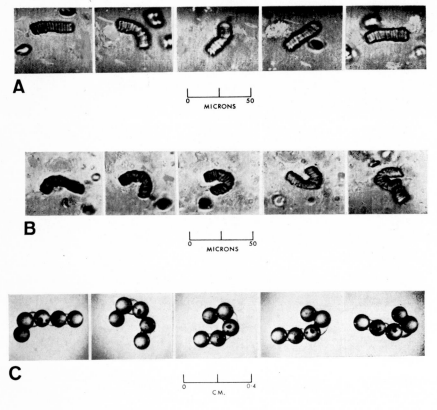

Fig. 7. Photomicrographs of the bending of rouleaux during clockwise rotation in the flow from left to right, at $\bar{u} = 0.03$ cm. sec.$^{-1}$ in a tube of 120 μm. diameter. The nearest tube wall, below the particles, is not shown in the photographs. A. "Springy" orbit, in which a rouleau of 13 cells buckles in one quadrant and straightens out again in the next. B. "Snake" rotation, in which the ends of the particle (20 cells long) are able to bend independently, and which is strikingly similar to C, the rotation in an oil of a chain of polystyrene spheres linked by water menisci (Zia, Cox and Mason, 1967). (After Goldsmith, 1967.)

1967), although here the particles continually rotated and there was no obvious visible deformation.

In oscillatory and pulsatile flow, the deformation and migration of liquid drops could also be observed, although when $\lambda > 10$, time-dependent effects entered which led to deviations of particle behaviour from theory (Takano, Goldsmith and Mason, 1968a).

In the case of a rotating rod, pulpwood fibre or linear rouleau, the compressive and tensile fluid stresses lead the particle to buckle or bend in one quadrant and then tend to straighten out again in succeeding quadrants of the orbit (Forgacs and Mason, 1959; Goldsmith, 1967). The flexibility of the particle depends on its bending modulus and axis ratio; it was found that for a given r_p there exists a critical value of the product (ηG) above which buckling set in. Some modes of deformation of rod-like particles are illustrated in Fig. 7. As did deformable liquid drops, these particles also migrated in tube flow toward the axis.

(c) Inertial effects

The phenomena described above, first observed at very low Reynolds numbers, continue to be exhibited in suspensions at higher flow rates and/or at lower viscosities, where, owing to inertia of the fluid, other effects now enter.

The most important of these is the two-way radial migration of rigid particles to an eccentric equilibrium position, as illustrated in Fig. 8, first studied with neutrally buoyant spheres by Segré and Silberberg (1962) and termed the "tubular pinch" effect. Since then it has been shown that rigid rods and discs behave in the same way and further that the equilibrium radial position in a vertically mounted tube depends on b/R and is shifted toward the wall or the axis, depending on whether the particle sedimentation velocity is of the same or opposite sign to the fluid velocity (Brenner, 1966).

Whereas in the creeping flow region rigid rods and discs in the tube continued to rotate in the orbits and radial positions of initial release, inertial effects at higher Reynolds numbers led the cylinders to drift into rotational orbits in which the energy dissipation was a maximum, as shown in Fig. 8 (Karnis, Goldsmith and Mason, 1966b). These phenomena have also been observed in oscillatory and pulsatile flow although here, owing to the changing velocity and velocity gradient distribution with changes in α, there are, at sufficiently high values of α, a number of positions at which the radial velocities are zero (Takano, Goldsmith and Mason, 1968a).

Experimentally, it was found that in suspensions at the same values of b/R and tube Reynolds number, deformable drops migrated inwards in both

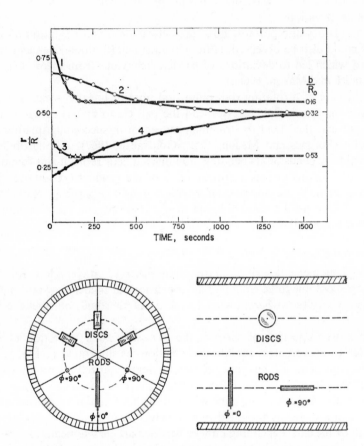

FIG. 8. Inertial effects in steady flow through tubes. *Upper part:* Two-way radial migration of rigid spheres in a tube of 0·2 cm. radius showing the effect of increasing particle size on the equilibrium position. The points of inflection in curves 1 and 2 indicate that the radial velocity is a maximum at a value of r/R intermediate between the initial and equilibrium value. *Lower part:* The final orbits achieved by rods and discs after drifting to an equilibrium radial position, viewed in the median plane of the tube, right, and along the tube axis, left. The faces of the discs are lying in the median plane and spin about their own axis of revolution; the rods have their long axes lying in the median plane and rotate without spin of their axis of revolution.

steady and oscillatory flow, with velocities considerably higher than those observed with rigid spheres or discs. Observations made with normal red blood

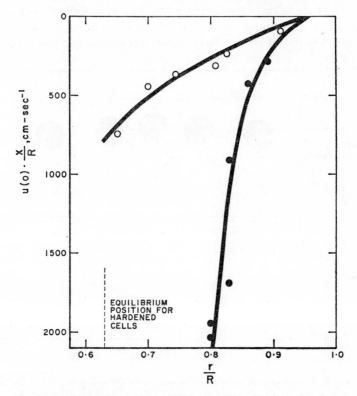

FIG. 9. The trajectories of normal human red blood cells (open circles) and cells hardened with glutaraldehyde (closed circles) in a tube of 40 μm. radius for particles initially at the tube wall (centre of rotation at $r/R = 0.94$). Plotted is the function $u(0).(x/R)$ against r/R where x is the distance down the tube from the initial position of release. It is evident that the red cells already rapidly migrate inward at values of $u(0).(x/R) < 100$. The hardened cells exhibit inward migration at much higher values of $u(0).x/R$ and were observed to go to an equilibrium position at $r = 0.63R$. The solid lines drawn are the best fit of the experimental points obtained by measuring the distribution of cells in the tube at various $u(0)$ and x at $c < 0.2$ per cent (Goldsmith, forthcoming publication).

cells and cells rendered non-deformable by hardening with glutaraldehyde (but still biconcave in shape) have shown a similar difference, as illustrated in Fig. 9 (Goldsmith, forthcoming publication).

THE KINETICS OF FLOWING SUSPENSIONS

(a) Collisions

Because of the velocity gradient in a liquid undergoing laminar tube flow, suspended particles are at times brought into close proximity and interact. Experiments in model systems have shown that two-body collisions between

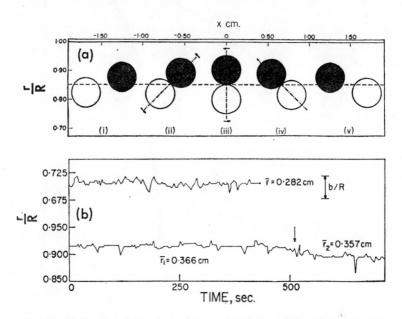

FIG. 10. (a) Tracings from photomicrographs of the collision doublet formed from rigid polystyrene spheres in the median plane of a tube during approach (i), collision (ii) to (iv), and recession (v). The spheres and their separation distance are drawn to scale with reference to the r axis; the X axis, drawn coincident with the tube at rest, has been expanded.

(b) Variation of radial distance r with time for tracer spheres in a dilute suspension, $c = 2$ per cent, due to collisions of the type shown in (a). The arrow shows a 3-body collision which resulted in a shift in the mean value, $\bar{r}$.

rigid and deformable spheres (Goldsmith and Mason, 1964), and between rigid cylinders (Anczurowski and Mason, 1967), are well-defined, since there is a marked change in the translational and rotational motion of each particle and they are in apparent contact for a time (Fig. 10a). From the observations, a kinetic theory of flowing suspensions was developed and, for rigid spheres of radius b in a suspension containing n single particles/cm.[3] at a volume concentration c, the number of two-body collisions/cm.^{3}, f, was calculated to be

$$f = \frac{32}{3} nGb^3 = \frac{8cG}{\pi} \tag{12}$$

and the steady state concentration of doublets c' to be

$$c' = \frac{20}{3} c^2 \tag{13}$$

The mean free path for a particle at a radial distance r in the tube is

$$l = \frac{3(R^2 - r^2)}{64rnb^3} \tag{14}$$

which may be compared to that of a molecule in a gaseous system containing only one species of n molecules/cm.^{3} having radius b

$$l = \sqrt{2} \cdot \frac{\pi nb^2}{4} \tag{15}$$

The difference in power of b in equations (14) and (15) and the presence of the coordinate r in equation (14) are related to the nature of the shear flow and to the two different collision mechanisms.

It follows from equation (13) that, considering only doublets, at $c = 15$ per cent, all the spheres at any given instant will be in collision. When applied to platelets in blood ($c \sim 0 \cdot 3$ per cent) the equation shows that, if the presence of other blood cells is ignored, only $0 \cdot 005$ per cent of platelets would be in collision at any given instant.

However, when the concentration exceeds 2 per cent the number of three-body and higher order collisions rapidly increases, which together with the depletion of singlet species in the system invalidates the simple calculations made above. Moreover, red blood cells, as may be seen on a microscope slide (Fahraeus, 1929), on making contact may form a permanent aggregate or rouleau. The frequency of particle radial displacements due to collision (Fig. 10b) also increases, and for cylindrical particles, red cells and rouleaux the freedom to rotate in the orbits predicted by Jeffery's theory is restricted by the crowding of the particles. These effects have been studied at particle volume concentrations up to 70 per cent and are now briefly described.

(b) Concentrated suspensions

Despite the frequent collisions between particles at concentrations greater than 2 per cent, the mean measured translational velocities $u'(r)$ in the median

118

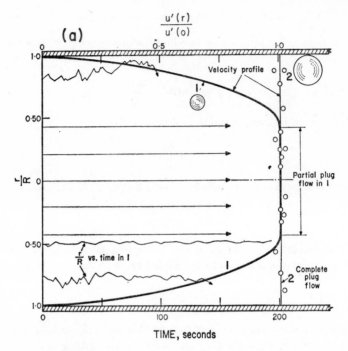

(a)

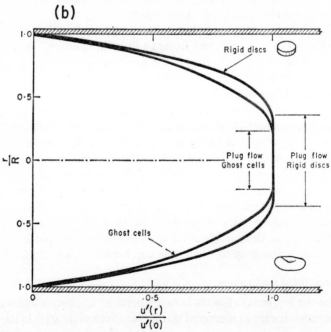

(b)

plane of the tube showed the velocity distribution to be still parabolic, as given by equation (1). When the concentration was further increased, however, a point was reached at which the profile deviated from the parabolic, becoming blunted in the tube centre with a region of plug flow in which $u'(r)$ was constant. In the transparent suspensions of rigid spheres and discs (Karnis, Goldsmith and Mason, 1966a) the region of constant velocity increased with increasing b/R while c was kept constant, spreading to the periphery of the tube until complete plug flow set in (Fig. 11a). In the transparent ghost cell suspensions (Goldsmith, 1967) the degree of blunting of the profile was much less marked, as shown in Fig. 11b. A further difference between the two systems was that the velocity distributions plotted in the dimensionless form of $u(r)/u(0)$ against r/R, as in Fig. 11, were independent of the centre line velocity, $u(0)$, provided the Reynolds number was low enough to preclude inertial effects. In the ghost cell suspensions, however, the velocity distribution became more parabolic as the flow rate was increased. In both suspensions the distributions of marker particles (spheres, discs or cells) in the tube were uniform and this fact, coupled with the observed dependence of the profile on c and b/R, suggested that the plug flow phenomenon was a wall effect of the kind postulated by Vand (1948). In the rigid particle system, measurements both in the tube and in a rotational viscometer confirmed this view by showing the suspensions to be Newtonian—that is, the apparent viscosity was independent of the velocity gradient. But as the velocity profile became increasingly blunted with increasing b/R, so the apparent viscosity decreased—an effect which had been known for some time in a variety of suspensions (Schofield and Scott Blair, 1930; Higginbotham, Oliver and Ward, 1958) and in blood (Fahraeus and Lindquist, 1931).

In the ghost cell system, the non-Newtonian behaviour, already well documented for whole blood where the apparent viscosity decreases with increasing rate of shear (Merrill et al., 1965), appears to be connected with the deformability of the cells which was clearly visible, especially at concentrations above 30 per cent. Thus, as with the rigid particles, the red cells at $c < 20$ per cent

---

FIG. 11. Velocity profiles in transparent concentrated suspensions plotted in the dimensionless form of equation (16).

(a) Rigid spheres suspension of $c = 33$ per cent in a tube $R = 0.4$ cm. at $u(0) = 0.16$ cm.sec^{-1}. As the ratio b/R was increased from 0.056 in curve 1 to 0.112 in curve 2, the partial plug flow became complete plug flow. The lines drawn are the best fit of the experimental points, shown only for curve 2. The variation in radial distance r with time for the tracer spheres, from which the profile in curve 1 was obtained, is also shown.

(b) Relative deviations from the parabolic profile in suspensions of rigid discs $b/R = 0.078$ and ghost cells, $b/R = 0.12$ at $c = 30$ per cent, flowing at $u(0) = 1$ tube diameter/second. The solid lines drawn are the best fit of the experimental points, not shown. Despite the higher b/R in the ghost cell suspension there was a markedly smaller region of plug flow.

5

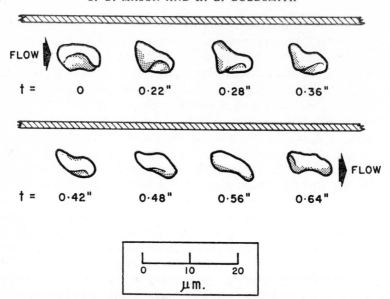

FIG. 12. Tracings of photomicrographs showing the distortions of the shape of a human erythrocyte flowing in a 70 per cent ghost cell suspension contained in a tube, $R = 47$ μm., from left to right at 200 μm./second. The sequence of shapes shown, with the time t from the first position indicated, were traced from 16 mm. ciné film.

were found to rotate with angular velocities which, although not obeying equation (8) because of frequent collisions causing radial displacements, did result in mean periods of rotation T in accord with equation (9). At higher concentrations, however, the cell rotations were markedly inhibited with the erythrocytes being continually deformed as they collided with the adjacent ghost cells, as illustrated in Fig. 12. The deformability of the red blood cells, which enables the suspension to flow even at concentrations of 98 per cent, is reflected in the much lower apparent relative viscosity, η_r' = suspension viscosity/suspending medium viscosity, compared to model systems, even emulsions of deformable water or oil droplets (Fig. 13).

(c) Inertial effects: two-phase flow

At higher tube Reynolds numbers the effect of particle size and concentration continues to be responsible for the partial plug flow; but an additional effect may now be superimposed on it which leads to even greater blunting of the velocity profile. This was observed in suspensions of rigid spheres and deformable drops where, either in steady or in oscillatory flow, a particle-free zone developed at the wall, whose width fluctuated about a mean value and

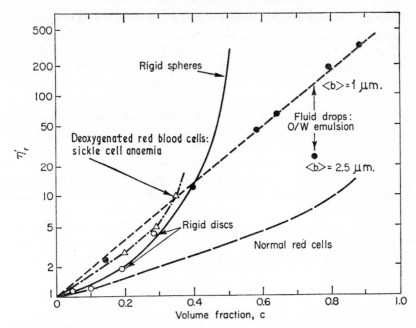

FIG. 13. The apparent relative viscosities η_r' of a red blood cell suspension from a normal dog as a function of concentration compared with that of suspensions of small rigid spheres, oil in water emulsions and rigid discs. Over the whole range of concentration, the blood cells have a considerably lower viscosity, a fact which is connected mainly with their deformability, as illustrated by the strikingly higher η_r' of the stiff sickled cells in which, as in rigid disc suspensions, flow is impossible at $c > 45$ per cent. (After Goldsmith and Mason, 1967.)

increased with time to an equilibrium value (Karnis, Goldsmith and Mason, 1966b; Takano, Goldsmith and Mason, 1968b). It resulted in the two-phase flow of a particle-rich core of relatively high viscosity surrounded by a particle-poor annulus of relatively low viscosity which acted as a lubricating layer.

Whether such a layer exists in flowing blood at high velocities is still a matter of debate. The available evidence *in vivo* (Phibbs and Burton, 1968) and *in vitro* (Bugliarello, Kapur and Hsiao, 1965) would indicate that its mean thickness is only of the order of half a cell diameter. Nevertheless, even such a small layer can cause an appreciable decrease in the energy dissipation of the flow in the vessel, as measured by the apparent viscosity (Thomas, 1962).

CONCLUSION

This account of the investigations of the microrheology of model suspensions and of blood has of necessity been brief, encompassing as it does a decade of work in this laboratory. Nevertheless it is hoped that we have shown the advantages, indeed the necessity, of working with simple model suspensions before embarking on the much more complex biological system. In this way it was possible to analyse the rotational and translational behaviour of the single human erythrocyte in terms of the previous quantitative experimental and theoretical study of the flow of suspensions of rigid discs. Similarly, it would have been difficult to interpret the motions of the red cells in the concentrated ghost cell suspensions had not the results of a parallel study in concentrated dispersions of model particles been available. Moreover, in each system it was first necessary to explore the movements of the isolated particle in Poiseuille flow at various tube Reynolds numbers before embarking on experiments concerned with interactions in dilute and concentrated suspensions.

Thus also it is expected that future work, especially that concerned with the pulsatile flow of blood cell suspensions, will be helped by the existing data on rigid and deformable model particle systems.

SUMMARY

This paper deals with the steady and oscillatory laminar flow of suspensions of rigid and deformable spheres, discs and rods in rigid circular tubes at volume concentrations from $0 \cdot 1$ to 50 per cent. An extension of this study to the Poiseuille flow of suspensions of human (disc-like) red blood cells and (rod-like) rouleaux is also described. The studies with model particles and blood cells have been carried out over a range of Reynolds numbers extending from the creeping viscous flow regime to that where inertia of the fluid plays an important part in determining particle behaviour.

Observations on single particles at very low Reynolds numbers include the steady rotation of rigid spheres, the rotation with variable angular velocity of discs and red blood cells, rods and rouleaux in spherical elliptical orbits as predicted by theory, the deformation and internal circulation of fluid drops and the buckling of flexible filaments and rouleaux. A consequence of the particle deformation and interaction with the wall is its migration to the tube axis. At higher Reynolds numbers, because of inertial effects, rigid spheres and cylinders also migrate laterally, but to an eccentric radial position.

The rotation, deformation and radial migration of model particles in oscillatory and pulsatile flow at values of Womersley's α parameter from $0 \cdot 5$ to 10 is similar to although more complex than that in steady flow.

In dilute suspensions, collisions of spheres and cylinders lead to the formation of doublets having a finite life-time and rotating as a unit. Their number in the tube increases very rapidly with increasing particle concentration.

At concentrations over 20 per cent by volume of rigid spheres or cylinders the velocity distribution becomes blunted in the centre of the tube although the suspensions still exhibit Newtonian behaviour. With concentrated transparent suspensions of reconstituted biconcave ghost cells containing normal red cells as marker particles, the blunting of profiles is less marked, the dispersions are non-Newtonian and the cells are considerably deformed.

At higher Reynolds numbers in steady flow, and in oscillatory and pulsatile flow, spheres in concentrated suspensions migrate inwards from the tube wall. This results in a two-phase flow of a central more viscous core surrounded by a thin peripheral, particle-depleted and less viscous zone, with an attendant decrease in the power dissipated in the tube.

Acknowledgements

The authors wish to thank the National Heart Institute of the United States Public Health Service (Grant HE 05911) and the Medical Research Council of Canada (Grant MT 1835) for their generous support of the work.

REFERENCES

ANCZUROWSKI, E. A., and MASON, S. G. (1967). *J. Colloid Interface Sci.*, **23**, 533–546.

BRENNER, H. (1966). *Adv. chem. Engng*, **6**, 287–438.

BUGLIARELLO, G., KAPUR, C., and HSIAO, G. (1965). *Proc. 4th int. Congr. Rheol.*, pp. 351–370, ed. Lee, E. H., and Copley, A. L. London: Wiley.

CHAFFEY, C. E., BRENNER, H., and MASON, S. G. (1965). *Rheol. acta*, **4**, 64–72 and correction *ibid.*, **6**, 100 (1967).

FAHRAEUS, R. (1929). *Physiol. Rev.*, **9**, 241–274.

FAHRAEUS, R., and LINDQUIST, T. (1931). *Am. J. Physiol.*, **96**, 562–568.

FORGACS, O. L., and MASON, S. G. (1959). *J. Colloid Sci.*, **14**, 457–472.

GOLDSMITH, H. L. (1967). *Fedn Proc. Fedn Am. Socs exp. Biol.*, **26**, 1813–1820.

GOLDSMITH, H. L. (1968). *J. gen. Physiol.*, **52**, 5S–27S.

GOLDSMITH, H. L., and MASON, S. G. (1962). *J. Colloid Sci.*, **17**, 448–476.

GOLDSMITH, H. L., and MASON, S. G. (1963). *J. Colloid Sci.*, **18**, 237–261.

GOLDSMITH, H. L., and MASON, S. G. (1964). *Proc. R. Soc. A*, **282**, 569–591.

GOLDSMITH, H. L., and MASON, S. G. (1967). In *Rheology: Theory and Applications*, IV, pp. 86–250, ed. Eirich, F. R. London: Academic Press.

HIGGINBOTHAM, G. H., OLIVER, D. R., and WARD, S. G. (1958). *Br. J. appl. Phys.*, **9**, 372–377.

JEFFERY, G. B. (1922). *Proc. R. Soc. A*, **102**, 161–179.

KARNIS, A., GOLDSMITH, H. L., and MASON, S. G. (1966a). *J. Colloid Interface Sci.*, **22**, 531–553.

KARNIS, A., GOLDSMITH, H. L., and MASON, S. G. (1966b). *Can. J. chem. Engng*, **44**, 181–193.

KARNIS, A., and MASON, S. G. (1967). *J. Colloid Interface Sci.*, **23**, 164–169.
MERRILL, E. W., BENIS, A. M., GILLILAND, E. R., SHERWOOD, T. K., and SALZMANN,
    E. W. (1965). *J. appl. Physiol.*, **20**, 954–967.
NORRIS, R. (1869). *Proc. R. Soc.*, **17**, 429–436.
PHIBBS, R. H., and BURTON, A. C. (1968). In *Proc. 1st int. Congr. Hemorheology*,
    pp. 617–632, ed. Copley, A. L. London: Pergamon Press.
SCHOFIELD, R. K., and SCOTT BLAIR, G. W. (1930). *J. phys. Chem.*, **34**, 248–262.
SEGRÉ, G., and SILBERBERG, A. (1962). *J. Fluid Mech.*, **14**, 136–157.
SHAH, P. N. (1967). M.Sc. Thesis, McGill University, Montreal.
SHIZGAL, B., GOLDSMITH, H. L., and MASON, S. G. (1965). *Can. J. chem. Engng*,
    43, 97–101.
TAKANO, M., GOLDSMITH, H. L., and MASON, S. G. (1967). *J. Colloid Interface Sci.*,
    23, 248–265.
TAKANO, M., GOLDSMITH, H. L., and MASON, S. G. (1968a). *J. Colloid Interface Sci.*,
    24, 253–267.
TAKANO, M., GOLDSMITH, H. L., and MASON, S. G. (1968b). *J. Colloid Interface Sci.*,
    24, 268–281.
TAYLOR, G. I. (1932). *Proc. R. Soc. A*, **138**, 41–48.
TAYLOR, G. I. (1934). *Proc. R. Soc. A*, **146**, 501–523.
THOMAS, H. W. (1962). *Biorheology*, **1**, 41–56.
VAND, V. (1948). *J. phys. Colloid Chem.*, **52**, 277–313.
WOMERSLEY, J. R. (1955). *J. Physiol., Lond.*, **127**, 553–563.
ZIA, I. Y. Z., COX, R. G., and MASON, S. G. (1967). *Proc. R. Soc. A*, **300**, 421–441.

DISCUSSION

Burton: As I mentioned in my paper, R. Phibbs in our laboratory has obtained pictures of freely flowing blood that has been frozen in the rabbit femoral artery, and Fig. 5 (p. 74) showed a section through the middle of the artery. The great crowding of cells is evident although the haematocrit is only 36 per cent. Of particular interest in this context is the preferred orientation of the red cells. Whereas an isolated cell tends to move at right-angles to the stream, in these crowded conditions the cells are practically all "edge on" to the observer (looking at a cross-section).

Another feature, not shown in Fig. 5, is that whereas the cells are oriented at all angles in the middle of the vessel, towards the walls they are lined up parallel to the wall, except for a two- or three-cell layer near the wall where they are rather scrambled—a "tumbling" layer, perhaps. Does this picture agree with what you observe in your model systems?

Mason: In general, yes. In our model systems, when looking along the axis of the tube one tends to see rods head on, and to see the edges of discs. This can be predicted theoretically for isolated particles, from the theory of G. B. Jeffery ([1922]. *Proc. R. Soc. A*, **102**, 161–179). The angular velocity of the disc is least in this orientation and thus the face of the disc spends most of the time in the direction of flow. At higher concentrations there is no theory, but we have confirmed visually that the preferred orientation of the face of the disc in the direction of flow is even more marked, which agrees with your observations. However it is not true that isolated particles tend to move down the tube with their faces at right-angles to the direction of flow if the particle is small relative to the tube, say less than one-fifth of its diameter.

As to the orientation of the peripheral red cells in parallel to the vessel wall in your femoral artery section, this is probably because their rotations are inhibited very close to the wall.

Burton: We have also measured statistically the distribution of cells, and we find a very thin layer close to the wall with a deficit of cells, compared to the middle of the artery, which agrees with your findings (pp. 112, 120).

Caro: Professor Mason, you said that in Poiseuille flow fluid stresses deform liquid droplets into ellipsoids and cause flexible particles to bend or buckle as they rotate. You also mentioned that in the liquid drop tangential stresses are transmitted internally to produce circulation patterns within the ellipsoid, and one wonders whether a similar circulation of the contents of the red cell occurs and how much it contributes to mixing the contents.

Mason: Internal convective circulation can be seen in rotating liquid drops, which is in accord with theoretical predictions (Rumscheidt, F. D., and Mason, S. G. [1961]. *J. Colloid Sci.*, **16**, 210), and we have demonstrated that this results in considerable mixing. I would predict that the same would occur in red cells provided that they are rotating and deforming at the same time; but unambiguous experimental proof is not yet available. The theory would be greatly complicated by the presence of the red cell membrane which would prevent transmission of the shear stresses generated at the outside surface to the fluid contents of the cell.

Burton: It would be very useful if you would extend the theory to the red cell, by applying the restriction that the surface area must not change during deformation. This would give a good approximation to what happens to a red cell in a shear gradient. The red cell has such a high Young's Modulus that once the area is increased, it will do everything to prevent further increase in area.

Mason: We have not done this; but we could readily do it experimentally using our artificial cells with nylon membranes (Chang, T. M. S., MacIntosh, F. C., and Mason, S. G. [1966]. *Can J. Physiol. Pharmac.*, **44**, 115) which would have the property you refer to.

Burton: Your artificial cells are spherical, however, and so cannot be deformed at all without increasing their surface area and running into their elasticity. Also, your microspheres have at least a thousand times the inter-facial tension of the red cell, from the experiments of A. W. L. Jay and M. A. Edwards ([1968]. *Can. J. Physiol. Pharmac.*, **46,** 731) so the membrane is much more rigid. The red cell, being non-spherical, can be deformed without eliciting its elasticity, so to extend the calculation for the unenclosed regime to the red cell you must include the requirement that the surface area be unaltered.

Philip: There is little profit in trying to modify these straightforward con-siderations of the convective distortion of a liquid sphere to Professor Burton's problem, because the convective distortion of a liquid sphere involves preservation of volume, *but its surface area increases more or less linearly with time.* On the other hand, solving the problem of the distortion of a body with a skin around it in a steady flow amounts to finding an *equilibrium* configuration of the body (with an equilibrium surface area, even if not the original one!). This involves the correct relationship between the pressure distribution and shearing stresses on the skin arising from the flow around the body and the distortions thus produced in the skin. There is a subtle interplay between the mechanics of the fluid and the mechanics of the body. [See also discussion, pp. 99–100.]

Owen: Professor Mason, have you observed any gross circulatory motion on the average among particles in a liquid flowing through a tube, such as has been observed in a cluster of particles falling freely through an unbounded gas?

Mason: There is no gross circulation in either tube flow or Couette flow. If we take Couette flow with one of the boundaries stationary, an isolated particle will move in a straight line, parallel to the direction of liquid flow; a number of particles at a low enough concentration (less than 1 per cent by volume) to produce only two-body interactions will maintain a constant mean position, relative to the direction of flow. If the concentration is increased so that three-body and four-body collisions occur, any one particle starts to wander about from one wall to the other, but there is no net motion. We have followed this up to concentrations of 60 per cent by volume. Yet an individual particle could be said to be diffusing, but in such a way that the diffusion is reversible.

Saffman: Do you see a layer of fluid near the wall which is free of particles, when you have interactions between many particles at these high concen-trations?

Mason: At high concentrations and at Reynolds numbers less than 10^{-3} we have never been able to detect net migration of particles, with spheres, rods or discs flowing through tubes. Of course with spheres there cannot be any particle centres nearer to the wall than the radius of the sphere, which auto-matically defines a certain plasma layer, but apart from this geometrical restriction there is no measurable change in concentration of particle centres across the tube. However, if one increases the Reynolds number to about unity, inertial effects come into play and particles are pushed away from the wall to produce a particle-free layer having a measurable thickness δ_n (Karnis, A., Goldsmith, H. L., and Mason, S. G. [1966]. *Can. J. chem. Engng*, **44**, 181–193) which increases with decreasing concentration. The effect also depends on the ratio of the particle radius to the tube radius and, as stated, on the Reynolds number.

Owen: What mechanism have you in mind for the interaction between rigid particles and the wall that will account for the plug flow in your Fig. 11 (p. 118)?

Mason: The mechanism is largely one of hydrodynamic interaction between the particles and the wall which produces a pseudo slip and in this way invalidates the classical Poiseuille equation which, of course, predicts a parabolic distribution. For this reason one must be cautious about using capillary viscometers for suspensions.

Saffman: In blood vessels is there a layer close to the wall which is free of red cells? I was under the impression there was, but doubts have been expressed about this.

Burton: The only data we have on the distribution of blood actually flowing derives from the quick-freezing of a rabbit femoral artery with blood rushing through at physiological rates. Statistically speaking there is a layer next to the wall which has a deficit of red cells, but it is very small, 2 or 3 μm. thick at most.

Taylor: One does not really need a cell-free layer of more than 5 μm. to produce a very powerful effect on viscosity. Dr. R. H. Haynes ([1962]. *Biophys. J.*, **2**, 95–103) could explain most of the radius-dependent viscosity effects of blood by a layer about 3 or 4 μm. thick. Everyone would agree that there is a statistical mean reduction in density; when one looks down a microscope there is no *constant* cell-free layer, but there is an average reduction in cell concentration. I believe C. A. Wiederhielm has done the same kind of quick-freezing experiments with similar findings, and my own experiments on optical density changes in glass tubes also showed a reduction in concentration (Taylor, M. G. [1955]. *Aust. J. exp. Biol. med. Sci.*, **33**, 1–16). But a layer only 3 or 4 μm. thick would affect the viscosity of a suspension.

Burton: As I said earlier (p. 81), Dr. Haynes discussed the two theories, the "graininess" or "sigma" theory and the plasma layer theory, and at the ends of the haematocrit range the plasma layer theory is not plausible (Haynes, R. H. [1962]. *Biophys. J.*, **2**, 95–103).

Taylor: The various values which Haynes calculated for the so-called sigma thickness or shell thickness in the different haematocrits required a large variation in apparent shell thickness from one haematocrit value to another;

over the range studied, the calculated thickness of the shell varied by a factor of 10 or 20, a quite implausible requirement. The thickness of the effective cell-free layer near the wall, on the other hand, varied by a factor of about two over the whole range of haematocrits. So the plasma layer theory seemed the more plausible explanation of the reduced viscosity of blood in narrow tubes. But it is a complex situation and one should also consider the shearing effects and whether or not they have reached their asymptotic values, and so on.

On a different point, Professor Mason said that Couette flow and flow in a tube are effectively equivalent. Professor Saffman and I discussed this matter of the migration of particles in 1956, and I wonder if he would like to comment on the problem of whether the forces acting on a particle in shear flow are the same as in Couette flow where the shear is constant at all points, or whether additional forces are present in parabolic flow where the shear effect is varying. In one case, Couette flow, the particle spins without migrating, and in the other case it both spins and migrates. Professor Saffman's treatment showed that in a parabolic velocity field there is an extra force.

Saffman: There definitely should be an extra migratory force in parabolic flow, but I have been so far unable to calculate it!

Lighthill: Professor Mason, will not the fact that there is a gradient in the average speed of rotation produce a different amount of pressure from collisions on one side of a particle from the other?

Mason: It is true that the higher gradient on the wall side of the particle produces more collisions than on the axis side. In practice, however, the effect is small (Goldsmith, H. L., and Mason, S. G. [1964]. *Proc. R. Soc. A*, **282**, 569–591). In connexion with Professor Taylor and Professor Saffman's comments, we have concluded that the main factor causing inward migration of fluid drops in Poiseuille flow is interaction with the wall; and that the variation in velocity gradient across the particle plays a minor role (Chaffey, C. E., Brenner, H., and Mason, S. G. [1965]. *Rheol. acta*, **4**, 64–72; [1967]. *Ibid.*, **6**, 100).

Mead: Will a small enough deformable particle at some distance from the wall migrate toward the centre?

Mason: Yes; the interaction with the wall extends right across the tube so that an isolated fluid drop will continue to migrate inwards, asymptotically approaching the tube axis where the velocity gradient is zero; in this position the drop is not deformed and does not rotate.

Muir: Is this likely to have more than a minor effect when one is breathing liquid aerosol droplets of the order of a micrometre in diameter?

Mason: I cannot say without knowing more about the velocities and the diameters of the tubes, but some of these phenomena are very pertinent to what happens when an aerosol goes through a respiratory filter where the velocity gradients can be very high indeed.

Owen: I have estimated the magnitude of the force on aerosol droplets associated with the shear flow and found it to be very small in the trachea. For example, a spherical particle, 1 μm. in diameter, falling vertically under gravity very near the wall of the trachea experiences a force, directed away from the wall, roughly equal to 10^{-3} times the particle weight, at inspired airflow rates of 40 l. min.$^{-1}$ or so.

FLOW OF HUMAN BLOOD IN GLASS AND PLASTIC FIBRES: A FILMED STUDY

E. W. Merrill,† H. J. Meiselman, E. R. Gilliland, T. K. Sherwood
AND E. W. Salzman

*Department of Chemical Engineering, Massachusetts Institute of Technology,
Cambridge, Massachusetts*

The purpose of the film is to show how, in the presence of fibrinogen (as in blood plasma), red cells undergo reversible aggregation and dissociation, whereas when they are suspended in isotonic saline solution there is virtually no association between cells, at least at normal levels of haematocrit.

The "structure" originating at low rates of flow from reversibly aggregating red cells evolves into a continuous network of cells capable of supporting a shear stress without flow. This is the *yield stress*, which is approximately proportional to the square of the fibrinogen concentration and the cube of the haematocrit, being about $0 \cdot 04$ dynes/cm.^{2} in normal human blood. The red cell aggregates evolve into rouleaux if given sufficient time either at very low rates of flow or in stasis.

"Blood" (that is, red cells in plasma or red cells in saline solution) was studied in hollow transparent fibres of which the internal diameters (50 to 120 μm.) are comparable to those of living microcirculatory vessels. Studies were made in conditions of starting, stopping, and flows at velocities relevant to the microcirculation, especially the venules. The fluid dynamic and rheological aspects of these studies are summarized by Merrill and co-workers (1965) and by Meiselman and co-workers (1967). The film is an abstract of the cinephotomicrographic documentation carried out in parallel with the quantitative fluid mechanical studies.

In parts of the film the percentage volume of red cells (haematocrit) was reduced to 33 per cent the better to permit visualization of the flows; in other parts the haematocrit was 40 per cent. Sequences were recorded through a microscope, either looking down on a horizontal fibre from above, or in side view.

† Professor Merrill was unable to attend the symposium but provided a copy of his film *Flow of Human Blood in Glass and Plastic Fibres*, to which this description and the following discussion relate.

We use the notation $\bar{U}$ to indicate the mean velocity, expressed as tube diameters per second. Thus if the internal diameter of the tube is 120 μm. and $\bar{U}$ is 5, the absolute mean velocity is 600 μm./sec.

The principal phenomena shown by the film are:

(1) The rapid aggregation of red cells in the presence of fibrinogen at low flows ($\bar{U} = 2$ to 3 or less), leading to plug flow of immobile packs of cells through an annular layer of clear plasma. Aggregates, rouleaux and single cells are all seen at medium flows ($\bar{U} = 7$).

(2) The collapse of fibrinogen-induced aggregates of red cells when rapid flow ($\bar{U} = 50$) succeeds slow flow, followed by reformation of aggregates at rest.

(3) The absence of aggregates of red cells in the absence of fibrinogen—that is, when the cells are suspended in saline solution.

(4) The curious result that at a normal erythrocyte sedimentation rate of a few millimetres per hour, red cells settle after only three minutes into a bed that fills little more than half the fibre. When flow is restarted, in the presence of fibrinogen the bed of red cells crumbles into gross aggregates that eventually disperse, filling the entire cross-section of the fibre. In isotonic saline solution, by contrast, the bed of red cells rapidly disperse when flow recommences.

REFERENCES

MERRILL, E. W., BENIS, A. M., GILLILAND, E. R. *et al.* (1965). *J. appl. Physiol.*, **20**, 954-967.

MEISELMAN, H. J., MERRILL, E. W., GILLILAND, E. R. *et al.* (1967). *J. appl. Physiol.*, **22**, 772-781.

DISCUSSION

Mason: In this film Professor Merrill is demonstrating the importance of rouleaux. I am always surprised by the neglect of these interesting structures in the haemodynamics literature, when they may have considerable importance.

Comparable structures to rouleaux occur in many systems over a wide range of dimensional scales. They form in the first place because of the regular geometry of the unit. Rouleaux would not form without the uniform dimensions and plate-like structure of the red cell, although possession of this structure by a unit does not guarantee the formation of rouleaux. Comparable ordered arrays occur on a molecular scale in soaps, where the micelles are ordered arrays of small molecules, generally in two or more layers, and in liquid crystals. On a larger scale, pulpwood logs cut to a standard length of four feet and floating down rivers aggregate into two-dimensional crystal lattices which are often preferentially oriented, depending upon the direction in which the rivers flow.

About a hundred years ago R. Norris ([1869]. *Proc. R. Soc.*, **17**, 429) speculated on the formation of rouleaux in blood and constructed a model system from corks cut to the same size and weighted to float on edge on the surface of water. When the system of packed floating corks was vibrated the corks started to form rouleau-like arrays. A similar system can be made from a series of roller bearings on a vibrating surface.

The red cells in rouleaux are held together by attractive forces which act over distances considerably greater than those encompassed by normal inter-molecular forces like van der Waal's attractive forces. Professor Burton has already mentioned (p. 99) what he thinks these forces may be.

Once a rouleau is formed it has an appreciable structural strength, and my colleague H. L. Goldsmith ([1967]. *Fedn Proc. Fedn Am. Socs exp. Biol.*, **26**, 1813) has tried to measure the force needed to disrupt it.

The amount of aggregation in a suspension of regular particles is influenced by several factors. As the mean shear stress is decreased the amount of aggregation increases, as has been demonstrated with wood pulp suspensions and by the aggregation of fibres in dispersions such as latex paint or printing inks, where aggregation can be reversible. By decreasing the velocity gradient of the medium one can increase aggregation and this gives rise to thixotropic flow properties in the system.

Burton: The formation of rouleaux is not something which happens within the physiological range of blood flow, however. With even the slightest flow the rouleaux are broken up. We should not over-emphasize the physiological importance of rouleaux.

Lighthill: Professor Merrill shows aggregation at $\bar{U}$ (that is, mean velocity divided by diameter) = 2 to 3, which is a very low rate of shear in relation to those normal in the blood flow.

Mason: Some physiologists say that rouleaux form only in a pathological state and that they do not normally occur.

Davies: Surely when plug flow is taking place, $\bar{U}$ can be less than one over a large part of the radius in the centre of a tube. One would therefore expect to find rouleaux there, in normal conditions.

Caro: There seemed to be a great inhibition of movement in the centre of the tube in Professor Merrill's film.

Mason: Yes, what you saw was plug flow, with a near zero velocity gradient and no rotation of particles or aggregates. Incidentally Professor R. Fahraeus considers that rouleaux are quite "normal" and states that one can see very strong rouleaux in horse's blood and also *in vivo* in the conjunctiva in man.

However, M. H. Knisely ([1965]. In *Handbook of Physiology, Section 2: Circulation*, pp. 2249–2292, vol. III, ed. Hamilton, W. F., and Dow, P. Washington, D.C.: American Physiological Society) considers that they occur in pathological conditions. He says that they are not found in blood from horses reared in relatively disease-free conditions.

Burton: However, if you watch the microcirculation you see stasis from time to time in the capillaries with the red cells stacked up in rouleaux, but where such a capillary joins one in which blood is free flowing, you see the red cells peeling off perfectly freely. I don't consider this abnormal.

Cumming: There is some confusion here in the use of the words "pathological" and "normal", from which disagreement seems to arise. An animal shielded from all infections so that it had no immune globulins in its circulation would be in a highly abnormal situation, in that it would be uncommon, but it would not be "pathological". On the other hand all of us are ordinarily infected by childhood diseases and so develop immune globulins to them. This is entirely "normal", but you might also say that it is pathological.

Mason: Professor Knisely uses "pathological" in a very restricted sense because if you press him he will agree that after a cocktail or a cigarette, rouleaux appear in the human conjunctiva—hardly a pathological state!

Burton: In infection, where the attraction between the red cells greatly increases, as shown by the sedimentation rate going up 50 times, there is agglutination of red cells. Bessis has made electron micrographs of red cells from group A blood mixed with anti-A serum to illustrate this (Bessis, M., and Bricka, M. [1950]. *Revue Hémat.*, **5**, 396–427). This aggregation is not readily reversible, as is normal rouleaux formation.

Stuart: The point of interest of rouleaux for blood flow studies would seem to be the difference that rouleaux make to the physiological properties of flow, and to discover how to describe this.

Burton: The physiological importance of rouleaux is that our picture of the microcirculation as a steady, very slow flow through the capillaries that can be speeded up is unrealistic; when one looks at the microcirculation it is instead a process of "stop and go". Similarly for our picture of diffusion equilibration. It is much more the case that capillaries fill up, and then flow stops and the vessel is washed out, in the backward as often as the forward direction; a "rinsing" mechanism in fact. Mathematically of course the result may be the same as if we treat it, as we do, as a steady flow. I suspect that rouleaux are important in affecting the force required to get flow started from nothing to a very small amount, in the terminal vascular bed where there is this process of stop and go independently all over the bed. In the larger vessels I doubt if rouleaux are important because they are broken up there by the shear gradient.

Lighthill: Professor Merrill gave $\bar{U} = 7$ as approximately the highest rate of flow at which rouleaux are formed, in normal human blood (he states that the upper limit could be significantly higher, however, if the fibrinogen concentration were above normal). $\bar{U} = 7$ would presumably be low compared with the shears that would be found in vessels of any size (for example, it implies a speed of only 840 μm./sec. for a diameter of 120 μm.). In other words, thixotrophy occurs only under conditions of stasis, and not under conditions of normal flow, in any tube. One would not expect to obtain *in vivo* the extreme plug situation shown in the film, where the whole mass of cells went along together.

Mason: Except at the centre of the vessel.

Burton: Physiological velocity in capillaries is about 0·5 mm./sec.; divided by the diameter of a capillary this gives a huge value of $\bar{U}$, so $\bar{U} = 7$ is certainly very low. So on the *average* blood flow is far too rapid for rouleaux to have an effect on the total rate of flow. But because the actual flow of the microcirculation is a matter of "stop and go", rouleaux will play some part in the detailed pattern of blood flow in a capillary bed.

Lighthill: How long must the blood stop before rouleaux form?

Burton: *In vitro*, rouleaux appear in a drop of blood within 30 seconds. I do not know how soon they appear *in vivo*.

Mead: Professor Burton, have you used your quick-freezing technique to examine blood flow in the smallest capillaries?

Burton: We have not examined capillary blood by this method. Whenever you stop blood in any vessel larger than a capillary where red cells *can* aggregate, rouleaux always form very quickly. Professor Lighthill's results suggest that even during the intermittent "stop and go", the effect of rouleaux on blood flow is negligible.

What is striking about a rouleau, and suggests that there is an attraction of one red blood cell membrane for another, is the fact that the diameter of a rouleau is considerably greater than that of a single red cell and the width of a red cell seen edge on is reduced when it is in a rouleau; the whole cell appears flattened as if it is not just touching at the rim. In addition the apposition of the cells is extremely regular, and when a cell sticks out, it does so symmetrically all round; in other words it is simply a larger cell. But red cells are never out of place as Professor Mason's logs often are. Some highly specific attraction evidently determines that red cells come together in accurate correspondence. Branching can happen, but it does not disturb the correspondence.

Mason: If the cells were in true mathematical contact one could never pull them apart. This follows from lubrication theory. But in Professor Merrill's film we do see them being pulled apart and coming back together again. So the cells are not in true physical contact.

Burton: If there are no long-chain molecules in the medium the cells have no tendency to stick together, which suggests that chains of oriented macro-molecules play a part in joining the cells together in rouleaux. The film showed that rouleaux did not form in isotonic saline solution. They will form in solutions of synthetic macromolecules such as polyvinylpyrrolidone as well as in plasma fibrinogen.

We should very much like to know what the configuration of the two membranes is, whether the cells are really parallel, and I have tried to persuade electron microscopists to make serial sections of rouleaux, but so far no one has done it. I suspect that the gap would be about 150Å (15 nm.) and per-haps something like "desmosomes" (bridges) would be seen, because we think that at certain points on the membrane there are charges, and there the proteins of the medium would presumably line up between the cells.

Caro: To return to the topic of a cell-free plasma layer discussed earlier (p. 127), in the transient studies recorded in Professor Merrill's film the cell-deficient layer of fluid near the wall seemed to widen and then to narrow again as the rate of flow increased.

Owen: The layer certainly appeared to be much more marked initially than later on when it tended to fluctuate in width. Is this something to do with the initial acceleration of the flow?

Stuart: It has been stated that the plasma layer is due to an inertial affect, and since acceleration is another form of inertia, it would be expected to be effective in the transient state, and then to disappear.

Merrill (by subsequent letter): The cell-deficient layer near the wall is observed to widen, then narrow, and ultimately disappear when the flow is observed from directly overhead (or from underneath) the fibre. Simultaneous observation of the flow through a *horizontally* placed microscope shows no such effect, but rather the expansion of the previously settled bed of red cells toward the "roof" of the fibre. One must conclude that the effect observed from overhead is the consequence of sweeping of cells upward and inward from the walls by the rapidly moving plasma flowing over the packed bed, a process which ultimately results in uniform re-dispersion of the cells.

THE OPTIMUM ELASTIC PROPERTIES OF ARTERIES

M. G. TAYLOR

Department of Physiology, University of Sydney, Australia

SINCE this symposium is concerned with the transport of materials in the body, it is relevant to examine the efficiency with which this transport occurs; in particular I shall consider some properties of the arteries which appear to contribute to the efficient operation of the circulatory system. To place the matter in perspective, let us recall that at rest a man's heart takes about five per cent of the cardiac output and accounts for about ten per cent of the total oxygen consumption. In heavy exercise, indeed, the heart alone may consume as much oxygen as does the whole body at rest. The heart is not a particularly efficient machine, and less than twenty per cent of its energy consumption appears as mechanical work in pumping blood around the body. Since, however, the body as a whole operates at about the same low level of mechanical efficiency, the heart is required to expend an appreciable amount of energy in supporting the performance of a physical work load. From this point of view, therefore, we see that anything which contributes to the efficiency of the cardio-vascular system is of value to the animal.

One way of attempting to establish an optimal design for the arterial system is to formulate a "cost function" and then seek the combination of physical properties and dimensions which will minimize it. The difficulty is, however, that at present we have no basis for assigning the proper physiological or biological "weights" to the various terms in the function, even if we knew all the terms that ought to be included. However, even in the absence of such a unified approach to the problem, it is still possible to obtain some useful appreciation of the various features of the system by considering them separately.

Previous studies of the pulsatile events in the arterial system (Taylor, 1964; O'Rourke and Taylor, 1967; O'Rourke, 1967) have concentrated on the connexions between the elasticity and architecture of the arterial tree and the pressure–flow relations which confront the heart. In this paper we shall be mainly concerned with the properties of the arterial system in relation to relatively slow changes of pressure within it, with a time-scale sufficiently slow for the events to be regarded as effectively simultaneous, so that a simple Windkessel model is acceptable.

The earlier work was based on a fairly detailed model of extended, bifurcating elastic tubes; it was shown that the elastic properties influence the amount of work which the heart must perform in pumping blood into the aorta. The external work of the heart can be expressed as a combination of "steady work" and "pulsatile work". The steady component arises from the work done in driving the mean flow against the mean aortic pressure; the pulsatile component similarly arises from the products of the pressure and flow terms oscillating around their mean values. The pulsatile component can be regarded as the cost imposed on the system by the fact that the flow of blood from the heart is intermittent and not continuous. It normally amounts to about ten per cent of the total external work of the left ventricle, and rather more for the right ventricle.

As far as pulsatile work of the heart is concerned, it has been shown that an optimum design for an arterial system would be one in which the input impedance was as low as possible, and relatively insensitive to change in the operating frequency. It is clear, however, that although very distensible arteries would provide such a desirably low input impedance, there would be other and undesirable consequences. For example, if there were a change in mean arterial pressure it would necessarily be accompanied by a large change in arterial blood volume.

There appear to be at least two main features which enable a branching assembly of elastic tubes, such as an arterial tree, to achieve a low and stable input impedance, and at the same time to maintain a relatively low overall distensibility. These have been explored in previous papers (Taylor, 1966a, b) and can be summarized as follows:

(i) Elastic non-uniformity in the system, such that the characteristic impedance increases peripherally; this is certainly the case for the mammalian system, where the wave-velocity increases progressively in peripheral arteries.

(ii) The presence of terminations lying at widely scattered distances from the origin so that, provided the frequencies are sufficiently high, the reflected waves from the terminations interfere at the origin and no sharp maxima or minima of input impedance are generated. Attention was directed to this feature of the arterial system by von Kries as long ago as 1892.

(iii) Other factors such as fluid viscosity and the viscosity of the wall material contribute to the stability of the impedance, but cannot influence the overall distensibility of the system.

In addition to the properties listed above, it has been known for many years that the distensibility of arteries is not constant, but decreases as they are further inflated. Most studies of wave propagation, pressure–flow relations and similar topics have avoided the complications of this non-linearity by assuming that the system is linear when operating with small displacements about a reference level. It is interesting, however, to speculate upon the physiological or biological significance of this non-linearity, and some of the calculations which follow are an attempt to assess this. We shall show that (*i*) subject to certain conditions, the minimum overall distensibility of a branching system of elastic tubes can be achieved by a suitable relationship between wave-velocity and vessel radius, regardless of the number of branchings or their lengths; and, (*ii*) if the distensibility of the arterial Windkessel decreases at higher distending pressures, then (a) the "response time" of the system is decreased and (b) less elastic work is "stored" in the system for a given increase in distending pressure.

OPTIMUM DISTRIBUTION OF ELASTIC PROPERTIES IN A BIFURCATING ASSEMBLY OF TUBES

Let us consider a set of branching elastic tubes, where L_i, R_i and c_i represent respectively the length, internal radius and wave-velocity of vessels of the i'th order of branching. We shall see that the lengths L_i are not important except that this model assumes that all branches of the same order have the same length. We seek first to determine what distribution of elasticity will give minimum distensibility of the assembly as a whole, subject to the constraint that the transit time for disturbances to travel from the origin to the terminations is a given quantity T. We shall show that minimum distensibility is attained when the wave-velocity is suitably related to the radius. We shall further combine this result with the relationship which Cohn (1955) obtained in his analysis of the similar problem of determining the relationship between the radii of successive vessels, such that the resistance to steady flow through the assembly was minimized. Cohn obtained his solution with the condition that there was a fixed total amount of material available to constitute the walls of the assembly; but, as pointed out previously (Taylor, 1967), his equations take the same form if the more realistic condition of fixed total volume of the system is imposed.

The reasons for choosing the condition that the transit time shall be a fixed quantity were based on a consideration of the input impedance of the system. Although we are here concerned with the behaviour of slow events in the Windkessel, our solution must also be an appropriate one when the pulsatile events are considered, and in particular the pulsatile work of the heart. We know that if the relations between the length of the system, wave-velocity and operating frequency are such that there is quarter wavelength resonance, then the input impedance will be at a minimum. We can express this condition in another way, by saying that if the "operating frequency" is $f' = 1/T'$, then the minimum input impedance will be achieved if disturbances take approximately $T'/4$ to travel from the origin of the system to its terminations.

We employ the simple expression which relates the wave-velocity c in an elastic tube to its distensibility and the fluid density ρ:

$$c^2 = \frac{\Delta P . V}{\Delta V . \rho}$$

where ΔP represents the increment in pressure resulting from an increment ΔV in the volume V of unit length of the vessel. In what follows we shall eliminate the density term by making it equal to unity.

If we take one of the branches in our assembly, we see that for a given pressure change ΔP_1 the volume change will be

$$\frac{\pi R_i^2 L_i}{c_i^2} . \Delta P_1$$

If there are N orders of branching, the total distensibility $\Delta V_1/\Delta P_1$ of the assembly is given by the summation of the volume increments

$$\frac{\Delta V_1}{\Delta P_1} = \sum_{i=0}^{N} 2^i . \frac{\pi R_i^2 L_i}{c_i^2}$$

We now make use of our condition on the transit time, namely

$$\sum_{i=0}^{N} \frac{L_i}{c_i} = T$$

and if we proceed along the lines followed by Cohn, we note that

$$\frac{1}{c_0} = \frac{1}{L_0}\left(T - \sum_{i=1}^{N} \frac{L_i}{c_i}\right)$$

so that

$$\frac{\Delta V_1}{\Delta P_1} = \pi R_0^2 . \frac{1}{L_0}\left(T - \sum_{i=1}^{N} \frac{L_i}{c_i}\right)^2 + \sum_{i=1}^{N} 2^i \frac{\pi R_i^2 L_i}{c_i^2}$$

Now, for $\Delta V_1 / \Delta P_1$ to be a minimum we require

$$\frac{\partial}{\partial c_i}\left(\frac{\Delta V_1}{\Delta P_1}\right) = 0 \qquad \text{for } i > 0$$

Thus we have

$$\frac{\partial}{\partial c_i}\left(\frac{\Delta V_1}{\Delta P_1}\right) = \frac{2\pi R_0^2}{L_0}\left(T - \sum_{i=1}^{N}\frac{L_i}{c_i}\right)\left(\frac{L_i}{c_i^2}\right) - 2.\frac{2^i \pi R_i L_i}{c_i^3} = 0$$

or

$$\frac{2}{c_0}.\frac{L_i}{c_i^2} = 2.2^i.\left(\frac{R_i}{R_0}\right)^2.\frac{L_i}{c_i^3}$$

whence

$$c_i = c_0.2^i\left(\frac{R_i}{R_0}\right)^2$$

We may now use this relationship to find

$$\text{Min}\left(\frac{\Delta V_1}{\Delta P_1}\right) = \sum_{i=0}^{N} 2^i.\frac{\pi R_i^2 L_i}{c_i^2}$$

$$= \sum_{i=0}^{N} 2_i.\frac{\pi R_i^2}{c_i}.\frac{L_i}{c_i}$$

$$= \sum_{i=0}^{N} 2^i \pi R_i^2.\frac{2^{-i}}{c_0}\frac{R_0^2}{R_i^2}.\frac{L_i}{c_i}$$

$$= \frac{\pi R_0^2}{c_0}\sum_{i=0}^{N}\frac{L_i}{c_i} = \frac{\pi R_0^2}{c_0}.T$$

We see that this value is independent both of the length of the branches and of the number of branchings in the assembly.

We may now combine our result with that of Cohn for the ratio of successive radii which gives minimum resistance to flow through the system, namely, $R_i = R_0.2^{-i/3}$. We find that the ratio of wave-velocities which would give minimum distensibility in this case is $c_{i+1} = 2^{i/3}.c_i$

We thus see that for a system with minimum resistance to steady flow, the optimum distribution of elastic properties is one which provides a wave-velocity which increases exponentially along the system. In general, however, all that is required is that the wave-velocities on either side of a bifurcation should be related as

$$c_{i+1} = c_i . 2 . \left(\frac{R_{i+1}}{R_i}\right)^2$$

Reflections in the optimum branching system

In addition to the favourable properties just discussed, the optimal distribution of elasticity has some interesting influences on the behaviour of disturbances travelling in the system.

We may define the reflection coefficient at a bifurcation as

$$\frac{1 - \left(\dfrac{Z_{0,\,i}}{Z_T}\right)}{1 + \left(\dfrac{Z_{0,\,i}}{Z_T}\right)}$$

where $Z_{0,\,i}$ is the characteristic impedance of a branch of order i, and Z_T is the characteristic impedance of a pair of branches of order $i + 1$, taken in parallel, being equal to $\frac{1}{2} . Z_{0,\,i+1}$.

For our present purposes we assume that the two branches of higher order have no reflections arising at their terminations, and we use the Waterhammer formula to find the characteristic impedances; thus,

$$\frac{Z_{0,\,i}}{\frac{1}{2} . Z_{0,\,i+1}} = \frac{\rho . c_i}{\frac{1}{2}\rho . c_{i+1}} . \frac{R_{i+1}^2}{R_i^2}$$

where it will be observed that the change in cross-section of the $i + 1$'th branch from that of the i'th has been taken into account, since this formulation of the characteristic impedance is in terms of the linear velocity of flow and not in terms of volume flow. If we now substitute for the ratio of c_{i+1}/c_i, we find that

$$\frac{Z_{0,\,i}}{\frac{1}{2} . Z_{0,\,i+1}} = 1$$

and hence the reflection coefficient at the bifurcation is zero. Since this is true for all values of i, we can see that a pressure pulse will travel centrifugally without reflection, until it encounters the terminations.

CONSEQUENCES OF ELASTIC NON-LINEARITY OF THE WINDKESSEL

In the previous sections we dealt with the disposition of elastic properties along a distributed system, and have tacitly assumed that while the pressure–volume relation may be a function of the order of branching it is independent of other factors. It is known that in the arterial system the distensibility is indeed variable from artery to artery, and shows a decrease in the more peripheral arteries; it has also been observed, however, that all arteries show a progressively decreasing distensibility as they are inflated. When one speculates upon the possible physiological significance of non-linearity it appears to confer two useful properties upon the system.

(*i*) It will reduce the amount of external work of the heart required to be "stored" as potential energy when the blood pressure is raised from one level to another, and

(*ii*) It will reduce the time taken for the pressure to increase after a change in peripheral resistance, the cardiac output remaining constant.

Work done in raising the blood pressure

Let us express the situation in terms of the model shown in Fig. 1. We have a storage element or Windkessel, with capacitance C, which, initially, we shall

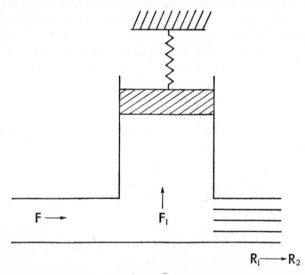

WINDKESSEL

FIG. 1. Windkessel model: the capacitance of the storage element is defined as C ml./mm. Hg.

take to be a constant. The capacitance discharges through a resistance R. We hold the inflow F constant, and change R; our problem is to compute the work done in bringing the pressure up to the new level. At first the pressure $P_1 = FR_1$, and after the Windkessel has charged up to its new level we have $P_2 = FR_2$. We know that if blood is being accumulated in the Windkessel at the rate F_1, then we have

$$F_1 = C \cdot \frac{dP}{dt}$$

Furthermore, the work being done per unit time in charging up the Windkessel is proportional to the product of the pressure and the flow into it, namely

$$dW = F_1(t) \cdot P_1(t) \cdot dt$$

Thus, if the Windkessel is charged up from time zero to time T, we have

$$W = \int_0^T F_1 \cdot P_1 \cdot dt = \int_0^T C \cdot \frac{dP}{dt} \cdot P \cdot dt = C \int_{P_1}^{P_2} P \cdot dP = \tfrac{1}{2} C(P_2^2 - P_1^2)$$

and thus, if the capacitance is a constant, the work done is proportional to the difference of the squares of the initial and final pressures, and is independent of the time taken for the change.

We now examine a more realistic model of the situation, in which the capacitance is made a function of the pressure, so that

$$C = \frac{C_0}{(1 + \alpha(P - P_0))}$$

where C_0, P_0 and α are appropriate constants.

If this form of capacitance is inserted into the integral above, we have

$$W = C_0 \int_{P_1}^{P_2} \frac{P}{(1 + \alpha(P - P_0))} \cdot dP$$

$$= \frac{C_0}{\alpha^2} \left\{ 1 + \alpha(P_2 - P_1) - (1 - \alpha P_0) \log \left(\frac{1 - \alpha(P_2 - P_0)}{1 - \alpha(P_1 - P_0)} \right) \right\}$$

In Fig. 2 we see the graphical representation of some computations of this function. It will be noted that the greater the amount of non-linearity, the less is the work required to move the system from one level of pressure to another. The values used were $c_0 = 1$ ml./mm. Hg, $P_0 = 100$ mm. Hg. For the largest value of α used ($\alpha = 0 \cdot 02$) we see that C_{200} is $\frac{1}{3}.C_{100}$, which is not at all an unrealistic value.

Time-course of pressure changes in a non-linear Windkessel

We see from Fig. 1 that if the total flow into the system is F, while the rate of storage in the Windkessel is F_1, the pressure in it is given by

$$P = (F - F_1)\,R$$

and thus

$$F_1 = \left(F - \frac{P}{R}\right)$$

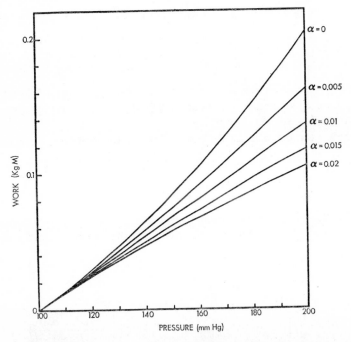

FIG. 2. Computed values of the "stored work" performed in raising the mean blood pressure. The initial value was 100 mm. Hg and the final values lie on the abscissa. The capacitance of the system was as defined in the text, with $C_0 = 1$ ml./mm. Hg, this being approximately the value for the human arterial system. The effect of increasing α, the parameter of non-linearity, is seen to be a reduction in the work needed for any increase in mean blood pressure.

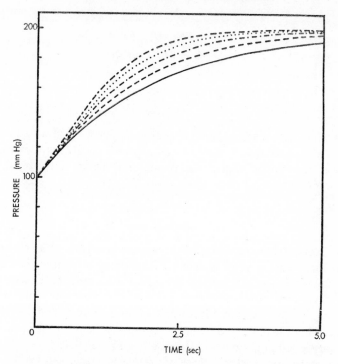

FIG. 3. Computed examples of the time-course of mean arterial pressure in response to a doubling of the peripheral resistance, cardiac output being constant at 100 ml./sec. The arterial capacitance was as defined in the text, with $C_0 = 1$ ml./mm. Hg. The solutions for various values of α are indicated as follows: 0·00 ———; 0·005 ------; 0·01 -.-.-.-.; 0·015 ......; 0·02 --------.

Considering the rate of change of pressure in the non-linear Windkessel, we have

$$\frac{dP}{dt} = \frac{F_1}{C} = \frac{(F - P/R)(1 + \alpha(P - P_0))}{C_0}$$

This equation can be integrated, with the conditions

$$F = \text{constant}$$
$$P = FR_1 \quad (t = 0)$$
$$R = R_2 \quad (t \geqslant 0)$$

to give

$$P(t) = \frac{FR_2 - A.R_2.e^{-\beta t}.(1 - \alpha P_0)}{1 + \alpha.A.R_2.e^{-\beta t}}$$

where

$$A = \frac{F(1 - R_1/R_2)}{1 + \alpha(FR_1 - P_0)}$$

and

$$\beta = \frac{1 + \alpha(FR_2 - P_0)}{R_2 C_0}$$

In Fig. 3 are shown some results of computations of $P(t)$ for various values of α. It will be seen that, as would be anticipated, the greater the progressive decrease of the distensibility of the Windkessel, the faster the pressure rises to its new level.

DISCUSSION

The results obtained above (pp. 138–141) are in accord with previous work (Taylor, 1965) on the input impedance of a single tube in which the wave-velocity increased along its length. It was shown there that such a disposition struck a favourable balance between low overall distensibility and high input impedance; we now see that this is true for a branching system. It remains to be shown what the optimal distribution is in a system where the branches are of arbitrary length, but no doubt the result will be similar.

As far as the non-linear elasticity of arteries is concerned, we see that this leads to two useful properties of the system. In the first place, if the arteries become progressively stiffer as they are further distended, there is a reduction in the amount of work which the heart must perform simply to inflate the Windkessel. Even quite a modest increase in stiffness can have a useful effect. In the second place, we see that an increasing stiffness of the Windkessel leads to a reduction in the time required for the pressure to rise after an increase in peripheral resistance. One may surmise, therefore, that a second benefit would be an increase in the speed of response to reflex adjustments of the peripheral resistance.

Acknowledgement

This work was supported by The National Heart Foundation of Australia.

REFERENCES

COHN, D. L. (1955). *Bull. math. Biophys.*, **17**, 219–227.
KRIES, J. VON (1892). *Studien zur Pulslehre.* Freiburg: Mohr.
O'ROURKE, M. F. (1967). *Cardiovascular Res.*, **1**, 312–326.

O'Rourke, M. F., and Taylor, M. G. (1967). *Circulation Res.*, **20**, 365–380.

Taylor, M. G. (1964). In *Pulsatile Blood Flow*, pp. 343–372, ed. Attinger, E. O. New York: McGraw-Hill.

Taylor, M. G. (1965). *Phys. Med. Biol.*, **10**, 539–550.

Taylor, M. G. (1966a). *Biophys. J.*, **6**, 29–51.

Taylor, M. G. (1966b). *Biophys. J.*, **6**, 697–716.

Taylor, M. G. (1967). *Gastroenterology*, **52**, 358–363.

DISCUSSION

Lighthill: Professor Taylor, I want to query your assumption of quarter-wavelength resonance. This seems to depend on having a closed end or a high impedance (or, better, low admittance) end. I suppose you have to have a total admittance at the downstream end which is less than that of the upstream end, to get a closed-end type of reflection. Bearing in mind that we are talking about admittances, which are flow amplitudes divided by pressure amplitudes, when we reach the small vessels it is difficult to see that at a typical branching there would be a very considerable total drop in admittance. It depends on radius³, and one finds at a typical branch that there is reduced total admittance downstream only if the area ratio is less than $\sqrt[3]{2}$; but this, actually, is thought to be about a typical value of area ratio. In other words I am arguing that even in the high resistance part of the circulation you should be getting quite good continued propagation, just as you are in the big vessels. Of course you may say that the distensibility goes on changing, but it seems to be agreed that peripheral reduction in distensibility occurs in the larger vessels but not also in the microcirculation.

Taylor: It obviously must reach an end somewhere. There are many points of evidence in favour of a closed end to the system. Of the two main points, one is that the input impedance comes down to a minimum from a very high value, and here the experimental facts are not easily explainable in terms of an open-ended system; in that case the impedance should be going up rather than coming down. The other point is that the phase velocities in the peripheral vessels are extremely high and this is consistent, and all the model interpretations are consistent, with approaching a closed end; that is, approaching a node and getting a positive reflection. If you track the amplitude of a harmonic from the heart out to the foot, the successive amplitudes all behave as if counting backwards from an anti-node at the periphery. The lowest frequency probably has a node right up near the heart; the second harmonic has a node half-way down the system, and the third harmonic has a node still further down. The whole interpretation makes sense only on that basis.

Lighthill: But on your own argument where you have admittance matching and an area ratio of $\sqrt[3]{2}$, all the energy goes through, so there is perfect transmission at those branches.

Taylor: This is only in the vessels with muscular walls. There are no accurate figures for the smaller vessels. On your basis you will have a problem explaining the input impedance that is found experimentally, which indicates approximately quarter-wavelength resonance. If you have an open end you must assume half-wavelength resonance.

Lighthill: I agree that this assumption of a closed end helps you to explain observed waveforms. I am only questioning whether the assumption is tenable.

Cumming: May I comment on the branching system and this figure of $\sqrt[3]{2}$? In a dichotomous branching system such as the lung airways there is a close approximation to $\sqrt[3]{2}$; but in the pulmonary circulation, dichotomous branching occurs in the larger vessels but branching becomes monopodial with occasional trichotomy in subsequent branchings, and furthermore the ratio of the sum of the daughters to the parent branch is often less than unity.

Lighthill: This would completely satisfy me. There seems to be a contradiction between the kind of area ratios described for example in *Blood Flow in Arteries* by D. A. McDonald ([1960]. London: Arnold) which would be typically 1·2 in the larger arteries and becoming larger peripherally, and the assumption, also from McDonald's book, that there is a closed-end type of reflection. These two are not logically compatible. If ratios are getting down to one or less than one, there can be no logical objection to closed-end reflection.

Caro: How did you arrive at these ratios, Dr. Cumming?

Cumming: We followed all the branches from the main trunk of the pulmonary artery of the human lung. This can be divided into two areas, pulmonary arteries down to branches of about 800 μm. diameter, and branches from 800 μm. down to about 50 μm. in diameter. For each branch, we determined by inspection whether it was monopodial, dichotomous or trichotomous. We then allocated to each branch a unique number and using a computer retrieved how many unique numbers showed each kind of branching. Of about 12,500 branches, more than two-thirds are monopodial. Then we plotted on a scatter diagram the surface area of the two daughter vessels compared with the parent vessel (if the two were the same it would have a value of unity). The mode is just above unity but there are many branchings where the two daughters have a smaller cross-section area than the parents from which they stem. The mean ratio was 0·6, but there were some ratios of 0·4.

Caro: Some years ago (Caro, C. G., and Saffman, P. G. [1965]. *J. Physiol., Lond.,* **178**, 193–210) we studied the rabbit pulmonary circulation in isolated lungs, visualizing the arteries by means of a radio-opaque oil. Vessel diameters were measured at branches, static intravascular pressure being 10 cm. water. In ten branches, selected because there was apparently dichotomy, the area coefficient ranged from $0 \cdot 86$ to $1 \cdot 48$, mean $1 \cdot 21$. The diameter of the daughter vessels ranged from $0 \cdot 08$ to $0 \cdot 02$ cm.

Burton: I still remain sceptical about treating the arterial system as though it has reflections that are significant. If you try to produce reflections and standing waves in your bath-tub you can only do so as long as you push your hand rhythmically; if you change the rhythm as the heart does in respiration, by as much as 15 to 20 per cent, you cannot produce a nice standing wave. In other words it has no relation to this analysis if the frequency is not very constant.

Taylor: It might be difficult to have a bath in an arterial system—there are too many branches for one thing!—but if you did and you made even random movements and analysed the amplitude transmission from point to point, as we have done with spectral analysis, you would find that the transmission ratios behave in a perfectly reasonable way on the basis of reflected waves and so forth. The steady state analogy, however, will work quite well.

Burton: Should you be using Fourier analysis in a non-linear case at all?

Taylor: The proof of this pudding is, like all mathematical puddings, in the eating. We can get sufficient superposition if we take different pulse waves of different frequencies and compare the ratios of transmission, say from the femoral artery at different heart rates; the first harmonic of one wave behaves very much like the second harmonic of a wave at half that frequency, and so on. There is indeed non-linear interaction but in most instances it is very small. For most cases we find that the linear model will do. I admit that in making detailed analyses of pressure–diameter relations with a very sensitive caliper, we got into trouble because of the elastic non-linearity (unpublished observations). The pressure–diameter relations were difficult to interpret and we had to use a non-linear model and fit non-linear relationships to make the interpretation. But for the pressure–flow relations and pulse-wave transmission the non-linear effects are extremely small. Results presented at Reykjavik ([1968]. *Proc. 1st int Conf. Hemorheology.* Oxford: Pergamon) on pulse wave transmission in non-linear elastic tubes also showed very little difference whether a linear model or a non-linear model was used.

Lighthill: The fact that propagation is over only a small number of wavelengths (less than one) helps; you could handle the non-linearity by a small perturbation on the Fourier series, showing that its main function would be to transfer a small amount of the energy from the first harmonic to the second.

Burton: Is it so small? The pulse pressure is 120/80; the distensibility of the arterial system at 120 is at least 30 per cent less than it is at 80 mm. Hg.

Lighthill: On the other hand the propagation over the harmonic is going less than a wavelength; this makes it a small perturbation.

Burton: The amplitude does increase; towards the femoral artery the pulse pressure is a lot bigger. I have never been convinced that that can be explained in terms of reflections, whereas the classical "breaking-wave" phenomenon explains it. The big amplitude disturbances travel faster; that is why a wave breaks as it comes to the shore.

Taylor: That is an entirely different system. It is very hard to explain this on that basis; the phase velocity differences are very small.

Burton: You could prove your theory experimentally by removing the piece of the vascular bed that you think is reflecting and replacing it with a tube system.

Taylor: If vasodilatation is produced in the femoral bed and the impedance is measured, the phase angle goes almost to zero. If vasoconstriction is produced by an injection of noradrenaline the phase angle increases further and you can follow the impedance as a function of time quite easily. It behaves exactly as a model would do in these circumstances.

Cumming: A possible experimental approach is to measure the femoral artery waveform in a person about to have a mid-thigh amputation.

Taylor: This was done, in effect, by people who measured the period of the standing wave in patients with cuffs applied to the thighs or in patients who had had amputations. They found some increase in the "resonant frequency", as they called it, of the arterial system. It behaves exactly like a resonating system, for a certain frequency.

Lighthill: But with the cuff it behaves more like a closed-end system than the real system?

Taylor: It behaves a bit more so. In fact the femoral pulse wave when the cuff was on was much the same as before; it just shortened the effective resonating length of the system.

Philip: Professor Taylor, are there independent observations of the elastic non-linearity of arteries?

Taylor: There is independent evidence of elastic non-linearity. One can plot the variation of Young's Modulus of different vessels as a function of the distending pressure (actually it is a function of the diameter at which they are being measured). But elastic non-linearity is a consequence of the peculiar constitution of blood vessels, which are made up of variable amounts of elastin and collagen and become considerably stiffer as they are stretched, because the collagen within the walls comes to bear more and more of the load.

Burton: Another completely different line of evidence is the pulse-wave velocity from the heart to the brachial, subclavian and other arteries.

J. O. Doupe ([1952]. *Can. J. med. Sci.*, **30,** 125–129) studied this in hypertensive patients, who have a much faster overall arrival than normal. He asked whether the faster rate was because the high pressure was distending the artery and making it stiffer, or whether it was stiffer because of the disease. He therefore lowered the blood pressure of hypertensive patients to normal, and the pulse-wave velocity also became normal. Doupe obtained a series showing how by varying the degree of distension of the artery, one can increase pulse-wave velocity considerably, which is evidence that overall elasticity is non-linear. The other work is usually done on excised arteries, but they are not very different from in life, because in the large arteries the fibres are mostly elastic fibres. (The only difference which can be detected in the elastic arteries is in the hysteresis loop, which does seem to depend upon the vitality of the smooth muscle.)

Taylor: We have soaked arteries in cyanide, adrenaline and so forth and made elasticity measurements after a week at 0° C. It makes surprisingly little difference. This makes one wonder what the smooth muscle of the thoracic aorta is really doing. One speculates that it may be sitting there making elastin.

Burton: Even in the femoral artery where there is a lot of smooth muscle and the vessel is contractile, the smooth muscle seems to be there merely to bedevil us, by going into spasm in unfortunate cases! But it is hard to see how the contraction of the lumen even to half its size would affect total peripheral resistance very much. I was interested that Dr. R. Buck (University of Western Ontario; personal communication), making electron microscope studies of muscular arteries, felt that the smooth muscle was there not to contract but to be the source of the elastin and collagen fibres.

Lighthill: When distensibility and pulse-wave velocity have been measured, have they been found to be in reasonable agreement?

Burton: In excellent agreement.

Schultz: Professor Taylor, do any of your models account for, or show, the dicrotic notch?

Taylor: This depends on what you mean by the dicrotic notch. If you mean the little jiggle that follows the closure of the aortic valves, this does not appear in my models because I have not put in a waveform with all the high-frequency flow components that would be needed to produce it. One can see it experimentally. It is a very high frequency component that damps out very fast. If I put a square-wave flow pattern into my calculations with enough harmonics I would probably see it, but that is a very fine detail.

Burton: The dicrotic notch is related to the closure of the valves?

Schultz: Yes, but the pressure minimum in the dicrotic notch seemed to

6

correspond to the maximum reverse flow velocity, and this was observed with a pressure cannula inside the aorta.

Taylor: This makes sense, because the valves are shut by the reversed flow. In most classical diagrams the pulsewaves in the aorta have been recorded with under-damped rather low frequency manometers, and one sees the manometer ringing; it is not the aorta because with a catheter-tip manometer that train of oscillations is not seen.

PRESSURE–FLOW RELATIONS IN
SMALL BLOOD VESSELS

C. G. CARO, M. F. SUDLOW, T. H. FOLEY AND A. UR

Department of Aeronautics, Physiological Flow Studies Unit, Imperial College of Science and Technology, London

DESPITE a large literature on the mechanics of peripheral blood flow there is still uncertainty on several aspects of this subject. The variation of static pressure along the length of resistance vessels and the related topic of the extensibility of these vessels remain incompletely understood.

There appear to have been few measurements of static pressure at different sites in arterioles. Wiederhielm (1967) reported that pressure in terminal arterioles and metarterioles in bat wings was pulsatile and ranged from 50 to 75 mm. Hg, as compared with 60 to 100 mm. Hg in terminal arteries and arterioles. However pressure in arterial capillaries, beyond the precapillary sphincter, was 10 to 25 mm. Hg with the sphincter closed and 50 to 55 mm. Hg with it open.

Permutt and Riley (1963) have suggested the presence in systemic vascular beds of a "waterfall" mechanism.† This was conceived to be due to active tension in arteriolar smooth muscle, which produced a pressure related to Burton's critical closing pressure. The theory predicted that blood flow would become independent of static pressure downstream of the "waterfall" when this pressure was lower than "waterfall" pressure. The theory is important in that it may render suspect calculations of vascular resistance. Such calculations are usually criticized on grounds that blood is a non-Newtonian fluid, having a viscosity which may alter under various conditions of flow. But an additional complication arises if the "waterfall" theory is validated. The downstream end of the pressure difference causing flow may then not be known. Permutt and Riley's (1963) theory appears to have been tested so far only on data obtained from excised animal ears perfused with Ringer solution.

There is also little unanimity on the extensibility of resistance vessels. As noted by Folkow and Löfving (1956), Whittaker and Winton (1933) and others concluded that resistance vessels were practically indistensible. However Green and co-workers (1944), again using pressure–flow relations in

† See pp. 274–275 for discussion of use of this term.

perfused vascular beds, produced equally convincing evidence that resistance vessels are quite distensible. More recently, direct visual observations of the dimensions of small vessels by Baez, Lamport and Baez (1960) and Wieder-hielm (1965) show these vessels to be almost indistensible at pressures above those normally prevailing. Folkow and Löfving (1956) suggested that contra-dictions between studies on the extensibility of resistance vessels might be reconciled if there were in different studies differences in smooth muscle active tension.

Studies have been made of the relationship between blood pressure and flow in the intact human forearm, using perfusion pressures ranging from normal to lower than normal (Burton and Yamada, 1951). But in a recent study Caro, Foley and Sudlow (1968) proposed a method for measuring blood flow in intact man during the course of an acute increase of perfusion pressure. A segment of forearm was abruptly exposed to subatmospheric pressure. There was no retrograde venous flow and by making appropriate control measurements account could be taken of the motion of soft tissue and probably that of interstitial fluid. These studies showed that acutely applied suction caused a large increase of blood flow. Assuming the downstream end of the pressure difference for flow to have been venous pressure, and blood viscosity to have been constant, a suction pressure of −90 mm. Hg reduced calculated resistance to 36 per cent of its control value. Such a finding is strongly sugges-tive of resistance vessels being extensible or subject to recruitment.

However other difficulties arise in the study of resistance vessel extensibility. Several investigations, including those of Folkow (1952), have shown blood flow to fall and then to increase shortly after perfusion pressure is lowered and to increase and then to fall after perfusion pressure is raised. These findings are open to the criticisms listed earlier. However Bayliss (1902), and Klemensiewicz (1921) (quoted by Folkow, 1952), observed vessel dimen-sions directly and noted constriction followed by dilatation, shortly after lowering vascular pressure, and dilatation followed by constriction after vascular pressure was raised. Such later changes can, it would seem, only be explained by active relaxation or shortening of contractile wall elements.

The nature of the mechanisms underlying these changes remains in dispute. Myogenic (Bayliss, 1902; Folkow, 1952), metabolic (Lewis and Grant, 1925), or myogenic and metabolic mechanisms (Walker, Mackay and Van Loon, 1967) have been proposed. Meanwhile, it is important to recognize that a change of vascular pressure may cause passive as well as active changes in the dimensions of or tension in wall elements. It would therefore seem important to determine whether there is some period of time, after a change of vascular pressure, during which changes of length are predominantly passive. During this time there should be negligible active change of tension in elements in the wall. Such information is needed for an understanding of the passive mechanics of a vascular bed. It may also aid the elucidation of the mechanisms concerned in the active response of vessels to change of pressure.

The work we report was undertaken as an extension of the study on forearm blood flow when the limb was exposed to subatmospheric pressure (Caro, Foley and Sudlow, 1968). The main objective was to determine whether there is a "waterfall" in the systemic circulation. The investigation was again on the intact human forearm (and not on individual resistance vessels). As such it is open to the criticisms already levelled. In addition resting blood flow would have been partitioned between muscle and skin approximately in the ratio $0 \cdot 7/0 \cdot 3$ (Cooper, Edholm and Mottram, 1955). Moreover only some 60–70 per cent of the vascular resistance would, under resting conditions, have been due to flow through the arterioles. It is however believed that the study, while inevitably lacking in precision, may have gained because measurements could be made with a minimum of interference to the circulation. Moreover very large changes of flow were seen in some of the experiments, suggesting that these changes were due to alterations in the region of the resistance vessels.

METHODS

We assumed the presence of a "waterfall" in the forearm circulation and tested for it in ways appropriate to testing for model "waterfalls", such as those described by Permutt and Riley (1963) and de Bono and Caro (1963). Because there is only a very small rise of mean upstream arterial blood pressure when the brachial artery is obstructed, the forearm was assumed to be perfused by a constant head of pressure, rather than a constant flow. We therefore monitored flow and attempted to determine the particular level at which venous pressure began to influence flow.

A full description of the study is given elsewhere (Sudlow et al., 1969). We examined, as a first step, the validity of measuring forearm flow by venous occlusion plethysmography, at raised levels of venous pressure.

We assumed that a simple lumped model of the forearm circulation, having linear elements, would be adequate. Inertial forces were ignored (see Sudlow et al., 1969, Appendix II). We further assumed, on the basis of results reported below, that any "waterfall" would be inoperative at venous pressures exceeding 20 mm. Hg. Thus, when venous outflow was obstructed, blood was conceived to flow from a constant pressure source (arterial pressure) through a resistance (resistance vessels) and to accumulate in the compliant veins. Study of this model showed that flow, during a small fraction (say the first tenth) of the time constant (product of compliance and resistance), is virtually independent of venous compliance. Flow then depends on the initial levels of arterial and venous pressure and on the value of the resistance. Venous occlusion plethysmography appeared therefore to be applicable at raised levels of venous pressure and even some degree of non-linearity of venous compliance appeared tolerable.

In experiments on man, forearm volume was monitored with a mercury-in-rubber strain gauge and pressure was measured in superficial forearm veins by means of indwelling plastic catheters attached to strain gauge pressure transducers. The reference plane for venous pressure measurement was the middle of the horizontal forearm, which was supported level with the right atrium. An arterial cuff was applied at the wrist and a second cuff was applied above the elbow. This second cuff was used both to measure flow and to raise venous pressure to chosen levels. When venous pressure had stabilized at a particular level (requiring up to two or three minutes) the cuff was inflated to 70 mm. Hg for about five seconds and blood flow was recorded at this level

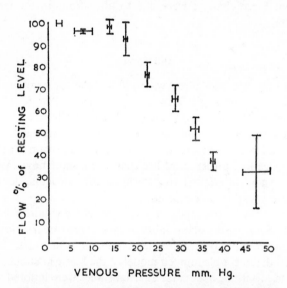

FIG. 1. Average values for forearm blood flow (eight subjects). Flow is expressed as a percentage of the preceding resting flow. Venous pressure is averaged at intervals of 5 mm. Hg. Bars indicate ± 1 s.e. When venous pressure was less than 17·6 mm. Hg flow exceeded 90 per cent of the resting level. Flow fell progressively at higher levels of venous pressure.

of venous pressure. Measurements were also made of post-congestion flow.
Venous congestion was abruptly released and, from as soon as one second
later, the cuff was inflated to 70 mm. Hg to record flow.

RESULTS

Shown in Fig. 1 are average findings for eight subjects on forearm flow
during congestion. Average resting venous pressure was 2·3 mm. Hg. Blood
flow is expressed as a percentage of the immediately preceding resting flow.
Up to a venous pressure of 17·6 mm. Hg, flow during congestion exceeded
90 per cent of resting flow. But flow became progressively smaller at higher
levels of venous pressure.

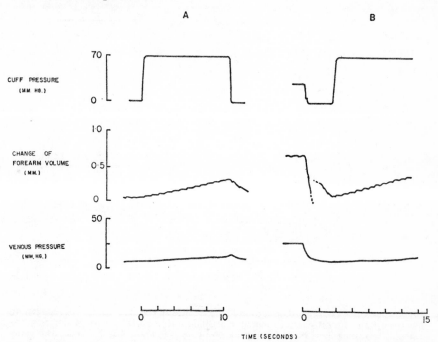

FIG. 2. A. Resting blood flow for one subject. B. Post-congestion flow measured from 3 sec.
after release of venous congestion at 20 mm. Hg. Post-congestion flow was constant and
closely similar to resting flow. Interruptions indicate where the strain gauge was rapidly
rebalanced between deflation of the congesting cuff and its reinflation to 70 mm. Hg.

As a preliminary to measuring post-congestion flow, pressure was recorded
in two superficial forearm veins while venous pressure was being raised to
30 mm. Hg and when venous congestion was released. The results are not
shown, but pressure was equal in the two veins after two minutes. Moreover

the decay of pressure was closely similar in both veins. It was 90 per cent complete in one second.

In Fig. 2A resting blood flow is shown for one subject and Fig. 2B shows flow measured from three seconds after the release of venous congestion at 20 mm. Hg. Post-congestion flow was constant and closely similar to resting flow. Similar results were obtained in five subjects studied in this way. Mean resting flow in these subjects was 3·2 ml./min. per 100 ml. (s.e. 0·3). Mean post-congestion flow was 3·6 ml./min. per 100 ml. (s.e. 0·5) when mean congesting pressure had been 18·2 mm. Hg.

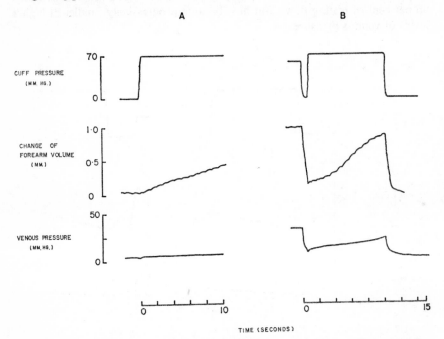

FIG. 3. Studies on the same subject as in Fig. 2. A. Resting blood flow. B. Post-congestion flow from 1 sec. after release of congestion at 30 mm. Hg. Early post-congestion flow was similar to resting flow, but delayed peak post-congestion flow was 2·9 times as great.

Fig. 3 shows results from the same subject as in Fig. 2. In A resting blood flow is plotted. In B flow has been recorded from one second after the release of venous congestion at 30 mm. Hg. During the first two seconds post-congestion flow was similar to resting flow. However between three and five seconds after the release of congestion, flow was 6·4 ml./min. per 100 ml. (1·98 times the resting value). Peak flow occurred five to six seconds after the release of congestion. The peak value was 9·4 ml./min. per 100 ml.

The results shown in Fig. 3 are extended in Fig. 4, recorded on the same subject. In A flow was recorded from one second after release of venous congestion at 40 mm. Hg; in B from three seconds and in C from five seconds. The early post-congestion flow is again low while the two later records show flows similar to those seen at comparable times on the first trace.

Results obtained from two other subjects (Fig. 5) summarize the preceding findings. Forearm blood flow was measured in the resting state (X) (averaged

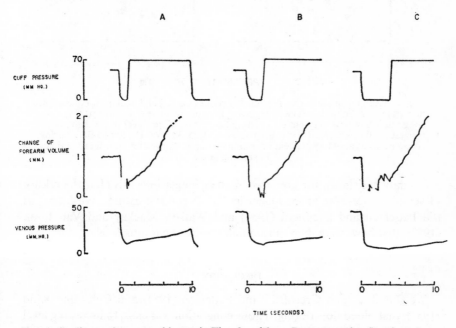

FIG. 4. Studies on the same subject as in Figs. 2 and 3. A. Post-congestion flow from 1 sec. after release of congestion at 40 mm. Hg. B. The same, from 3 sec. C. The same, from 5 sec. The records made from 3 sec. and 5 sec. show flows similar to those recorded at comparable times on the first trace. The strain gauge was rebalanced.

values for several determinations) and during venous congestion at various levels of pressure (open circles). Peak post-congestion flow (filled circles) is plotted at the relevant level of venous congesting pressure. Below 15 mm. Hg resting pressure, flow during congestion and post-congestion flow are closely similar. At 25–30 mm. Hg, flow during congestion was about 85 per cent of the resting level, but peak post-congestion flow was 300–500 per cent of the resting level. Similar results were obtained in seven subjects so studied.

6*

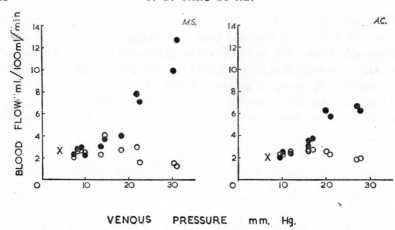

FIG. 5. Mean resting flow (X), flow during congestion (○) and peak post-congestion flow (●) in two subjects. When congesting pressure was less than 15 mm. Hg, post-congestion flow was very close to resting flow. Above this level of pressure, post-congestion flow exceeded the resting value. At 25–30 mm. Hg (when flow during congestion was about 85 per cent of resting flow) post-congestion flow was 3–5 times the resting level.

No data are shown for flows recorded at longer intervals after the release of venous congestion, at the higher levels of venous pressure. We found, as did Patterson and Shepherd (1954) and Walker, Mackay and Van Loon (1967), that flows were then substantially below the resting level.

DISCUSSION

We found, as had Greenfield and Patterson (1954) and Coles and Kidd (1957), that blood flow during venous congestion was close to its resting level until venous pressure was made to exceed 15–20 mm. Hg. Thereafter flow fell progressively with increase of venous pressure. Two points follow from these findings. The first is that if there is a "waterfall" in the forearm circulation when venous pressure is raised, "waterfall" pressure must be less than 15–20 mm. Hg. We have argued that flow through a "waterfall" depends on downstream pressure only when this exceeds "waterfall" pressure. From this argument it follows that venous pressure must be the downstream end of the pressure difference causing flow, when this pressure exceeds 15–20 mm. Hg. Moreover, this information permits us to calculate vascular resistance, at various levels of venous pressure, if flow is known.

We found the average flow in eight subjects to be 52 per cent of resting flow at a venous pressure of 33·4 mm. Hg, and 56 per cent of resting flow at a venous pressure of 22·3 mm. Hg. Mean arterial blood pressure was 83 mm. Hg. Vascular resistance calculated as ([mean arterial − mean venous pressure]/ flow as percentage resting value) was 0·95 at a venous pressure of 33·4 mm. Hg, and 0·71 at 22·3 mm. Hg. Assuming venous pressure to have been operative also in the resting state, resistance would then be 0·82. A minimum value of resistance was therefore found at about 22 mm. Hg, while resistance at 33 mm. Hg exceeded the resting value. Studies of blood flow in the finger (Shanks, 1955) and in the toe (England and Johnston, 1956) similarly showed that vascular resistance was normal or slightly above normal at higher levels of venous pressure.

It cannot however directly be assumed that the near-constancy of vascular resistance at higher venous pressures indicates constancy of the dimensions of the vascular bed. It seems probable that venous congestion would to some extent dilate, and reduce the resistance of, the capillary and post-capillary vessels; in which case there would have to be some constriction of pre-capillary vessels to keep resistance almost constant. It is, however, still not permissible directly to relate resistance to geometry, for resistance is a function both of geometry and of blood viscosity. This type of study gives no independent measure of either.

Some clarification is gained from considering the high delayed post-congestion flow. Presume for purposes of discussion that venous congestion had distended the resistance vessels. Presume further, as suggested by Patterson and Shepherd (1954), that these vessels once dilated require some time to regain their resting dimensions, and that their sustained dilatation accounted for the high level of post-congestion flow. For simplicity we assume that the dimensions of the resistance vessels are identical during congestion and at the height of the post-congestion flow. To account for the normality or slight increase of resistance during congestion, blood viscosity would then have to be considerably higher during congestion than in resting conditions. Consideration of the influence of rate of shear on blood viscosity helps to show whether any large changes of blood viscosity can be expected.

Conceive of the resistance vessels as a single tube, through which there is a Poiseuille type of flow of blood. Our data permit us to make some predictions about the changes of dimensions of this tube and of the velocity of the blood during venous congestion and after its release. The mean rate of shear in small vessels is given by Whitmore (1967) as approximately 500 sec.$^{-1}$ At such rates of shear, viscosity is approaching its asymptotic value. Thus for the peak post-congestion flow to be three times the resting level, for the same pressure difference, the radius of the imagined tube would have to be greater than its resting value by a factor of 1·32. Blood velocity would be increased by $1 \cdot 73$ and the mean rate of shear by $1 \cdot 32$. The reduction of blood viscosity would be immeasurably small.

Consider also the hypothetical case where, during congestion, resistance vessels are dilated (radius increase of $1 \cdot 32$) but flow has (as at a venous pressure of 35 mm. Hg) fallen to 50 per cent of the resting value. Mean velocity is now 30 per cent of the resting value and the mean rate of shear is 22 per cent of its control value, or approximately 100 sec.$^{-1}$ Whitmore's data suggest that blood viscosity will then be less than 10 per cent greater than normal. Yet to account for the volume flow measured with perfusion pressure reduced during congestion from 80 to 45 mm. Hg and geometry identical to that in the post-congestion state, blood viscosity would have to be increased by 333 per cent.

There is another possible way in which blood viscosity might increase during venous congestion. Filtration of plasma might have been increased, leading to an increase in the haematocrit. However such changes would presumably be confined largely to the capillaries, which normally contribute only a small fraction of the total vascular resistance.

We submit therefore that the observed slight increase of resistance seen during congestion is explicable in terms of slight constriction (and not dilatation) of resistance vessels. Support for this argument comes from the direct visual observations of Bayliss (1902) and Klemensiewicz (1921). They found that vessels tended to constrict some time after their internal pressure was raised.

We had been concerned that it had required two to three minutes to raise venous pressure when venous outflow was obstructed. This would presumably give ample time for compensatory active change of active tension in the smooth muscle of resistance vessels. It seemed therefore logical to raise venous pressure and then to lower it rapidly in an attempt to study the immediate (and presumably more passive) effects of change of venous pressure.

We found, as had Lewis and Grant (1925), Patterson and Shepherd (1954) and Walker, Mackay and Van Loon (1967), that post-congestion flow was considerably higher than the preceding resting flow. However two new findings emerged from our study. The first was that post-congestion flow exceeded resting flow only if congesting pressure had been greater than 15–20 mm. Hg. The second finding was that one to two seconds after release of venous congestion flow was, even at higher levels of venous pressure, not much different from resting flow. It was only after two to three seconds that flow began to rise, and peak flow was not seen until four to six seconds after the release of congestion.

It seems useful in attempting to explain these findings to consider the results

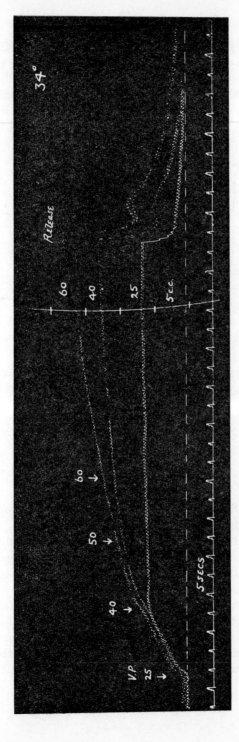

FIG. 6. Reproduction of records of decay of forearm volume after release of venous congestion.
The first (lowest) curve shows the effect of throwing a pressure of 25 mm. Hg on to a shoulder and then runs horizontally until, at the end of 2 minutes, the pressure is released, when the curve speedily falls to its original base line. The second curve is similar except that the pressure is raised to 40 mm. at 20 seconds. The third is similar to the second except that the pressure has been further raised to 50 and finally to 60 mm. Arm volume, about 600 ml. (Reproduced from Lewis and Grant, 1925, by permission of *Clinical Science*.)

of earlier workers and proposals advanced by them. Lewis and Grant (1925) had suggested that active vasodilatation occurred during the course of venous congestion, as the result of retention of metabolites. But, as in the studies of Patterson and Shepherd (1954) who favoured not active dilatation but passive stretching of vessels, and Walker, Mackay and Van Loon (1967), flow was not

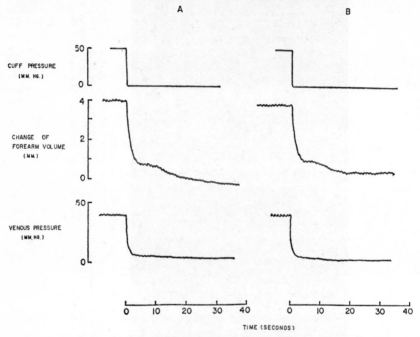

FIG. 7. Decay of forearm volume after release of venous congestion at 40 mm. Hg. The decay was delayed at 2–3 sec. with (A) or without (B) an arterial cuff on the wrist.

measured until about five seconds after the release of venous congestion so that low early post-congestion flows were not seen.

The arguments we have presented make us unable to accept that vasodilatation (whatever the mechanism) had occurred during venous congestion. It is our belief that vasodilatation did occur, but not until venous congestion had been released for two to three seconds.

Findings by Lewis and Grant (1925), though not so interpreted by them, seem to support this contention. Their results, reproduced in Fig. 6, show that the decay of forearm volume immediately after the release of venous congestion was not smooth but was interrupted at two to three seconds by a hump. We repeated their experiment (Fig. 7) and found that this hump was present whether there was an arterial cuff on the wrist (A), as in their studies, or not (B). This hump seems to us to indicate that arterial blood inflow began to increase two or three seconds after the release of venous congestion. Moreover the abruptness of the inflexion seems counter to what would be seen were this a manifestation of mechanical delay in the onset of increased flow, through an already dilated vascular bed.

Consider again events in the forearm circulation after relief of venous congestion, in order to gain further insight into the mechanisms responsible for the various rates of post-congestion flow seen. At congesting pressures below 15–20 mm. Hg, when flow during congestion was normal, there was no difference between post-congestion and resting flow. In these circumstances it would seem difficult to argue that there had been any retention of metabolic products. Moreover it could be argued that pre-capillary vessels were not exposed to any increase of distending pressure, either by virtue of the presence of a "waterfall", or more simply because these lower levels of venous pressure caused distension of post-arteriolar vessels and hence permitted the same volume flow rate for a reduced perfusion pressure.

However at venous pressures exceeding this apparently critical level by only a few millimetres of mercury, and when flow during congestion was reduced by as little as 15 per cent, peak post-congestion flow was as high as 300 per cent of the resting level. Nonetheless, even in these experiments, post-congestion flow during the first two seconds after release of congestion was closely similar to flow in the resting state. Such findings might be explained by transmission delays preventing the onset of higher rates of flow through a bed previously dilated by venous congestion, although our arguments relating to blood viscosity fail to support such a hypothesis. It is however of interest to examine the mechanical processes in the development of an increased rate of flow in the forearm when a new driving pressure is applied.

After the release of venous congestion a new rate of flow cannot be established until a wave of pressure release has been propagated upstream along the veins, through the capillaries and resistance vessels, to the arteries. We have not attempted to determine experimentally the rate of propagation of such a pressure wave. The static pressure drop per unit length of any accessible artery is normally so small as to make it unlikely that such a measurement would be meaningful. Landis (1930) reported that two to three minutes were required for capillary pressure to return to normal after the release of venous congestion, but this seems an excessively long time.

Our measurements of flow during and after release of venous congestion appear, however, to provide useful information. Flow during congestion, at higher levels of venous pressure, was considerably less than the resting flow (approximately 50 per cent reduction at 35 mm. Hg). Nevertheless re-application of the cuff one second after release of congestion showed that flow was restored to its resting level during the first second. It would seem difficult to explain such an increase of the rate of arterial inflow other than by an increased pressure drop per unit length of artery. And this would require arrival of the wave of pressure release in the artery in less than one second.

Lighthill (Appendix II, Sudlow *et al.*, 1969) has analysed the mechanics of propagation of a wave of pressure release in the forearm circulation and estimated the mechanical lag to be at most one second. Inertia is of little consequence. The process is dominated by the compliance of each vessel against the resistivity of the same vessel. The calculation is based on apparently conservative estimates of the components of the mechanical lag.

From this theoretical evidence, together with the experimental finding of restoration of resting flow in one to two seconds after the release of congestion, it seems reasonable to conclude that the mechanical lag in the forearm is shorter than the delay seen between the release of venous congestion and the onset of increased post-congestion flow. Furthermore, assuming the arguments about blood viscosity to be correct, a mechanism may be provided to explain active vasodilatation after release of venous congestion.

The argument here is necessarily speculative. Let it be assumed that higher venous pressures failed to dilate the resistance vessels. These vessels are apparently capable of being dilated by an abrupt increase of pressure (Green *et al.*, 1944; Caro, Foley and Sudlow, 1968). Hence it must be presumed that they developed, during venous congestion, sufficient active tension to balance the increased distending pressure.

Let it further be assumed that the wave of pressure release reaches the resistance vessels within one second of the release of venous congestion. Since they already have increased active tension in their walls, the vessels will passively constrict. We speculate that shortening of wall elements (or inappropriateness of length to tension) is in some way sensed and in some way leads to abrupt and excessive relaxation of active tension. With active tension now being inappropriately low in relation to distending pressure, passive dilatation and a fall of vascular resistance ensue.

We are thus advancing a myogenic type of mechanism to explain the findings. But high post-congestion flows were seen when flow during congestion had been reduced by as little as 15 per cent, making it unlikely that a significant metabolic debt had been incurred. However, in advancing this theory we are conscious that there seem to be no data on the rate at which human resistance vessels are able to relax their active tension.

These findings, and those of our earlier study (Caro, Foley and Sudlow,

1968), are usefully viewed against observations by Folkow (1952). His results on perfused animal limbs show that the increase of flow that follows reduction of perfusion pressure occurs more quickly than the reduction of flow that follows raising of perfusion pressure. In our earlier study we had been able to increase forearm blood flow for 10 to 20 seconds by exposing the limb to subatmospheric pressure. Our present results suggest that relaxation of active tension was occurring in the space of two to three seconds. It seems therefore legitimate to ask whether active tension in vascular smooth muscle can be reduced more rapidly than it can be developed.

Further studies are clearly needed to confirm these various findings. Ideally, direct observations should be made of the dimensions of small vessels suddenly subjected to change of static pressure. It must also be recognized that the change of flow we detected after the release of congestion may have been due not simply to change of active tension in vascular smooth muscle but to alteration of the rate of vasomotion at pre-capillary sphincters (Wiederhielm, 1967). We also want to discover whether changes of flow occur uniquely after the release of venous congestion, or whether they are also seen on abrupt reduction of normal static vascular pressure.

SUMMARY

A study was made to test whether there is a Poiseuille type of pressure gradient along resistance vessels in the forearm circulation, or a vascular "waterfall". In the latter case flow would be independent of venous pressure when this was less than "waterfall" pressure.

Forearm flow was measured by venous occlusion plethysmography at normal and raised venous pressures. Below 15–20 mm. Hg flow was normal. Above this level flow fell progressively with increase of venous pressure. Such a finding could be explained by a "waterfall" or by dilatation of post-arteriolar vessels. However a "waterfall", if present, could not be set at a pressure exceeding 15 to 20 mm. Hg.

Vascular resistance was at a minimum at a venous pressure of 15 to 20 mm. Hg, but it exceeded this, and, to a small extent, the level of resting resistance, at higher levels of venous pressure. Data in the literature on the relationship of blood viscosity to rate of shear suggest that the increase of resistance during congestion cannot be explained by an increase of blood viscosity compensating for dilatation of resistance vessels. Rather does it appear that there was slight active constriction of resistance vessels.

In an attempt to study the passive mechanics of the vascular bed, flow was also measured immediately after release of venous congestion. When venous pressure was lower than 15 to 20 mm. Hg post-congestion flow was equal to resting flow. At higher levels of venous pressure, flow one to two seconds after release of congestion was again similar to resting flow, but by four to five seconds flow was 200–300 per cent of the resting level.

Analysis of the components of the propagation of a wave of pressure release in the forearm circulation and the rapid restoration of normal flow after release of congestion suggests that the lag does not exceed one second. Active vasodilatation appeared therefore to be occurring, not during the course of venous congestion, but within two to three seconds after its release. These circumstances suggest that a myogenic mechanism is responsible for the vasodilatation.

REFERENCES

BAEZ, S., LAMPORT, H., and BAEZ, A. (1960). In *Flow Properties of Blood*, ed. Copley, A. L., and Stainsby, G. Oxford: Pergamon Press.
BAYLISS, W. M. (1902). *J. Physiol., Lond.*, **28**, 220–231.
BURTON, A. C., and YAMADA, S. (1951). *J. appl. Physiol.*, **4**, 329.
CARO, C. G., FOLEY, T. H., and SUDLOW, M. F. (1968). *J. Physiol., Lond.*, **194**, 645–658.
COLES, D. R., and KIDD, B. S. L. (1957). *Circulation Res.*, **5**, 223–225.
COOPER, K. E., EDHOLM, O. G., and MOTTRAM, R. F. (1955). *J. Physiol., Lond.*, **128**, 258–267.
DE BONO, E. F., and CARO, C. G. (1963). *Am. J. Physiol.*, **205**, 1178–1186.
ENGLAND, R. M., and JOHNSTON, J. G. M. (1956). *Clin. Sci.*, **15**, 587–592.
FOLKOW, B. (1952). *Acta physiol. scand.*, **27**, 99–117.
FOLKOW, B., and LÖFVING, B. (1956). *Acta physiol. scand.*, **38**, 37–52.
GREEN, H. D., LEWIS, R. M., NICKERSON, N. D., and HELLER, A. I. (1944). *Am. J. Physiol.*, **141**, 518–536.
GREENFIELD, A. D. M., and PATTERSON, G. C. (1954). *J. Physiol., Lond.*, **126**, 508–524.
KLEMENSIEWICZ, R. (1921). *Abderhaldens Handb. Biol. Arb. meth.*, **4**, 32.
LANDIS, E. M. (1930). *Heart*, **15**, 209.
LEWIS, T., and GRANT, R. (1925). *Heart*, **12**, 73.
PATTERSON, G. C., and SHEPHERD, J. T. (1954). *J. Physiol., Lond.*, **125**, 501.
PERMUTT, S., and RILEY, R. L. (1963). *J. appl. Physiol.*, **18**, 924–932.
SHANKS, R. G. (1955). *Clin. Sci.*, **14**, 285.
SUDLOW, M. F., FOLEY, T. H., UR, A., and CARO, C. G. (1969). Submitted for publication.
WALKER, R. L., MACKAY, I. F. S., and VAN LOON, P. (1967). *J. appl. Physiol.*, **22**, 889–899.
WHITMORE, R. L. (1967). *Nature, Lond.*, **215**, 123–126.
WHITTAKER, S. R. F., and WINTON, F. R. (1933). *J. Physiol., Lond.*, **78**, 339.
WIEDERHIELM, C. A. (1965). *Fedn Proc. Fedn Am. Socs exp. Biol.*, **24**, 1075.
WIEDERHIELM, C. A. (1967). *Fedn Proc. Fedn Am. Socs exp. Biol.*, **26**, 495.

DISCUSSION

Burton: Some years ago Peter Gaskell and I ([1953]. *Circulation Res.*, **1**, 27–39) studied the variation of blood flow in the limbs with posture, as a way of raising the venous pressure. We discovered that as the limb is lowered the driving pressure is the same but there is a very marked effect below a certain level; the arterial inflow decreases, which we called, perhaps mistakenly, a veni-vasomotor reflex. S. Yamada ([1954]. *J. appl. Physiol.*, **6**, 501–505) obtained the same result with negative pressure, on the fingers. There seemed to be a back effect of shutting down the arterioles, as a result of congesting the veins, which depended upon the degree of vasomotor tone.

Rosenberg did the same with the rabbit leg and ear (Rosenberg, E. [1956]. *Am. J. Physiol.*, **185**, 471–473; Burton, A. C., and Rosenberg, E. [1956]. *Am. J. Physiol.*, **185**, 465–470). In fact there is quite a literature that could be cited in support of Dr. Caro's findings. The name "veni-vasomotor reflex" was however a bad one, though the speed of the response suggested a reflex. I now realize that if the microlymphatic system were lobulated in the way the blood circulation is, such that the microlymphatics channelled as a cuff around the metarteriole coming in (although I can find no anatomical evidence in the literature that this is so), it might be a purely mechanical effect, and on this scale it could happen in a fraction of a second. When venous pressure is raised the lymphatic volume and flow increase immediately, and this could be compressing the arteriole.

This effect of congesting the veins on the arterioles can be demonstrated very readily with a finger plethysmograph. If the blood flow is cut off altogether by a high-pressure cuff and if the subject is cold, with high vasomotor tone, there is no circulation; if the venous occlusion cuff is inflated, the only result is that the finger volume decreases. If the subject is warm and vasodilated the effect is not seen.

Caro: I must point out that we, like others mentioned in my paper, did *not* find marked vasoconstriction during venous congestion. Rather do our results suggest that vascular resistance was perhaps 15 per cent greater during venous congestion than in the control state. And if, as seems likely, there was a 10 per cent underestimation of flow at higher levels of venous pressure, then vascular resistance during congestion would have been about normal. The crucial point with regard to attempting an explanation of the high post-congestion flow is that the bed was *not* significantly dilated during venous congestion.

We must study the response using blocking agents because we are not yet clear about mechanisms. However, G. C. Patterson and J. T. Shepherd

([1954]. *J. Physiol., Lond.,* **125,** 501) found hyperaemia after release of venous congestion in a man with traumatic denervation of the arm. Thus the mechanism would not appear to operate through a large-scale reflex pathway.

Renkin: Dr. S. Gray and I (unpublished observations) studied the effects of raising venous pressure in the isolated perfused gracilis muscle preparation, and we have evidence that the "veni-vasomotor reflex" is not a physical effect but must involve contraction of smooth muscle. The vascular smooth muscle is first relaxed completely by shutting off the blood flow for 3 or 4 minutes. Then flow is turned on again and venous pressure is suddenly raised. During the period in which full reactive hyperaemia is maintained there is no response, but actually a fall in resistance as the vessels become distended. During recovery of vascular tone, the vasoconstrictor response gradually reappears. It would be possible to do this experiment in man.

Caro: A point which is of great concern to us is to know if it is possible for vascular muscle to relax in, say, 2 seconds.

Burton: Full relaxation may take 15 seconds.

Caro: We found that full relaxation took about 5 seconds.

Lassen: We have made observations on the effect of venous stasis on muscle blood flow in man. Stasis is produced by changing the position of the leg from the horizontal to the leg-down position and blood flow is measured by recording the clearance of xenon-133 injected intramuscularly. In normal man the muscle blood flow decreases during venous stasis despite the unchanged arterio-venous pressure difference. On the other hand in patients with occlusive vascular disease of the leg and with a very low distal blood pressure the flow increases quite markedly in dependency. Apparently the vascular resistance of the hypotensive vascular bed is considerably reduced by the passive distension caused by the increased transmural pressure in dependency (Dahn, I. *et al.* [1967]. *Scand. J. clin. Lab. Invest.,* Suppl. 99, 160–165; H. Bossaert and A. Amery, personal communication, 1968).

Why does this distension not reduce vascular resistance in normal man? Since the normal response (moderate flow decrease) is seen not only at resting flow levels but also during maximal reactive hyperaemia we assume that nervous mechanisms are not directly involved and that autoregulatory constriction of the smooth muscle cells dominate.

In patients with a permanent low-pressure distal vascular bed due to severe occlusive vascular disease this constriction is evidently defective and here distension does occur. This vascular bed then behaves exactly like the pulmonary vascular bed, which is also a low-pressure system in which gravitational forces exert a prominent effect on the circulation.

Caro: Our studies were, as I noted, on normal subjects. However, Dr.

Lassen's finding of vascular dilatation in response to increase of transmural pressure, in patients with partial arterial obstruction, is very interesting.

I would like to add a rider to my comments on the apparent rates of constriction and relaxation of vessels. The latter rate seemed from our studies greater than the former (see also Johnson, P. C. [1968]. *Circulation Res.*, **22,** 199–212); but this could be accounted for by the operation of different control mechanisms in the two circumstances.

Note added by Dr. Caro in proof: It is of interest that A. J. Brady ([1968]. *Physiol. Rev.*, **48,** 570–600) reports effects of quick stretches or releases on cardiac muscle. In cardiac muscle these have to be applied during a twitch, since it cannot be tetanized. Stretches or quick releases applied after the first half of the rising phase of the twitch apparently tend to produce uncoupling, resulting in less peak tension development than when the muscle is fixed at the short length throughout the twitch. Brady suggests that a change in stress, applied at an appropriate time, results in bond fractures that tend not to be reformed.

VELOCITY DISTRIBUTION AND TRANSITION
IN THE ARTERIAL SYSTEM

D. L. SCHULTZ, D. S. TUNSTALL-PEDOE†, G. DE J. LEE†,
A. J. GUNNING‡ AND B. J. BELLHOUSE

*Department of Engineering Science, University of Oxford, † Cardiac Department,
Radcliffe Infirmary, Oxford, and ‡ Department of Surgery, Radcliffe Infirmary,
Oxford*

THE velocity with which blood is ejected from the left ventricle into the ascending aorta and its history as it passes into the first two major branches— the innominate and the brachiocephalic arteries in the dog, the carotid and innominate arteries in man—and thence to the descending aorta, have attracted many research workers. Although the volumetric rate in response to stimuli is probably more important in most physiological studies than the fluid velocity, techniques permitting direct velocity measurements are nevertheless of interest, particularly if the instrument used has a high frequency response. This is borne out by the literature on turbulence in blood flow and its relationship with the heart sounds (Rushmer, 1961), platelet deposition and red cell damage in prosthetic valves (Davila *et al.*, 1967).

Estimates of velocity can be obtained from volumetric flow studies if the diameter of the vessel is known, but much of the detail is lost. Spencer and Denison (1956) produced estimates of 112 cm./sec. in the upper thoracic aorta of dogs from electromagnetic flowmeter studies, and Prec and co-workers (1949) deduced a mean velocity of $21 \cdot 3$ to $87 \cdot 4$ cm./sec. in man. These values lead to the conclusion that the peak Reynolds number in dogs may reach 4,500 to 5,000 and in man could be as high as 12,000, a value well above that at which uniformly laminar flow would be expected, except in ideal fluid dynamic conditions certainly not encountered in the ventricle– valve–aorta geometry of man.

Two of the earlier attempts to measure blood velocity directly were those of von Deschwanden, Müller and Laszt (1956), who employed a Pitot tube, and Machella (1936), who used a hot-wire anemometer threaded transversely across the vessel to observe flow in the aorta and coronary arteries. We have used essentially the same technique as Machella, namely the measurement of dynamic heat transfer from a heat source in contact with blood and

172

small enough to be mounted in a fine hypodermic needle or catheter. Machella was apparently unaware of the frequency limitations of his device but in the event these were not great and it was possible to observe and estimate the major features of pulsatile blood flow. Later research workers have used cine-angiographic techniques (McDonald, 1952), ultrasonic flowmeters (Franklin et al., 1959) and flow-sensitive thermistors (Grahn, Paul and Wessell, 1968), and Ling and Atabek (1967) have reported preliminary results in dogs with thin metallic film anemometers. The transition from laminar to turbulent flow in pulsating flows has received attention from Combs and Gilbrech (1964), Cotton (1960), Yellin (1966), and Hale, McDonald and Womersley (1955), and while the vascular geometry is undoubtedly complex there has been insufficient direct evidence of the state of the flow at peak ejection velocity on which to base either a mathematical or a physical model.

The data presented in this paper are the preliminary results of an attempt to map the velocity distribution in the aorta and pulmonary artery of dogs and to obtain comparisons of the velocities in normal and diseased human aortas and pulmonary arteries.

EXPERIMENTAL TECHNIQUES

The thin-film anemometer we have used is an adaptation of a technique familiar to fluid dynamicists, in which the rate of transfer of heat from a small metallic element is determined electrically and is related to the fluid velocity by calibration. The more common type of anemometer has a hot wire as the heat source, as first described by King (1914). The advantages of a thin film as a heat source in haemodynamic studies lie mainly in the smooth surface presented to the bloodstream and in the small size, which enables the velocity-sensitive element to be built into catheters and hypodermic needles (Bellhouse et al., 1967).

The metallic surface film may be formed by vacuum evaporation, vacuum sputtering or the use of conducting paints. Vacuum sputtering is preferable to evaporation and is used for the commercial production of most thin-film anemometers (e.g. Disa Electronik, Denmark). The sputtering technique produces a dense uniform metallic film of controllable thickness to which lead wires can readily be soldered. The use of conducting paints demands little equipment and is probably most suited for making films on curved surfaces for inserting into catheters and hypodermic needles. Such a paint consists of a suspension of platinum and silver particles dispersed in an organic fluid of high viscosity to prevent settling (e.g. Hanovia Products

05-X). When this suspension is hand-painted on to glass, air-dried and baked in a furnace at 640° C for 30 minutes, it adheres firmly to the glass as a bright hard film about 1 μm. thick (Schultz, 1962; Vidal and Hilton, 1956). Up to seven coats are applied in order to obtain more stable calibration than can be achieved with single-coat films. The metallic film may be insulated electrically from the fluid in which it is immersed by a further series of coats of a mixture of oxides of titanium and silicon, as described by Vidal and Golian (1967).

In operation the film forms one arm of a self-balancing Wheatstone bridge (Fig. 1), and is normally maintained at approximately 5° C above blood

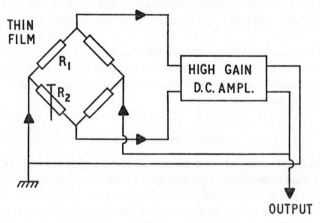

Fig. 1. Feedback bridge to achieve operation at constant resistance of thin-film probe.

temperature by setting R_2 at $1·01 \times R_1$, the temperature coefficient of the film material (05-X) being $0·002/°C$. Transfer of heat from the film to the blood cools the film, lowers its resistance and initiates an output signal from the bridge to the feedback power amplifier which restores the bridge to balance. Operation at constant temperature is essential if transient thermal waves in the substrate are to be avoided and high sensitivity is to be obtained at low operating temperatures. The frequency response of the whole system is limited by the gain and bandwidth of the feedback amplifier, since the thermal diffusion time in the film itself is of the order of 10^{-7} sec. (Schultz, 1962). A detailed analysis of the performance of such devices has been given by Bellhouse and Schultz (1967), who investigated their application to skin friction and velocity measurements in air and liquids.

Conduction of heat to the fluid from the heated film and from the substrate near it is governed by the equation:

$$Nu = A(Pr)^{1/3} (Re)^{1/2} + B(Pr)^{1/3} \tag{1}$$

where Nu = Nusselt number, $qL/k\Delta T$,

Re = Reynolds number, $UL\rho/\mu$, or UL/ν,

Pr = Prandtl number, $C\mu/k$,

A and B are constants.

Expressed in terms of the quantities measured:

$$\frac{V^2}{\Delta T} = C + D(U)^{1/2} \tag{2}$$

where V = film voltage,

ΔT = temperature difference between film and fluid,

U = fluid velocity,

C and D are constants, and it is assumed that the Prandtl number is constant.

The two dimensionless parameters which characterize the forced heat transfer, the Prandtl and Reynolds numbers, may be combined as

$$(C^{1/3} \rho^{1/3}/k^{1/3} \nu^{1/6}) (U^{1/2} L^{1/2})$$

and thus the major difference between whole blood and water, the kinematic viscosity, ν, is seen to have much less effect than the specific heat, density and thermal conductivity, which are not widely different in the two fluids. The physical properties of blood vary considerably with its temperature and composition, but if we assume that specific heat is $0 \cdot 87$ g. cal./°c (Mendlowitz, 1948), density is $1 \cdot 055$ g./cm.^{3} and thermal conductivity is $0 \cdot 00143$ $(1–0 \cdot 2\varphi)$, (where φ = haematocrit, Singh and Blackshear, 1967), that is, $0 \cdot 00129$ for whole blood, then the ratio of the physical properties of water to those of blood is $1 \cdot 039$ (assuming ν is $0 \cdot 038$ cm.^{2}/sec. for whole blood at 37°c). This difference of 4 per cent is likely to vary with shear rate, since the viscosity appears to be dependent on this, but it is not possible to allow for such variation in the dynamic calibration used. The exponent of U in equation (2) varies by approximately 5 per cent with probe geometry and in practice the exact value is determined by calibrating over a wide range of velocities in a towing tank in which the probe moves through a stationary fluid at a uniform speed.

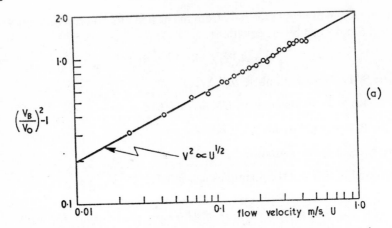

FIG. 2 (*a*). Calibration of thin film obtained in water in a towing tank, illustrating quadratic heat loss law. V_B: Bridge voltage at velocity U. V_0: Bridge voltage at zero velocity.

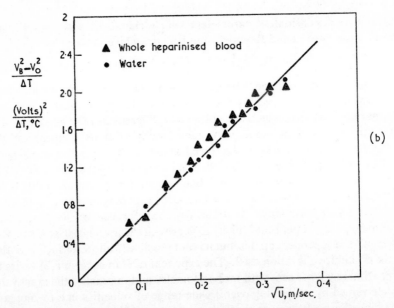

FIG. 2 (*b*). Calibration of thin film in water and whole, heparinized blood.

Such a calibration for a hypodermic mounted probe is shown in Fig. 2(*a*), where the exponent is seen to be 0·5. Fig. 2(*b*) compares calibrations obtained in water and whole heparinized blood.

A sketch of the thin film element before it is mounted in a hypodermic needle is shown in Fig. 2(*c*). The purpose of the two auxiliary films is discussed

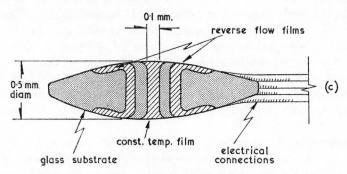

FIG. 2 (*c*). Construction of triple element thin-film probe for insertion in catheter or hypodermic needle.

later. The effect on the calibration of the distance of the heated element from the probe tip was studied by constructing a variable-geometry probe which was calibrated in water in a towing tank. For distances of 3·2, 5·7, 10·8 and 15·9 mm. from the tip the calibration followed equation (3), deduced from boundary layer considerations for steady flow:

$$\frac{i^2 R}{k\Delta T} = \frac{V_B^2}{Rk\Delta T} = A \Pr^{1/3} \operatorname{Re}^{1/2} \left(\frac{L}{x}\right)^{1/6} + B \tag{3}$$

where R, V = probe resistance and voltage,

L = probe length,

x = distance from tip of probe to sensitive element,

A and B are constants.

Since body temperature changes only slowly, the probe can be operated at a fixed ΔT. The voltage across the feedback bridge, V_B, is proportional to the film current, so the above equation reduces to equation (2).

Equation (2) will hold only if the parameter fx/U (where f is the frequency) is smaller than unity, otherwise time-dependent terms will affect the calibration. For $x = 0·5$ cm. and $U = 100$ cm./sec. the maximum frequency for which equation (3) will hold exactly is 200 Hz. Above this limit another calibration is required but this is not of great practical importance in blood flow. In an attempt to reduce the value of x, the heated elements were raised above the rest of the needle surface and faired in to make a smooth protuberance. This merely deflected the viscous boundary layer without improving the frequency range of equation (2). The probe was calibrated dynamically by oscillating it harmonically in a still bath of water. Frequencies of up to 10 Hz and peak-to-peak displacements from $0 \cdot 5$ to $2 \cdot 5$ cm. could be used, and in all cases the calibrations at peak velocity coincided with those obtained by towing. For a frequency f and peak-to-peak displacement $2A$, the peak velocity is $2\pi fA$ and $fx/U = x/\pi(2A)$, which is independent of frequency. For $x = 0 \cdot 5$ cm., the highest value of fx/U is obtained for the least value of $2A$, and $fx/U < 0 \cdot 32$. The frequency response of the film and its substrate alone have been examined in detail by Bellhouse and Schultz (1967) and Bellhouse and Rasmussen (1968).

The criterion $fx/U < 1$ was satisfied in the needle-mounted probes previously described. The tip of a 1 mm. needle is bent through a right-angle and the thin film is inserted in the centre of the short arm on the lower edge (Figs. 2(c) and 4). Since the distance of the films from either corner or tip of the

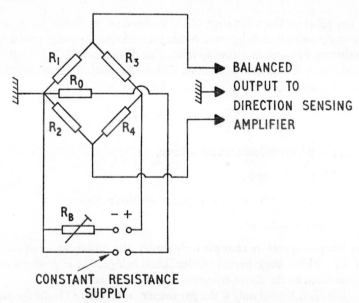

FIG. 3. Triple element thin-film bridge circuit for the detection of flow reversal. R_0: Film heated by constant resistance bridge (bridge not shown, see Fig. 1). R_1, R_2: Direction-sensitive films on same substrate as R_0, see Fig. 2 (c). R_3, R_4: Balancing arms of bridge.

needle was only about 3 mm. the responses of the probe to both forward and reverse flow were equal. Other advantages of this configuration were that the tip could be sharpened so that the needle could pierce blood vessels and the short arm could be brought into contact with the lower wall and the signal used to establish a zero flow baseline. When the film was inserted into a catheter the sensitivity to forward and reverse flow was not usually the same and allowance had to be made for this.

It is convenient to correct for the quadratic power law of the film response before the velocity signal is recorded; this may be done using a commercially available linearizing unit (Disa Elektronik), which allows the exponent of U to be altered in steps of $0 \cdot 1$ and includes amplifiers which permit the sensitivity of the probe to be set at a convenient value, say 50, 100, 150 cm./sec. per volt.

Since the probe essentially measures heat transfer rate it is insensitive to the direction of flow. The method adopted for indicating this important feature of arterial blood flow is shown in Fig. 3. In addition to the film R_0 operated at a constant temperature of 5°C above blood temperature, two further films, R_1 and R_2, one upstream and one downstream of R_0, are located in the arms of a Wheatstone bridge through which a low current, 5 mA, is passed. Such a low current has no effect on the operation of the central film but when fluid warmed by passage over the central film is swept by the flow over one or other of the two collateral films, an out-of-balance signal appears at the bridge terminal and the polarity of this signal indicates the direction of fluid flow. The frequency response of this system is of course limited to about 10 Hz by the transit time between the films and the thermal conductivity of the fluid and substrate, but it is adequate to detect the onset and termination of reverse flow. In practice one reversing film gives sufficient indication of flow reversal in laminar flow, but is less satisfactory in turbulent flow. Examples of the performance of this auxiliary film will be presented in context.

Since the performance of the thin film as a velocity sensor depends on maintaining a clean surface in contact with the fluid it is essential to avoid deposition of platelets. It has been found that the films may be operated at up to 15°C above blood temperature without deposition in heparinized dogs. However, in order to ensure complete freedom from surface contamination and cell damage we operate the film only 5°C above central blood temperature. At this temperature the film, and its associated electronics, still has very adequate sensitivity (50 cm./sec. per volt), and the leakage of current from the non-earthed end of the film to patient earth is less than 1 μA. This leakage current could be reduced still further by the application of an insulating coat as previously described, but our experience in both animals and man shows that the existing level is satisfactory. At such low overheat ratios it is necessary

180   D. L. SCHULTZ ET AL.

to check the blood temperature periodically so that a constant sensitivity is maintained throughout any prolonged series of measurements.

EXPERIMENTS IN DOGS

The purpose of the experiments in dogs was twofold: firstly to develop techniques for traversing the human aorta and pulmonary artery rapidly during surgery, in order to confirm by a more direct method the measurements of velocity obtained from diagnostic studies using catheter tip anemometers; secondly to use the dog to provide a fluid dynamic model of the human aorta to determine the velocity distribution at as many sites as possible so that the effects of vascular geometry and elastic properties could be studied in detail. A knowledge of the spatial velocity distribution properties is particularly important in interpreting data obtained from catheter studies in man with thin-film anemometers, since, being velocity-sensitive devices, they sample only the velocity over the catheter itself.

Method

Mongrel dogs weighing between 14 and 24 kg. were anaesthetized with Nembutal (pentobarbitone sodium). The dogs were ventilated through an endotracheal tube with room air, using a Palmer pump delivering an optimal tidal volume and having a maximum positive pressure of 15 cm. of water, regulated by a blow-off valve.

The femoral vein and femoral artery (in some cases) were catheterized. The aorta and pulmonary artery were approached by resection of the 4th left rib with the dog lying on its right side with a centre lift arching the body. The pericardium was then incised and the fat pad around the arch of the aorta and pulmonary artery were dissected away so that a perspex collar could be slipped around the relevant vessel (Fig. 4). This collar supported the needle velocity probe and enabled its location to be determined as it was traversed in steps across the vessel. A fine nylon catheter was inserted into the apex of the left ventricle and held in position with a purse string. This catheter was attached to a Statham P23Gb strain gauge transducer so that the left ventricular pressure could be monitored continuously.

The velocity probe was dipped in heparin and then inserted into the lumen of the aorta or pulmonary artery through a purse-string suture in the vessel wall. The probe had just previously been calibrated in a sinusoidal oscillatory vibrator and its sensitivity adjusted to a level such that the maximum anticipated velocity in the dog would not overload the recording system. After the probe was inserted into the vessel its resistance at central blood temperature

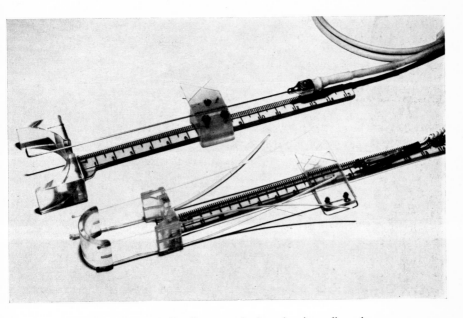

FIG. 4. Cuff and half-cuff supports for hypodermic needle probes.

[*To face page 180*

was measured. The overheat ratio was then set to be exactly 1·01, that used in the calibration procedure, and with the thin film held against the lower wall of the artery to produce a no-flow signal, the linearizer was set up to establish a zero flow baseline. There is generally no need to make large adjustments to the linearizer if care has been taken to establish the correct overheat ratio in both calibration and operation.

The probe was traversed by hand across the aorta or pulmonary artery and at each station between 20 and 40 cardiac ejection pulses were recorded on magnetic tape, together with signals from the left ventricular pressure

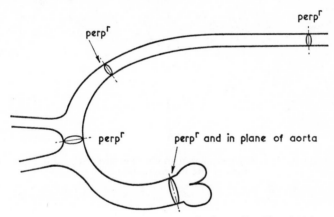

FIG. 5. Locations of aortic traverses in dogs. (See Figs. 6–12.)

transducer, femoral pressure where applicable, ECG, and ventilation. These signals were recorded on a tape recorder with a frequency response from d.c. to 1,250 Hz at 19·05 cm./sec. (7½ in./sec.). Subsequently the recorded velocity signal was replayed through an integrator to give the time-averaged velocity at each station of the traverse.

Velocity traverses have been made at the locations shown in Fig. 5, with minor variations in the relative dimensions, depending on the size of the dog. The effect of normalizing the average velocity in the ascending aortas, traversed perpendicular to the plane of the aorta, is shown in Fig. 6 for seven dogs. The profile of the average velocity is seen to be approximately flat with skewness towards the right lateral wall of the aortic arch. This skewness is not apparent on the profiles (Fig. 7) taken on a diameter in the plane of the aorta. Less data are available on this diameter of the aorta because, in general, the surgical preparation for a traverse in this direction precludes other measurements. The variation in velocity over the period of observation at each radial

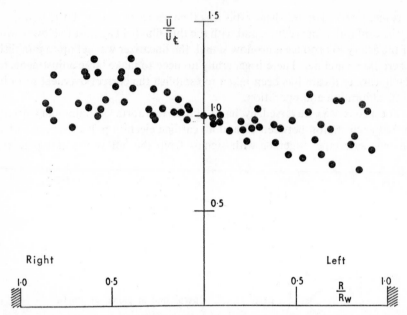

FIG. 6. Normalized velocity distribution on diameter perpendicular to plane of aorta in dogs. Results from seven dogs.

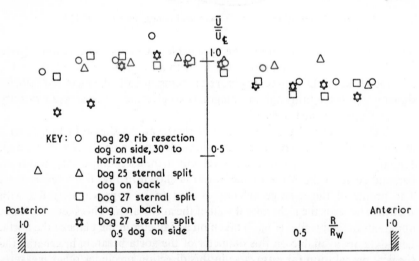

FIG. 7. Normalized velocity distribution on diameter in plane of aortic arch, showing effect of posture. Results from three dogs.

position was found to be small. Fig. 8 illustrates the systolic maximum and time-averaged velocities observed during approximately 20 beats per station (the time-averaged values are those in Fig. 7). A typical centre-line velocity is shown in Fig. 9 together with the ventricular pressure record. The velocity

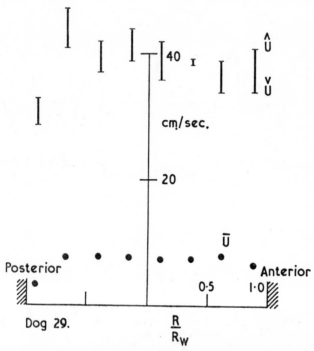

Fig. 8. Maximum and minimum systolic and time-averaged velocities in aorta of dog. Traverse in plane of aortic arch; dog on right side, rib resection.

profiles taken at the arch and in the descending aorta show no differences from those in the ascending aorta. It is difficult to obtain satisfactory traverses in the plane of the aorta at the mid-point of the arch with any normal technique of arterial exposure. Fig. 10 shows the velocity profile at the mid-point of the arch and 11 mm. distal to the subclavian artery and indicates that there is no significant fluid dynamic flow structure in the aortic arch. Steady viscous flow in a curved circular tube would normally induce secondary flow (two contra-rotating vortices) but there is as yet insufficient evidence that this occurs to any marked extent in the aortic arch, where the flow pattern is confused by two major branches.

7

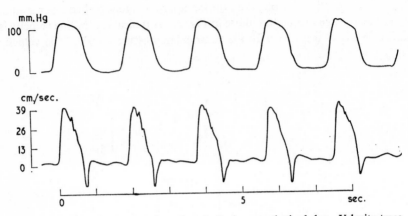

FIG. 9. Ventricular pressure and aortic velocity in anaesthetized dog. Velocity trace corrected for flow reversal.

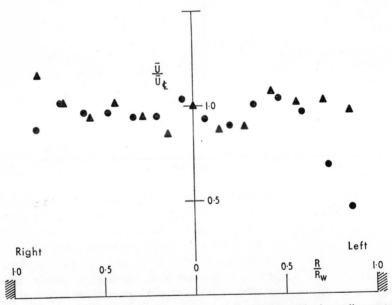

FIG. 10. Normalized velocity profile at mid-point of arch (●) and in descending aorta (▲) 11 mm. distal to subclavian artery in dog.

The essentially flat velocity profile in the ascending aorta finally must develop into a near-parabolic profile in the systemic arteries. In a circular pipe under conditions of steady flow the profile would be expected to become parabolic after an inlet length/diameter ratio of 0·058 Re for steady laminar flows. At a peak Reynolds number of 1,500 this ratio to a fully developed profile would be 87, or for the average Reynolds number of 465 for the same dog the ratio would be 27. Nevertheless the velocity profile in the thoracic aorta of a 25 kg. dog (Fig. 11) shows the development of such a profile with a

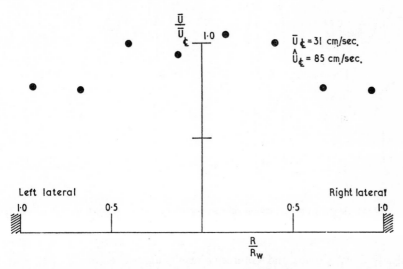

FIG. 11. Normalized velocity profile in thoracic aorta of dog. Diameter 0·7 cm. Variation of peak systolic velocity ± 7 per cent.

very high rate of shear at the wall. The probe at this location, in a narrow-bore tube, would produce a blockage of 18 per cent in the worst case (probe at far side of vessel) and the results should be taken only as an indication that transition to a parabolic profile is occurring within the arterial system. There is as yet little reported work on the development of velocity profiles in tapered tubes and although attempts have been made to allow for such branches as the intercostal by assuming a uniformly "leaky" wall in the model, no general conclusions are available for comparison.

It is clear from our records of pulsatile velocity that aortic flow is laminar and indeed, with peak Reynolds numbers not exceeding approximately 1,500 this would be expected. Coulter and Pappenheimer (1949) reported a transition Reynolds number of 1,760 in steady flow of whole blood in a vessel of 3·4 mm.

diameter (haematocrit 45 per cent). The effects of pulsatility on the transition phenomena have been studied by Combs and Gilbrech (1964) and Yellin (1966). Combs and Gilbrech did the most comprehensive set of experiments and found that the transition Reynolds number increased as the ratio of the unsteady to steady velocity ($u'/\bar{U}$) was increased until at values of $u'/\bar{U}$ of about 0·65 the trend was reversed and the transition phenomena again took place at a Reynolds number of 2,200, the value found for their apparatus in

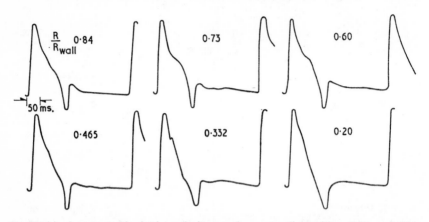

FIG. 12 (a). Average aortic ejection velocity waveforms at radial positions $R/R_W = 0·20$ to 0·84 in ascending aorta of dog. Average calculated from 10 beats.

steady flow. Combs and Gilbrech's results agreed reasonably well with a theoretical argument based on the non-linear generation and dissipation of turbulence, at least up to the values of $u'/\bar{U}$ at which the critical Reynolds number decreased. The ratio of u'/U in the dogs studied in the present series is approximately three and thus on the basis of Combs and Gilbrech's work it would be slightly *less* than the steady state value. This conclusion is, however, an extrapolation of their results and should not be regarded as indicative of the behaviour either (*a*) in non-sinusoidal flows or (*b*) in flows within the inlet length.

Pulsatile velocity profile

The flow of a viscous fluid through a circular pipe under the influence of a sinusoidal pressure difference has been studied theoretically and experimentally in some detail by Uchida (1956), Sexl (1930), Womersley (1957) and others. The parameter which characterizes the relationship between the oscillatory pressure gradient, $\partial p/\partial x = -\rho k \cos\omega t$, and the resulting flow is $\alpha = R\sqrt{\omega/\nu}$. At very low values of α the velocity $u(r,t)$ can be shown to be

$$u(r,t) = \frac{k}{4\nu}(R^2 - r^2)\cos\omega t$$

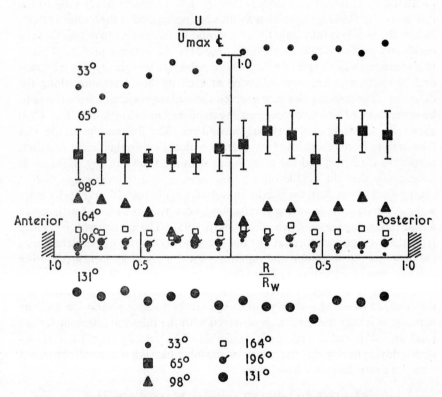

FIG. 12 (b). Fluctuating velocity profile in ascending aorta of dog deduced from Fig. 12 (a). 1 cardiac cycle = 360°. Maximum divergence from average occurs during deceleration phase at 65°. Maximum and minimum values observed during 10 cycles shown.

That is, the flow and pressure gradient are in phase and the velocity distribution is a parabolic function of the radius of the vessel. At very large values of α the velocity $u(r,t)$ tends to

$$u(r,t) = \frac{k}{\omega}\left\{\sin\omega t - \sqrt{\frac{R}{r}}\exp\left(-\sqrt{\frac{\omega}{2\nu}}\,\overline{R-r}\right)\sin\left[\omega t - \sqrt{\frac{\omega}{2\nu}}\,\overline{R-r}\right]\right\}$$

The velocity is now in quadrature with the pressure gradient. In man the fundamental frequency in the system can range between 0.9 and 1.2 Hz and α can thus have values between 13 and 17 (McDonald, 1952). Uchida (1956) has shown that an α of five can be regarded as an "intermediate" frequency parameter and presents results for the velocity distribution which have been tabulated by Gilbrech and Combs (1963). These remarks apply only to the flow after the inlet length, which may thus be approached in the femoral artery. Before the profile is fully established it would be reasonable to expect that the oscillatory profile would at all times resemble the average profile. To test this assumption the aorta of a dog whose pulse rate was steady was traversed and 20 ejection pulses were recorded at each of the 14 stations along the diameter. The steady pulse rate enabled the measured ejection waveforms to be superimposed and an average pulse established at each station. Fig. 12(a) shows six representative averaged waveforms. The fluctuating profile was then derived from this series of waveforms, which show no significant variation across the diameter, and the resulting profiles are shown in Fig. 12(b). It is noteworthy that the profile during flow reversal is a mirror image of that during systolic ejection, the maximum velocity again being found at the inner wall. A similar profile during reverse flow, occurring in a patient with severe aortic incompetence, is discussed later (p. 195). The maximum divergence from the average waveform at any one location occurs during deceleration of the flow and the maximum and minimum systolic velocities measured during this experiment are shown in Fig. 12(b).

When the aortic flow is determined with an electromagnetic flowmeter the deceleration phase of systole exhibits less stroke to stroke variation and the conclusion is that the variations observed with the thin-film anemometer are local and their radial average is negligible. The velocity transducer shows slight eddying during the latter phase of diastole which is not normally observed with the electromagnetic flowmeter.

CATHETER STUDIES AND ARTERIAL TRAVERSES IN MAN

The patients studied all required left side catheterization of the heart for diagnostic purposes. Access to the exposed aorta or pulmonary artery for the traverse studies presented here was obtained during surgery for the replacement of aortic or mitral valves or pulmonary valvotomy (one case).

The results of four studies are presented which include instances of:

(1) Mitral incompetence: aortic and pulmonary artery traverse.
(2) Pulmonary stenosis: pulmonary artery traverse.
(3) Aortic incompetence: aortic traverse.
(4) Aortic stenosis: aortic traverse.

During catheterization, access to the aorta was obtained by exposure of the brachial artery in the right antecubital fossa and a formal arteriotomy was performed. Through this a No. 7 or No. 8 velocity catheter was introduced into the ascending aorta under fluoroscopic control. Aortic pressure was recorded through the catheter whose orifice opened at its tip. The velocity sensor was located 5 mm. proximal to the catheter tip. All patients were conscious and unpremedicated except that some of the more nervous were given methyl pentynol (Oblivon), 750 mg.–1,000 mg. All patients were given 5,000 i.u. heparin at the time the catheter was inserted.

The catheter could be manoeuvred up towards the aortic valve or down-stream around the arch of the aorta. Readings were also taken within the left ventricle. Cineradiograms were taken at each of the catheter sites in order to locate the catheter tip with reference to the aortic valve cusps. In cases of severe aortic stenosis the jet issuing from the constriction deflected the tip of the catheter out of the jet but in some studies it was possible to keep the catheter in the jet by protruding only a short unsupported length of the catheter. As with the needle-mounted probes, the leakage current from the non-earthed end of the thin film to patient earth was kept low by restricting the total bridge voltage to 1·5 volts and the probe temperature to 42° C. The resistance of the film at central body temperature was determined in catheter studies with the film in the subclavian artery, since it was found that the peripheral artery temperature was lower than that in a central artery such as the aorta. When the linearizer had been correctly set up during calibration and the correct overheat ratio obtained it was not necessary to occlude an artery to obtain a zero flow signal.

Two particular catheter studies merit presentation for comparison with data obtained from the same patients during valve surgery. The relatively flat velocity profile in the ascending aorta was used to determine the average aortic velocity and the cine-angiogram was used to determine aortic diameter and catheter tip location.

A patient with the clinical signs of mitral incompetence, namely atrial fibrillation, enlarged left ventricle, a harsh pansystolic murmur heard best at the cardiac apex, and with a giant left atrium on X-ray, gave a typical aortic velocity waveform (Fig. 13(a)) during cardiac catheterization. The flow was laminar and a clear indication of flow reversal was obtained, shown in the lower trace. The peak systolic velocity observed was 68 cm./sec., and with an aortic diameter of 2·4 cm. measured during subsequent surgery the Reynolds number was 4,300. Since the patient was fibrillating it was not possible to obtain an average ejection pulse, although the waveform of the pulses tended to be similar. When the same patient was studied during surgery for mitral

valve replacement a detailed traverse of the aorta 4 cm. above the aortic valve
was possible. With a similar technique to that used in dogs a traverse was
made from anterior to posterior wall. A perspex half-cuff (Fig. 4) guided
and located the tip of the needle, which was again inserted through a purse

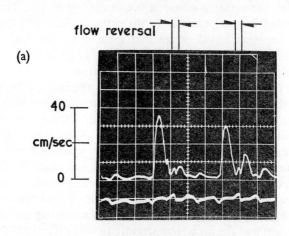

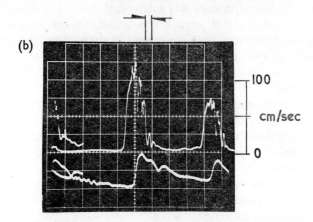

FIG. 13 (*a*). *Upper trace:* Aortic velocity recorded with
catheter tip probe. Male aged 42 years. Mitral incompetence, atrial fibrillation and heart failure. Note laminar
flow. Re = 4,300 for maximum observed velocity of 68
cm./sec. *Lower trace:* Signal from flow reversal detection
system.

(*b*) *Upper trace:* Aortic velocity in same patient recorded
1 month after (*a*) during an aortic traverse preceding valve
replacement. Turbulence at peak systole, Re = 7,800,
U = 130 cm./sec. *Lower trace:* Femoral pressure.

string. During the month between cardiac catheterization and surgery the patient had been under medical treatment with bed rest, digitalis and oral diuretics. The aortic velocity had increased to a peak of 130 cm./sec., Reynolds number 7,800, and there was evidence of transition to turbulence at peak systolic ejection velocities of 70 cm./sec. and above, Reynolds number 4,400 (Fig. 13(b)). It would be premature to take these figures as other than a guide,

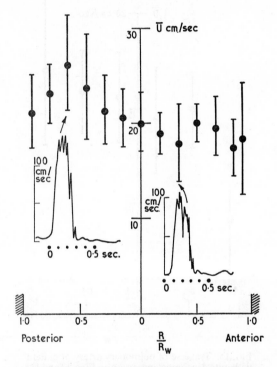

Fig. 14. Aortic traverse in adult male with mitral incompetence showing time-averaged velocity at each radial station ±1 standard deviation. Turbulence at peak systole across aorta. Maximum velocity 130 cm./sec., Re = 7,800.

especially as the patient had rheumatic heart disease which may have slightly damaged the aortic valve as well as destroying the mitral valve, but it is still significant that a Reynolds number of 4,300 can be accompanied by strictly laminar flow. The measured velocity profile, pre-operatively, is shown in Fig. 14. It displays the same general features as those reported in the earlier work on dogs. There is a region of higher average velocity at the inner radius

7*

of curvature of the aorta. Although atrial fibrillation affected the reproducibility of the ejection pulses, as seen by the large standard deviation, the trend is obvious. During the traverse peak systolic velocity varied between 130 cm./sec. and 50 cm./sec. During the operation but before replacement of the patient's mitral valve, a traverse was made of the pulmonary artery, diameter

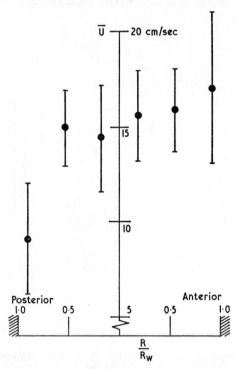

FIG. 15. Traverse of pulmonary artery of patient
with mitral incompetence; see also Figs. 13 and 14.
± 1 standard deviation.

35 mm., just distal to the pulmonary valve. The velocity profile (Fig. 15) was not as uniform as in the aorta and the average velocities are lower, 17–22 cm./sec. compared with 18–26 cm./sec. in the aorta. The pulmonary artery is more sharply curved at the point of measurement and this feature, together with its shortness before it branches into the right and left main pulmonary arteries, may be responsible for enhancing this asymmetry, coupled with the fact that the pulmonary artery in the open-chested state is easily deformed and collapsible when ventricular diastole and valve closure takes place. At this

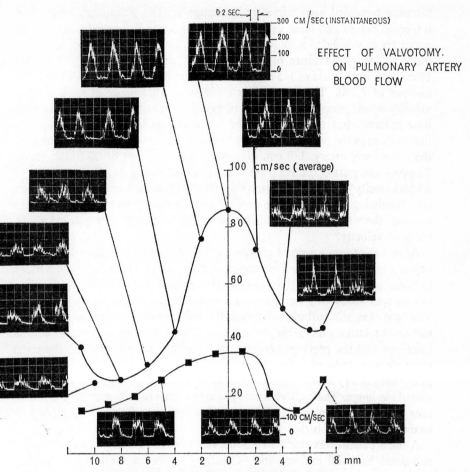

FIG. 16. Pre- and post-operative pulmonary artery traverses in patient with congenital pulmonary stenosis.

time the pulmonary artery wall might easily touch the thin film on the needle and momentarily prevent blood flowing past it when it was close to the wall.

The second study was made on a boy aged seven with congenital pulmonary stenosis. This child had an enlarged right ventricle and a loud pulmonary ejection systolic murmur with an absent pulmonary component to the second sound. On X-ray he had an enlarged right ventricle, ischaemic lungs and a small aorta. The pressure gradient across his pulmonary valve at operation was 53 mm. Hg before valvotomy and 13 mm. Hg after valvotomy (aortic pressure remained approximately unchanged). The pulmonary artery was traversed before and after valvotomy and the aorta before valvotomy. The aortic traverse yielded a uniform velocity profile with peak velocities at the inner radius of curvature of 70 cm./sec., a centre-line average velocity of 10 cm./sec. in an aorta of 1·5 cm. diameter, corresponding to a peak Reynolds number of 2,750. There was clear evidence of turbulence at peak systolic velocity which persisted to the end of systole and very little disturbance after flow reversal, but the contiguity of the two vessels could cause pressure fluctuations in the pulmonary artery to affect the aortic flow. The traverse of the pulmonary artery, 1·8 cm. diameter, was made just distal to the valve. The pre- and post-operative traverses are shown in Fig. 16. The presence of a high velocity jet with a maximum velocity of 275 cm./sec. and highly turbulent flow persisting throughout the cardiac cycle is clearly seen. As with aortic stenosis, the waveform rises slowly and is approximately symmetrical about the peak velocity.

After valvotomy a second profile was taken to ascertain the effect on the velocity of the procedure. This appeared (Fig. 16) to have resulted in a more uniform profile without the pre-operative central jet, although the cardiac output was necessarily decreased as a result of the length of the operation. The flow was still turbulent because the valve cusps, though resected, still remained relatively inflexible at the roots. The valve-open area was of course increased and the pressure gradient decreased so that the load on the right ventricle was reduced. The presence of turbulence in the post-operative pulmonary artery should have little effect on the fluid dynamics of the arterial side of the lungs. The highly elastic system branches rapidly and the increasing area at each junction would lead to a reduction in the Reynolds number and to the dissipation of turbulence.

A third patient was studied who had severe aortic incompetence following sub-acute bacterial endocarditis. Clinically he had a markedly collapsing pulse, a blood pressure of 155/50, a large left ventricle, and a long aortic early diastolic murmur, all suggesting aortic incompetence. Additionally there was an aortic ejection systolic murmur and absent aortic closure sound, suggesting valve damage. At catheterization severe aortic incompetence was confirmed with a left ventricle pressure of 152/39 (femoral artery pressure 156/50) and an aortogram demonstrated torrential incompetence. As could be deduced from the pressure measurements there was no significant aortic stenosis. Velocity measurements during catheterization showed that there were two regimes of flow—turbulence in the ejection phase followed by laminar regurgitation (Fig. 18). The maximum velocity during the forward ejection phase was approximately 88 cm./sec. and the Reynolds number was 7,350 (based on an

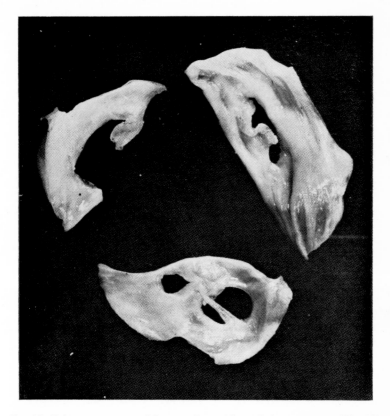

FIG. 17. Valve cusps removed from patient with aortic incompetence (Fig. 18).

aortic diameter of 3·1 cm. determined during subsequent surgery), high enough to cause turbulence even without the additional disturbance introduced by the defective valve (Fig. 17).

During surgery the aorta was traversed and the average velocity profile for both forward and reverse flow was determined (Fig. 18). The velocity profile in forward flow shows some degree of peaking in the centre, perhaps caused by restriction of the calcified valve cusps. The reverse flow profile was relatively

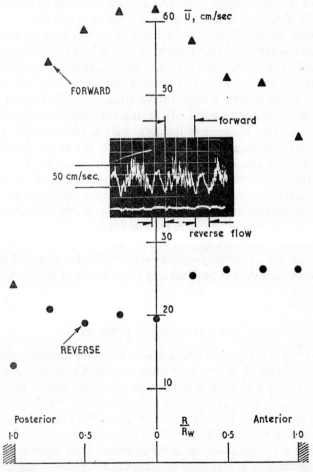

FIG. 18. Pre-operative traverse in patient with aortic incompetence. Profiles of forward and reverse flow shown separately. *Inset:* Catheter probe signal showing turbulent flow through perforated valve cusps followed by laminar regurgitation.

flatter, but both profiles gave similar results to those from previous catheter studies. The maximum instantaneous forward velocity at the centre line was 90 cm./sec., in close agreement with the catheter study; the maximum reverse flow velocity was 45 cm./sec., in reasonable agreement with the 50 cm./sec. derived from the catheter data.

From the forward and reverse flow profiles it was possible to estimate the ratio of volumetric ejection to regurgitation. The average forward velocity was found to be 55 cm./sec., the average reverse velocity 22 cm./sec. Using the ratio of forward systolic to reverse diastolic intervals of 0·765, the volumetric ratio of ejection to regurgitation was found to be 1·90.

The fourth patient illustrates the fourth common type of valve disease. The patient has calcific aortic stenosis, as shown by a slow-rising but regular pulse, blood pressure of 160/85, a large left ventricle, a single second heart sound, a third heart sound and an ejection systolic murmur radiating to the neck. The X-ray showed a large left ventricle, a calcified aortic valve and dilatation of the ascending aorta. An aortogram showed no significant aortic incompetence. Two traverses of the aorta were in fact made during surgery for aortic valve replacement, 35 mm. distal to the valve, the first on the posterior–anterior axis and the second at an angle of about 45° to this. On the first traverse there was little evidence of the expected jet. A second traverse showed markedly increasing turbulence towards the right anterior wall (Fig. 19). By manipulation of the probe it was possible to locate the jet and peak velocities of 220 cm./sec. were recorded in it.

The variation in the peak systolic velocity at each radial location was large, up to ± 35 per cent, especially near the vessel walls, but it tended to diminish as the jet approached. The peak velocity in the centre of the jet showed much less variation.

CONCLUSIONS AND SUMMARY

It is too early to draw any firm conclusions about the transition phenomenon in the aorta. Certainly a very wide range of velocities in anaesthetized dogs can be measured, with peak systolic values ranging from 25 to 75 cm./sec., isoprenaline being used at the latter value to restore the cardiac output to something approaching its normal resting value. The range of peak Reynolds numbers is thus between 790 and 2,370 (assuming $v = 3·8 \times 10^{-2}$ cm.^{2}/sec. and diameter $= 1·2$ cm.) and flow in the latter case is turbulent at peak systole.

The measurements in man have been confined to patients requiring cardiac catheterization and surgery because of valvular disease and once again a wide range of velocities has been measured, between about 70 and 440 cm./sec.,

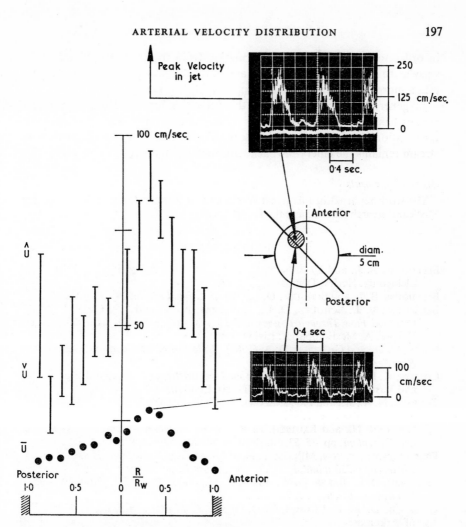

FIG. 19. Pre-operative aortic traverse in patient with aortic stenosis. Time-averaged velocities and maximum and minimum systolic instantaneous velocities shown. Aortic diameter =
5 cm.

the former laminar at a Reynolds number of 4,400 and the latter turbulent
throughout the cardiac cycle, because of severe stenosis.

It is possible to be more definite about the velocity profile. It appears that
the velocity profile in the ascending aorta, at the arch and in the first part of
the descending aorta is reasonably flat and this profile is maintained throughout
the cardiac cycle. There is some skewness in the velocity profile on the lateral
axis. Care must be taken to cause the minimum disturbance to the vasculature

in order to obtain consistent information from traverses of exposed blood vessels. In the lower thoracic aorta and in the femoral artery there is evidence that a more developed profile becomes established in dogs and man.

In general the information on the velocities measured during catheter studies has been well supported by subsequent traverses during surgery but the positioning of the catheter in a large blood vessel carrying a high velocity stream remains the chief drawback with such techniques.

Acknowledgements

The work reported in this paper forms part of a programme supported by the Medical Research Council and the Royal Society.

REFERENCES

BELLHOUSE, B. J., and RASMUSSEN, C. G. (1968). *Disa Information*, 6, 3–10. Disa Elektronik, Herlev, Denmark.

BELLHOUSE, B. J., and SCHULTZ, D. L. (1967). *J. Fluid Mech.*, 29, 289–295.

BELLHOUSE, B. J., SCHULTZ, D. L., KARATZAS, N. B., and LEE, G. DE J. (1967). In *Blood Flow Through Organs and Tissues*, pp. 43–54, ed. Bain, W. H., and Harpur, A. M. Edinburgh: Livingstone.

COMBS, G. D., and GILBRECH, D. A. (1964). *Univ. Arkansas Engng exp. Station Res. Rep. Ser.*, 4.

COTTON, K. L. (1960). The Instantaneous Measurement of Velocity of Blood Flow and Vascular Impedance. Ph.D. Thesis, London.

COULTER, N. A., Jr., and PAPPENHEIMER, J. R. (1949). *Am. J. Physiol.*, 159, 401–408.

DAVILA, J. C., PALMER, T. E., SETHI, R. S., DeLAURENTIS, D. A., ENRIQUEZ, F., RINCORN, N., and LAUTSCH, E. V. (1967). In *Heart Substitutes, Mechanical and Transplant*, pp. 25–53, ed. Brest, A. N. Springfield, Ill.: Thomas.

DESCHWANDEN, P. VON, MÜLLER, A., and LASZT, L. (1956). *Beitr. Haemodynamik. Abstr. comm. 20th int. physiol. Congr., Brussels*, pp. 930–931.

FRANKLIN, D. L., BAKER, D. W., ELLIS, R. M., and RUSHMER, R. F. (1959). *I.R.E. Trans. med. Electron.*, 6, 204–206.

GILBRECH, D. A., and COMBS, G. D. (1963). *Fluid Mech. Rep.* no. 1. University of Arkansas.

GRAHN, A. R., PAUL, M. H., and WESSEL, H. V. (1968). *J. appl. Physiol.*, 24, 236–246.

HALE, J. F., McDONALD, D. A., and WOMERSLEY, J. R. (1955). *J. Physiol., Lond.*, 128, 629–640.

KING, L. V. (1914). *Phil. Trans. R. Soc. Ser. A*, 214, 373–432.

LING, S. C., and ATABEK, H. B. (1967). In *Proc. 19th Ann. Conf. Engng in Med. and Biol.* New York: Institute of Electrical and Electronic Engineers.

McDONALD, D. A. (1952). *J. Physiol., Lond.*, 118, 328–339.

MACHELLA, T. E. (1936). *Am. J. Physiol.*, 115, 632–644.

MENDLOWITZ, M. (1948). *Science*, 107, 97.

PREC, O., KATZ, L. N., SENNETT, L., ROSEMAN, L., FISHMAN, A. P., and HWANG, W. (1949). *Am. J. Physiol.*, 159, 483–491.

RUSHMER, R. F. (1961). *Cardiovascular Dynamics*, 2nd edn. Philadelphia: Saunders.

SCHULTZ, D. L. (1962). In *Symposium on Some Developments in Techniques for Temperature Measurement*, paper 7. London: Institute of Mechanical Engineers.

SEXL, T. (1930). *Z. Phys.*, **61**, 349.

SINGH, A., and BLACKSHEAR, P. L. (1967). In *VIIth int. Conf. on Med. and Biol. Engng, Stockholm*, p. 400, ed. Jacobsen, B. Stockholm: Royal Academy of Engineering Sciences.

SPENCER, M. P., and DENISON, A. B. (1956). *Circulation Res.*, **4**, 476–484.

UCHIDA, S. (1956). *Z. angew. Math. Phys.*, **7**, 404–422.

VIDAL, R. J., and GOLIAN, T. C. (1967). *A.I.A. Aerospace*, **5**, no. 9, 1579–1588.

VIDAL, R. J., and HILTON, J. H. (1956). *Cornell Aero. Lab. Rep.* No. IM-1062-A-1.

WOMERSLEY, J. R. (1957). *Wright Air Dev. Centre Tech. Rep.* WADC-TR56-614.

YELLIN, E. L. (1966). *Circulation Res.*, **19**, 791–804.

DISCUSSION

Burton: Your probe is obviously most sensitive to the layer immediately touching it, but it must have some sensitivity to the velocity of layers further out. Do you know over what distance it averages?

Schultz: There is a viscous boundary layer on the surface of the probe and in addition a thermal boundary layer caused by the heat produced electrically in the film. Since we measure heat transfer, the probe is sensitive to the thermal boundary layer thickness. We operate these devices at 5° c above central blood temperature in order to avoid deposition of platelets as well as for safety reasons, and the thermal boundary layer thickness is then of the order of 0·1 mm. If the probe were very close to the wall conduction would increase a little, but we don't intend to make measurements closer than a millimetre.

West: How accurately can you measure the position of the probe? You are dealing with extremely small distances.

Schultz: We can position it to within a millimetre and can reproduce data to a millimetre. I believe that Ling and Atabek used something more complicated but I am suspicious of any mounting which cannot move with the vessel; that is why we make our devices and their mountings so light.

Caro: As you know, we are also working on a hot-film probe to measure blood velocity, and I wonder how you manage to keep the flow attached to the film during flow reversal? Can you be sure there is no separation in the region of the film, particularly when you are studying a patient with aortic regurgitation and have rather high velocities during the reverse flow phase?

Schultz: The design of the shape of the leading edge of the probe is important in this respect, in order to keep flow attached all the way along. In the direction of reverse flow we have a large radius of curvature so that there are no strong pressure gradients which would cause separation during this flow regime.

Philip: The transition to turbulence in the dog at a Reynolds number of 2,370 seems surprising, in view of the fact that you have no simple geometrical situation and no steady situation in the aorta.

Schultz: The nature of the ventricular wall and the outflow track may explain this result. There is no shear at the ventricular wall because it is collapsing; so it is really the best situation possible for producing high velocity flow. Also the ventricular walls are smooth, apart from the area of the mitral valve which is uneven, and I have been trying to relate these velocity gradients to the location of the mitral valve. We have made casts to find out where the mitral valve was in relation to our velocity peaks, and the answers as yet are rather unclear.

Lassen: What is your evidence for turbulence? Do you study the angiographic picture?

Schultz: We take simultaneous cine-angiograms during the catheterization solely to locate the tip of the probe. Certainly in torrential aortic incompetence you can see the turbulent flow on the angiogram but the frequency response of the sensing element is more than adequate to detect turbulence.

Stuart: I wonder whether the time-interval that you have when the velocity is near its maximum is enough for turbulence to develop?

Schultz: In one study on a dog in which turbulence was produced by giving isoprenaline we found that transition to turbulence occurred very rapidly at $Re = 2,300$, but we have as yet insufficient evidence to be sure there is no incubation period.

Saffman: In steady situations with straight tubes at these transition Reynolds numbers, turbulence is often intermittent. One finds alternating regions of laminar and turbulent motion, the regions being separated by a very sharp interface. Are there any signs of that?

Schultz: We have some evidence of a disturbance during the deceleration phase, but I am not sure whether it is just diffusion or true turbulence. The work of E. L. Yellin ([1966]. *Circulation Res.*, **19**, 791–804) and of G. D. Combs and D. A. Gilbrech ([1964]. *Univ. Arkansas Engng exp. Station Res. Rep. Ser.*, **4**) shows clearly this neutral stability; that is, if a disturbance is created, it neither grows nor decreases. We need to work in a glass system at this point, where we can observe more directly, and then try to simulate the situation in animals. There may well be bursts of turbulence in the descending aorta which are propagating downstream.

Brecher: This is very interesting work, Dr. Schultz, and I must congratulate you on it. When we developed the bristle flowmeter we ran across a phenomenon of turbulence which was beautifully recorded with that high frequency device (Brecher, G. A. [1959]. *I.R.E. Trans. med. Electron.*, **6**, 294). Turbulence was often observed when peak flow velocities were reached in arteries during ventricular ejection. At a critical velocity the onset of turbulence from non-turbulent flow took 2 or 3 msec. Once the flow had become turbulent it remained so, even as the flow rate declined below the level of the critical velocity at which the onset of the turbulence had occurred. The records depicting this phenomenon were never published because this was only a casual observation. An investigation of the cross-section of velocities in a vessel, as you can now make, should produce very interesting results.

Taylor: This is certainly most fascinating work. Would you say more about the entrance lengths? The entrance length for pulsatile flow is considerably less than that for established steady flow. What is the entrance length for pulsatile turbulent flow? Since you are starting with a flat velocity profile it might be very short.

Schultz: For steady laminar flow the entry length/diameter ratio is $0 \cdot 058$ Re. If we take the peak Reynolds number for a dog as approximately 2,500, then the entry length is about 180 cm.

Lighthill: There is surely a difference between the expected critical Reynolds numbers in the entry length region and the Poiseuille flow region, and generally the former would be higher. Putting it another way, you have to base the Reynolds number on the thickness of the boundary layer. So the difficulty is to explain the case of the dog in which transition took place at 2,370, as Dr. Philip said. Presumably, although you will ordinarily have a very nice uniform entry flow, there will, as you say, be conditions like aortic incompetence where it is not smooth; are you sure that your dog was not in some trouble of that kind?

Schultz: You may be right! I take that Reynolds number of 2,370 as indicative of a lower limit only. I do not regard it as significant until we have repeated the work in a rate-controlled dog and kept its pericardium intact.

Burton: How likely is it that at high flows you have an "Aeolian harp" phenomenon? The needle itself may be producing eddies.

Schultz: Particularly in cases of stenosis where the jet velocity is very high you can certainly feel the needle vibrating, but it is to some extent damped by the arterial wall and I would anticipate very little disturbance from this source.

Mead: Do you find disturbances downstream from the device which would be washed back by flow reversal? This would be easy to test *in vitro*.

Schultz: The probes are calibrated by oscillating them in a water bath and any remaining disturbance should be seen, but it is not.

Lighthill: You have presumably demonstrated your devices on known flow—ordinary Poiseuille flow—and shown that it does pick up, even quite near the wall?

Schultz: Yes.

Caro: Do you detect any peculiar flow patterns, for example separation of flow from the walls near branches?

Schultz: We compared velocities in the aortic arch with those in branches, expecting phase lags and secondary flow, but we have found no evidence of major secondary flows. The leading edges of the velocity waveform in the ascending aorta and in the carotid artery are coincident.

Caro: Does this mean that the arterial system is so well designed that it prevents flow separation occurring in the region of branches?

Schultz: Yes, at least at these early branches. However, further down, at the renal artery branching, there are divisions which go backwards. At these branchings it may well be a different story.

Lighthill: I would have expected the first sign of secondary flow to be a reduced velocity on the inside wall. The main effect of a secondary flow would be at the boundary layer, and so you would get a boundary layer accumulating on the inner wall. The main centrifugal force on the interior region would be entirely balanced by the pressure gradient, and that pressure gradient would be forcing fluid in the boundary layer back to the inside bend. You might therefore expect the main effect to be an accumulation of boundary layer fluid in the inside bend, and therefore fluid with a lower velocity, but you do not seem to see this.

Schultz: We have not observed this, but we have done only one dog.

Burton: A study of a young patient with a patent ductus arteriosus would be most interesting. You might pick up some unusual patterns in that situation.

Schultz: We have seen dogs with patent ductuses but we have not yet studied the problem.

SECTION III
MASS TRANSPORT IN THE LUNG

THE DISTRIBUTION OF GAS FLOW IN LUNGS

J. MEAD

*Department of Physiology, Harvard University School of Public Health,
Boston, Massachusetts*

MY purpose is to discuss what governs bulk flow of gas in lungs. Most of what is known has been discovered by physician-physiologists, who were not to be put off by its complexity. They found a ready-made framework for their analysis in electrical circuit theory. If one relates volumes of gas displaced into and out of the lungs by way of the airways to simultaneous variations in transpulmonary pressure, as measured for example between the mouth and oesophagus, one finds that for small tidal volumes—say 500 ml. or less—and ordinary variations in flow—say ± 2 l./sec.—the relationship between the pressure and volume events can be approximately described with an equation of motion identical in form to that for an electrical circuit made up of a capacitor, resistor and inductor in series.

Let me stress that this correspondence is not simply wishful thinking inflicted on the respiratory system. It is an experimental result, and one with remarkable significance. The air entering the lung by a common path, the trachea, is distributed via a branched system of airways to some millions of air spaces embedded in a tissue mesh. Nevertheless, the lung behaves mechanically as if it consisted of a single flow-resistance in series with a single volume-elastic element.

Electrical circuit theory tells us that the relationship between a sinusoidal voltage and current at the terminals of any electrical circuit composed solely of passive elements—that is, capacitors, resistors and inductors—no matter what their arrangement, can always be perfectly simulated with a circuit composed of a single capacitor, single resistor and single inductor arranged in series. In general, however, the values of these equivalent elements will change as the frequency of the applied sinusoidal voltage is changed. The important point about the lung is that over a range of frequencies from nearly zero to the highest attainable, the equivalent compliance, resistance and inertia change little, if at all. How can this be?

For an electrical network to have the same equivalent elements at all frequencies, the current in all branches of the network must bear a fixed relationship to that passing through the circuit terminals. For this to be so the relative impedance of the branches must remain constant. For the lungs, the observation that the equivalent compliance, resistance and inertia are constant indicates that the relative mechanical impedance to volume change of all the myriad separate pathways for gas flow and volume change within lungs remains the same for both slow and rapid events.

At this point it is helpful to introduce the concept of time constants. The mechanical inertia of the lungs is so small that at frequencies up to about 2 cycles per second it contributes negligibly to transpulmonary pressure. If we limit further considerations to frequencies less than 2 cycles per second we can ignore it. Our equivalent circuit is now simply a resistor and capacitor in series. A circuit made up of a fixed capacitor and resistor in series responds to a step change in voltage with a change of charge which is exponential in time. Thus,

$$\Delta q = e^{-\frac{1}{RC}t}$$

where RC, the product of the resistance and capacitance, is the time constant of the circuit.

It is easy to show that, provided the time constants of all of the branches of a circuit are the same, the relative impedance of all the branches will be the same at all frequencies. Such a network would have the same equivalent compliance and resistance at all frequencies.

The possibility that the lung is constructed with the flow resistance of airways matched to the compliance of air spaces so as to yield equal time constants throughout is an attractive one. Indeed the abundance of smooth muscle in airway walls, together with the presence of stretch receptors sensitive to distension, suggests the further attractive possibility that this matching might be controlled by way of appropriate changes in the flow resistance of the airways. But recently direct measurements of airway resistance at different levels of the branching system have largely obliterated this promising picture. In brief, for most of the lung, the frequency-independent behaviour indicates not equality of time constants, but simply shortness of time constants. For most of the lung, the time constants are so short that the air spaces never have time, at least at physiological breathing frequencies, to depart appreciably from their static configuration. They change volume dynamically with very nearly the same pattern of volume change that would be obtained for a series of static volume steps.

In other words, the resistance to gas flow offered by the airways has only a small influence on the distribution of gas flow in normal lungs. Bulk flow of gas within lungs is governed almost entirely by the elastic distensibility of the air spaces and the forces distending them.

That this is so is readily appreciated when the nature of the mechanical impedance to volume change is considered. The magnitude of the mechanical impedance, $|Z|$, is expressed by the ratio of the amplitude of applied pressure to the amplitudes of the resulting flow variation. For a pure flow resistance this ratio is fixed and defines the flow resistance, R. For a pure volume-elastic element this ratio is proportional to the product of the reciprocal of the compliance, $1/C$, and the reciprocal of the angular frequency, $1/\omega = 1/2\pi f$. Hence for a pure volume-elastic element $|Z|$ is $1/\omega C$. For a flow resistor in series with a volume-elastic element,

$$|Z| = \sqrt{R^2 + 1/(\omega C)^2}$$

Because of the frequency dependence of the volume-elastic part of the mechanical impedance, the nature of the mechanism on which the impedance depends changes with frequency. As frequency decreases the elastic properties dominate, and *vice versa*.

In the lung the nature of the mechanical impedance also varies along the airway. Virtually all the compliance of the lungs resides in the air spaces which terminate the airways. But the resistance to gas flow is distributed among the various generations of branching. Thus at normal lung volumes somewhat more than half of the total resistance is between the mouth and the lower end of the trachea, and more than half of the remainder is in the first six or so generations of the total of 20-odd generations of branching. As a result of this reduction in resistance the mechanical impedance becomes increasingly dependent on volume-elasticity at successive generations of branching. Thus at a particular breathing frequency there is a certain level of branching beyond which the mechanical impedance is almost entirely elastic, and beyond which the distribution of gas flow becomes almost solely dependent on the distribution of elastic distensibility of the air spaces and on the forces to which they are subjected. What is surprising is that during normal quiet breathing this point appears to be at the very first division of the airway. The mechanical impedance peripheral to the lower end of the trachea is in this case certainly more than 90 per cent elastic, and the same is true even during the increased ventilation accompanying exercise.

To summarize so far, the volume–pressure behaviour of the normal lung undergoing small volume excursions at normal lung volumes can be closely simulated by a mechanical flow-resistor in series with a mechanical compliance. The observation that the values of the resistance and compliance do not change over a wide range of breathing frequencies is taken as evidence that the distribution of volume change is independent of breathing frequency. This independence is not the result of equality of time constants of separate pathways within the lung, but rather relates to the shortness of these time constants relative to the interval of a breathing cycle. As a corollary of this, the mechanical impedance of the separate pathways within lungs, under physiological circumstances, is predominantly elastic in nature, and airway resistance plays almost no role in the distribution of gas flow to the various parts of the lung.

We have next to consider what governs the distribution of distension of air-spaces. So far we have treated the pressure difference between the mouth and the pleural surface as representative of the pressures to which all parts of the lung are exposed. Implicit in this has been the assumption that the pressure is the same at all points on the pleural surface, and that the air spaces deep within the lungs are exposed to the same distending pressure as those at the surface. For the latter assumption we have only indirect evidence. Since to a close approximation alveolar pressure is everywhere the same, the walls of air spaces, both sides of which are exposed to alveolar pressure, are not exposed directly to transpulmonary pressure. Indeed all the forces distending air spaces are applied by way of the tissues attached to them. It is at least possible that the stress concentration applied by tissue forces to the walls of air spaces is everywhere the same in normal lungs. If this stress concentration is also the same as that developed by the pulmonary parenchyma at the pleural surface, where by definition it must equal static transpulmonary pressure, then all air spaces are in effect exposed to static transpulmonary pressure at all times.

When lungs are fixed at constant volume, either chemically or by freezing, and then sliced, the uniformity of expansion of the air spaces can be examined. At a given height in the lung this uniformity is striking. Since air spaces throughout seem to be made of the same stuff, their uniformity of expansion can be taken as indirect evidence that they are subjected to similar distension.

We have direct experimental evidence on the topography of pressure at the external surface of the lungs. It has long been anticipated that because the lung has weight, the pressure at the lower surface should be greater than that at the upper one. This has now been demonstrated repeatedly—at least in experimental animals—and has been inferred from measurements of gradients of air-space distension in the gravity field, both by the use of radioactive gases and by morphological measurements. It appears that a pressure gradient of about $0 \cdot 25$ cm. water per cm. of vertical distance exists at the pleural surface. This corresponds quite closely to the hydraulic gradient one would expect for a liquid with the same density as the lung at normal volumes. But several points indicate that it is not simply a hydraulic gradient. First, it is not uniform—tending to be greater on surfaces which incline from the vertical. Secondly, it is not completely reversible with inversion, tending to be greater when the apices are uppermost. Thirdly, the gradient does not appear to change with lung volume despite the attendant changes in lung density. Finally, as an additional simplifying but puzzling feature, it does not change over a considerable range of change in shape of the lungs, such as can be produced at constant lung volume by compressing the abdomen while expanding the rib cage, and *vice versa*.

Although the exact basis for the gravity gradient in pleural pressure remains to be worked out, we already know that in a given posture it is relatively fixed, and this makes analysis of its implications for the distribution of lung distension comparatively simple. The oesophageal pressure at the highest point of a 30-cm. lung is approximately 4 cm. water less and that at the lowest point some 4 cm. water more than that measured at the mid-point. Thus at resting end-expiration, where oesophageal pressure might be −6 cm. water, pleural pressure at the apex is approximately −10 cm. water while that at the base is only −2 cm. water. Since the gradient is fixed, the change in pleural pressure during breathing is the same at all levels, and one might suppose that the associated change in distension would also be the same. But this disregards the non-linearity of lung distensibility. In speaking of pulmonary compliance as a constant I was careful to specify small volume changes around a given lung volume. But pulmonary compliance changes with lung volume, decreasing as lung volume increases. Accordingly, the compliance of the upper—more distended—parts of the lung is less than that of the lower, less distended regions. The volume change associated with a given change in distending pressure is less in the upper than in the lower regions of the lung. As a result, bulk flow of gas is distributed more to the lower than to the upper regions.

Parenthetically, we may return briefly to the matter of time constants. Airways are also distended when the lungs are distended and the flow resistance of the airways decreases as the lung volume increases. The time constants of pathways leading to upper regions are decreased, by reductions both in compliance and resistance, relative to those of lower regions. This distribution would favour gas flow in the upper regions and thus tend to make the distribution of gas flow more uniform. In actual fact, in normal lungs even the longest time constants of pathways to dependent regions appear to be too short to influence gas distribution, at least at normal breathing frequencies.

To summarize once again, although the distribution of gas flow is normally independent of the distribution of airway resistance, it is definitely influenced by the forces of gravity acting in combination with the non-linear volume-elasticity of lungs. As a result the upper regions of the lungs receive roughly half the bulk flow of gas per gram of lung tissue received by the lower regions.

Finally, a word about smooth muscle in the airways. What is its function?

In normal lungs at least, it does not appear to exert any appreciable influence on the distribution of gas flow. And certainly it is not without opportunity. A modest increase in airway resistance above that achieved passively in the lower, less distended, regions could make the distribution of gas flow in the lungs more uniform. But apparently this does not happen. Whatever the functions of airway smooth muscle may be, they do not include, under ordinary circumstances at least, an action equivalent to that of the vascular arterioles.

SUMMARY

Perhaps surprisingly, the distribution of gas flow to different regions of the lung depends hardly at all on the distribution of gas-flow resistance offered by the airways. This is because at ordinary breathing frequencies the main mechanical impedance to gas flow within the lungs stems from the elastic distensibility of the air spaces terminating the airways, the flow resistance of intrapulmonary airways being, comparatively speaking, extremely small. But air-space distension is not the same in all parts of the lung. There is a gradient of increasing distension from bottom to top because of the weight of the lungs. Because the lower, less distended regions are more compliant than the upper, more distended ones, there is a gradient of increasing gas flow from top to bottom.

BIBLIOGRAPHY

General

FENN, W. O., and RAHN, H. (eds.) (1963). *Handbook of Physiology, Section 3: Respiration*, vol. I. Washington, D.C.: American Physiological Society. (Chapters 13–17 deal with respiratory mechanics.)

Distribution of time constants

OTIS, A. B., McKERROW, C. B., BARTLETT, R. A., MEAD, J., McILROY, M. B., SELVERSTONE, N. J., and RADFORD, E. P., Jr. (1956). *J. appl. Physiol.*, 8, 427–443.

Distribution of airway resistance

MACKLEM, P. T., and MEAD, J. (1967). *J. appl. Physiol.*, 22, 395–401.
GREEN, M. (1964). *St Thom. Hosp. Gaz.*, 63, 136–139.
HORSFIELD, K., and CUMMING, G. (1968). *J. appl. Physiol.*, 24, 384–390.

Distribution of pleural pressure and of ventilation

KRUEGER, J. J., BAIN, T., and PATTERSON, J. L., Jr. (1961). *J. appl. Physiol.*, 16, 465–468.
MILIC-EMILI, J., HENDERSON, J. A. M., DOLOVICH, M. B., TROP, D., and KANEKO, K. (1966). *J. appl. Physiol.*, 21, 749–759.
WEST, J. B., and DOLLERY, C. T. (1960). *J. appl. Physiol.*, 15, 405–410.
GLAZIER, J. B., HUGHES, J. M. B., MALONEY, J. E., PAIN, M. C. F., and WEST, J. B. (1966). *Lancet*, 2, 203.

DISCUSSION

Lighthill: In abnormal forms of breathing like coughing, do the time constants and inertia of the lung become significant?

Mead: Yes, indeed. One can put the respiratory system through all sorts of gymnastics and apply the information learned to normal breathing. One can greatly influence the distribution of ventilation by making quick enough events. For example, during a very quick expiration there can be a quite uniform contribution from all parts of the lung as a result of the distribution of the resistance. This is very different from what is obtained statically. Some of the most interesting features of pulmonary mechanics have to do with the amazing degree of compression of the airways which occurs during coughing or simply during a forced expiration. The aerodynamicists may not have spent much time on the behaviour of compressible tubes. We could do with some help in that area.

Lighthill: Does the smooth muscle come in in coughing?

Mead: My guess is that the function of the smooth muscle may be to increase the effectiveness of expectoration, because in bronchial constriction the distribution of dynamic compression, which is an important part of the effectiveness of a cough, is influenced and more of the tracheo-bronchial tree can be compressed. First the upper parts are compressed and then compression extends further and further out; as Peter Macklem put it, you appear to sweep out the front hall first and then work backwards towards the rear of the house!

Burton: Alveolar ventilation must depend on the presence of the special surface-tension mechanism for looking after Laplace's Law.

Mead: I disagree a little. In the ordinary volume range of breathing the presence of surfactant permits virtually all the air spaces to remain open. The stability of the air spaces in this circumstance depends on the character of the tissue. Certainly if you were to allow the surface tension to go up to that of serum you would be in severe trouble, even at ordinary lung volume.

West: I was interested and surprised to learn that apparently the distribution of pressure over the lung does not alter over what you describe as a considerable range of change of lung shape. This behaviour would be expected if the lung were a semifluid, for example a foam of density $0 \cdot 25$. But we know that the lung is fairly solid; if you push an excised and inflated dog lung out of shape, it resists distortion; it has a good deal of intrinsic shape.

Mead: The distribution of pressure is certainly not entirely independent of shape; of course it can be exquisitely sensitive to it. But over a wide range of shape change, such as you can produce externally on a whole animal, the pressure appears not to change appreciably. The dog lung, which is highly lobated, can be made to take up a great variety of shapes, simply by slipping lobe upon lobe, and this has been proposed as an important function of lobation in lungs, that it permits some independent mechanical behaviour. But transpulmonary pressure is not appreciably altered. Certainly once you make local changes, even a small denting caused by the ribs makes quite substantial changes in local pleural pressure. Presumably the strain related to these changes extends only a very small distance; this would be an interesting point to pursue.

Caro: Are you saying that if we float a lung, as in John West's foam, for example, this is not very relevant to what is happening in the chest cage? Will the lung tend on inspiration to float up against the top of the container because its density has dropped?

Mead: I would suppose so.

Farhi: We have been able to study members of our department and teach them to shift their expiration from thoracic contraction of muscles to abdominal contraction. In this situation the same flow can be maintained, and at the same volume oesophageal pressure will change by as much as 1 or 2 cm. water, and at the same time the composition of the expired gas changes; so possibly what you found in the dog does not apply entirely to man. We were working at lung volumes 1·5 litres above functional residual capacity (F.R.C.).

Mead: That is very interesting. It is difficult to interpret oesophageal pressure at low lung volumes, but these are evidently in the same range.

West: How much change in shape were you getting in the dogs? How much did the diameter of the chest change at the bottom compared with the top?

Mead: It was a very striking change on the X-ray films, from a very thin lung to quite a plump one.

Caro: Presumably then a middle lobe would float up among the other lobes if it were better ventilated than they were?

Burton: What room is there for one lobe to float? There is no space between lobes.

Mead: A lobe moves up at the expense of the volume of the region above it; a bit of lung previously above it will be found below.

Stuart: May I return to Professor Mead's analogy with an electrical circuit. In electrical circuits there are many situations where non-linearities come in; a famous case is the van der Pol equation. Are there any situations in lung dynamics where violent changes occur which might bring in a non-linearity of volume flow or of the rate of change of volume flow?

Mead: As flow is increased the flow resistance of the airways becomes highly non-linear. Non-linearity is even more striking during forced expirations which are associated with large changes in geometry of the airways. The non-linearity of the lung's distensibility—and a good share of it is surface tension, as Professor Burton has emphasized—is very great; it is non-linear with respect to volume and time. When I said that pulmonary compliance and resistance are constant I did specify that this was for very small volume changes and low rates of flow. For ordinary breathing these linear approximations are reasonable.

Lighthill: We have this interesting contrast with the blood circulation, because in the lung the resistance is in the big airways. Would you consider that the resistance is in the big airways because that is where there is turbulent flow?

Mead: No, because the resistance is in the larger airways with simple laminar flow as well.

Burton: It is due to the difference in the branching geometry between the airway system and the vascular system.

Cumming: Fig. 1 shows the pressure drop over the bronchial tree, based on measurement of an airway cast followed by calculation using Poiseuille's Law. The bulk of the pressure drop occurs in tubes of diameters between 2 mm. and 5 mm., and is based on steady state, fully developed laminar flow.

Lighthill: Is it not so that in certain conditions, turbulence is present in the trachea?

West: We made some measurements in a hollow cast of the human bronchial tree some years ago (West, J. B., and Hugh-Jones, P. [1959]. *J. appl. Physiol.*,

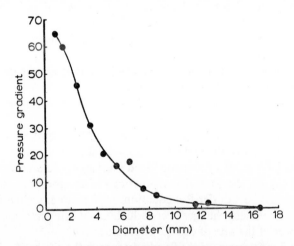

Fig. 1. (Cumming). The pressure drop over the bronchial tree. The pressure gradient is plotted as a percentage of the total pressure drop.

14, 753–759) and found turbulence in the trachea at expiratory flow rates of about 20 l./min. At 80 l./min. turbulence was also found in the segmental and lobar bronchi.

Farhi: Professor Mead, how do you reconcile the statement that flow is mainly laminar with a statement you made several years ago that when one goes from breathing air to breathing helium, airway resistance is essentially proportional to the gas density (Mead, J. [1955]. In *Proc. Symp. Underwater Biology*, pp. 112–123, ed. Goff, L. G. Washington, D.C.: National Academy of Sciences—National Research Council)?

Mead: That result remains a mystery to me! We changed the physical properties of the gas breathed by going from air to 100 per cent helium or to 100 per cent ethane—that is, to a gas that is very much less dense in the case of helium, and slightly more viscous, or to a gas which is about half as viscous as air and somewhat more dense, as is ethane. We appreciated that the distribution of turbulence—the Reynolds number—was going to change grossly because the kinematic viscosity was changed grossly, but we had thought that with ethane we would at least reduce the pressure for a given flow, at low flow rates. In fact, it was increased very slightly. For helium, we thought that we would influence matters at high flow rates, but that towards zero flow there would be little influence; but in fact all the way to zero flow there was a marked reduction in the pressure required for flow.

Cumming: We have some observations too on whether turbulence developed in the upper airways, in which we have measured the flow rate at the lips and plotted it against the volume flow rate at the lips, and apparently this depends to some extent on a little-considered phenomenon. We consider flow in the tracheo-bronchial tree normally as being in a dry situation, whereas in fact it is far from dry; and in patients with increased sputum it is a very notable phenomenon that at high flow rates, two-phase flow starts in the tracheo-bronchial tree and causes a marked perturbation as flow goes turbulent. That is, the air phase becomes turbulent at the same time as the layer of liquid between the tracheo-bronchial wall and the gas moves, going into little waves—the thin-film instability. This phenomenon occurs only at high flow rates, not in normal breathing. It will occur whether or not there is an excess of liquid, but when there is, it occurs more readily.

Lighthill: Professor Mead seems to be implying that resistance is fairly closely linear as a function of velocity, but I wondered whether, if it was an entry-length phenomenon, it would not be expected to vary with velocity to the power 3/2, and if it was turbulent, with velocity nearly squared? It is difficult to think of any circumstances, if the resistance is in the big airways, where one would expect it to vary linearly with velocity.

Mead: Let me quote some actual figures. If a parabolic description is given of the pressure–flow relationship, then pressure is proportional to $K_1 \times$ flow $+ K_2 \times$ flow^2; K_1 in a normal individual at normal lung volumes is about $1 \cdot 3$ for the total airway, and K_2 would be about $0 \cdot 3$.

Burton: How much do you have to increase the respiration for the second term to equal the first?

Mead: In ordinary quiet breathing at rest the peak flow is something like $0 \cdot 5$ l./sec., and during heavy exercise perhaps 10 times greater. At rest the first term is nearly 10 times the second. In heavy exercise the two terms are about equal.

Actually, about two-thirds of the K_2 value is in the larynx, so the actual K_2 for lung, at normal lung volumes, is about $0 \cdot 1$, which makes it a more linear relationship. I was not implying that the system is a fully linear one in terms of resistance, only that if you restrict the amplitudes it is nearly so.

Caro: Studies that we have made on John West's lung cast, allowing water to flow through it and injecting a filament of dye, show quite extensive secondary motion in the region of the division of the trachea and the lobar branches, at quite modest Reynolds numbers (Re = 300).

Lighthill: Resistance in secondary flow is not linearly related to velocity. There is a departure from linearity as the Reynolds number increases.

Philip: It would be illuminating if we could have a picture of the way in which the Reynolds number varies down the airways. It is clearly important to know whether there is a substantial region in which the Reynolds numbers are of the order of one.

TABLE I (Owen)

VARIATION OF VELOCITY AND REYNOLDS NUMBER IN THE UPPER AIRWAYS
Inspired volume flow, 40 l. min.$^{-1}$

Generation	Length/ diameter	Velocity cm. sec.$^{-1}$	Reynolds number
Trachea	6·7	263	3,100
Main bronchi	4·0	286	2,290
Lobar bronchi	2·3	314	1,710
Segmental bronchi	1·3	334	1,230

Owen: In the first four generations they are as shown in Table I. After that, the Reynolds numbers fall very rapidly: to about 500 in the fifth generation (the trachea being counted as zero), 50 in the tenth generation and unity in the fifteenth, subsequently decreasing further still.

BEHAVIOUR OF AIRBORNE PARTICLES IN THE RESPIRATORY TRACT

BERNARD ALTSHULER

*Institute of Environmental Medicine, New York University Medical Center,
New York*

THE motion of suspended particles (aerosols) in the respiratory tract is a difficult and necessary area for intensive study: difficult because the tract is complicated geometrically and mechanically, necessary because the site and amount of deposition are required to evaluate the tissue dose from inhaled particulates and because aerosols can be used to study pulmonary function.

The detail and accuracy that is acceptable or desirable depends on the use of the results obtained. As an example of a crude approximation, a Task Group on Lung Dynamics (1966) appointed by the International Commission on Radiation Protection has recommended that, in the absence of specific information, a worker breathing an environmental aerosol be considered to have 25 per cent deposited in his nose and pharynx, 8 per cent in his tracheo-bronchial tree, and 25 per cent in his deep pulmonary region. As an example of the need for finer distinctions, the evaluation of radiation dose to bronchial tissue in uranium miners requires detailed examination of almost all aspects of particle motion in the lung—relatively fine localization of deposition is required for categories of sizes extending over the complete range from molecules of the unattached radon daughter products to the coarsest dust to which daughter products may attach (Altshuler, Nelson and Kuschner, 1964).

The deviation of particle motion from gas motion is caused by Brownian motion, gravity and inertial force. This deviation is dominated by Brownian motion for particles with diameters less than $0 \cdot 2$ μm. and depends on the quantity $d^{-1}(0 \cdot 18 + d)^{1/2}$ where d is particle diameter in micrometres; its dependence on particle density is negligible. For larger particles with diameters greater than 1 μm., this deviation is dominated by settling and inertial displacement and its dependence on particle density ρ and diameter d is determined by the quantity $\rho d^2(1 + 0 \cdot 18 d^{-1})$. Thus, for a fixed respiratory pattern there is a diameter at which total deposition is minimized, which is near $0 \cdot 5$ μm. for unit density spheres (Altshuler *et al.*, 1957). Total deposition increases to near 100 per cent as size increases or decreases.

Most of the deposition with $0 \cdot 5$ μm. diameter particles is in the deep pulmonary region. As large particles increase in size or small particles decrease in size, deposition in the upper tract, including the bronchial tree, will increase, less particles will reach the deep pulmonary region and the portion of these deposited there will increase. Consequently deep pulmonary deposition as a function of particle size will have two maxima which can be roughly located around $0 \cdot 02$ and 2 μm. diameter (unit density). The larger size has special importance for environmental hazards and inhalation therapy. It depends on the kind of breathing and has too large an uncertainty: Davies (1964) suggested it may be as small as $0 \cdot 4$ μm. for miners and Altshuler, Palmes and Nelson (1967) suggested it could be as large as 5 μm. with quiet mouth breathing.

Aerosols are useful for the study of special aspects of pulmonary function. Particles of $0 \cdot 5$ μm. diameter are approximate tracers of air flow through the lungs and have been used to assess convective mixing in the lung (Altshuler et al., 1959; Altshuler, 1961; Altshuler and Briscoe, 1961; Muir, 1967). The measurement of deposition of aerosol during breath-holding holds promise of giving an index of the dimensions of the pulmonary spaces in life (Palmes, Altshuler and Nelson, 1967).

Another application occurs in the measurement of the clearance of deposited particles in the lung by the external counting of radioactive tagged insoluble particles (Albert et al., 1967a; Lippmann and Albert, 1968). The measurement is the combined effect of deposition and the movement of deposited particles on bronchial mucus, and independent knowledge of regional deposition would help us to evaluate regional mucus flow.

Experimental studies of regional deposition in the lungs are necessarily indirect because the pulmonary spaces are inaccessible, large in number, small in dimensions, and many features that are important for dynamic considerations are poorly understood. Thus theoretical analysis is required and is emphasized in this paper.

One experimental approach measures aerosol and volume during expiration. Such measurements can be used with a predictive theory that calculates both regional deposition and expired aerosol for the conditions of the experiment (Landahl, 1950, 1963; Landahl, Tracewell and Lassen, 1951, 1952; Beeckmans, 1965a, b; Task Group on Lung Dynamics, 1966). Other estimates of regional deposition have been obtained by regarding the respiratory tract as a series of filters whose penetration characteristics are determined by the measured concentrations and these in turn determine regional deposition (Brown et al., 1950; Altshuler, Palmes and Nelson, 1967).

Another experimental approach mentioned above uses external scintillation counting of deposited particles tagged with a gamma-emitting isotope. Deposition in the pulmonary region without mucus flow has been inferred from the clearance of particles moving with bronchial mucus (Albert *et al.*, 1967*b*; Lippmann and Albert, 1968). The procedure has potential for more refined regional deposition as more knowledge is obtained about regional mucus flow.

Other work on deposition is reviewed by Hatch and Gross (1964) and discussed by Davies (1967).

The studies involve gross simplifications which are based more on plausibility and necessity than on rigorous inference but give estimates which are required and useful. Typically, however, the magnitudes of the uncertainties are not stated and these can be large, making the results unreliable. This, combined with the use of different conditions, makes it difficult to judge and compare the studies.

The theoretical problem is difficult and awkward with a multiplicity of complications whose relative importance is hard to evaluate. Existing theory has generally been primitive, justified by the circumstance that all first-order effects are not reliably established. The situation calls for a more rigorous theoretical treatment of the individual features and their incorporation into a computer programme which evaluates their separate effects in relation to the rest of the system.

The second section of this paper is a critical review of existing theory with suggestions for improvement. The third section discusses unpublished work on aerosol mixing in forced expiration single breaths that was done with William A. Briscoe of Columbia University. The fourth section discusses some partially published work on deposition during breath-holding by E. D. Palmes and co-workers.

THEORY

The behaviour of an aerosol in a system of passageways representing the respiratory tract was first calculated by Findeisen (1935). His analysis was modified by Landahl (1950, 1963) and further extended by Beeckmans (1965*a*, *b*). Their published papers give rather complete descriptions and have been the basis of other published calculations. Detailed calculations of regional deposition with additional considerations of nasal deposition and of large molecules and small nuclei have been published by a Task Group on Lung Dynamics (1966) and by Altshuler, Nelson and Kuschner (1964).

All these treatments are closely related. With perhaps a few exceptions, their modifications generally show no great quantitative changes but they are valuable by increasing credibility. Indeed it might be appropriate to speak of one predictive Findeisen-Landahl-Beeckmans theory. Even the tubular filter-bed approach used by Altshuler, Palmes and Nelson (1967) as a deductive theory to go with continuous measurements of expired aerosol is closely tied to the Findeisen-Landahl-Beeckmans predictive theory, which was used to determine certain essential quantities.

Beeckmans (1965*a, b*) has incorporated most refinements. Two of these add much to the credibility of the calculations: (1) he considered convective mixing which causes aerosols to recycle and accumulate beyond the tidal penetration; (2) he did the calculations for two different models of the respiratory tract—for the relatively crude Findeisen-Landahl model and for the more detailed regular dichotomy model of Weibel—and found little quantitative changes. We shall review the theory with primary attention to Beeckmans' papers.

Model of the respiratory tract

Weibel (1963) has made careful and extensive morphometric measurements of excised lungs fixed at three-quarters maximum inflation, of a cast of the larger airways in the bronchial tree, and of bronchograms. Regularities in

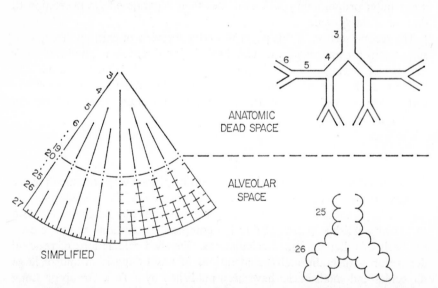

FIG. 1. Sketch of branching airways in the lungs. It indicates decreasing diameters, expanding total cross-section, smooth-wall dead space, and the contrast between the alveolated walls of the alveolar space and the simplified model that puts all alveoli at the end of the terminal duct (alveolar sac). The numbers correspond to the regions of Table I.

these measurements were summarized in his regular dichotomy model "A" and some of the irregularities were also described.

Horsfield and Cumming (1967, 1968) have made more extensive measurements on bronchial casts and describe the branching angles. The static and dynamic structure in life is considerably more irregular (Glazier *et al.*, 1967; Dollfuss, Milic-Emili and Bates, 1967).

This structure has generally been considered as fixed in size with rigid walls. However, the system works as a flexible elastic structure, although little is known about the elastic properties of the tissue. It should always be kept in mind that the walls are distensible.

Table I

WEIBEL'S REGULAR DICHOTOMY MODEL OF RESPIRATORY TRACT AT 3/4 MAXIMUM INFLATION

As used by Beeckmans

Region α	Number of elements	Diameter mm.	Length mm.	Volume ml.	Fraction alveolated	Volume in alveoli, ml.
				Conductive		
1†	1	20	70	20		
2†	1	30	30	20		
3	1	18·0	120	30·5		
4	2	12·2	48	11·2		
5	4	8·3	19	4·0		
6	8	5·6	7·6	1·5		
7	16	4·5	12·7	3·5		
8	32	3·5	10·7	3·3		
9	64	2·8	9·0	3·5		
10	128	2·3	7·6	3·8		
11	256	1·86	6·4	4·4		
12	512	1·54	5·4	5·2		
13	1,024	1·30	4·6	6·2		
14	2,048	1·09	3·9	7·6		
15	4,096	0·95	3·3	9·8		
16	8,192	0·82	2·7	12·4		
17	16,384	0·74	2·3	16·4		
18	32,768	0·66	2·0	21·7		
19	65,536	0·60	1·65	29·7		
				215		
				Transitory		Respiratory
20	131,072	0·54	1·41	42	0·12	6
21	262,144	0·50	1·17	61	0·25	21
22	524,288	0·47	0·99	93	0·50	63
23	1,048,576	0·45	0·83	140	1·00	220
24	2,097,152	0·43	0·70	224	1·00	436
25	4,194,304	0·41	0·59	350	1·00	882
26	8,388,608	0·41	0·50	591	1·00	1,502
				1,500		3,150
				Respiratory		
27‡	300 × 10⁶	0·26		3,150		

† Landahl (1950) dimensions
‡ Equivalent to making region 26 the only alveolated region

The Weibel model and its modification by Beeckmans are schematically illustrated in Fig. 1 and quantitatively described in Table I.

Regions 1 to 27 with only the first five columns represent the model used by Beeckmans (1965b). Regions 3 to 26 with all columns comprise the Weibel regular dichotomy model of the lung. Regions 1 and 2 are added to the Weibel lung model to represent the mouth and pharynx. They are crude representations which are expected to be poor for extreme breathing and extreme particle sizes but unimportant for the lung with near-normal breathing and more stable sizes.

Regions 1 to 19 represent the *anatomical dead space*, called the *conductive zone* by Weibel. The Weibel regions 20 to 26 are called the *alveolar space* here, sometimes alveolar region or pulmonary compartment (Task Group on Lung Dynamics, 1966). It consists of the passageways which comprise the *transitory zone* of Weibel and the alveoli which comprise the *respiratory zone* of Weibel. *Alveolar deposition* means deposition in the alveolar space. Regions 23 to 26 are completely alveolated and an element is called an *alveolar spatial unit*. It consists of the alveolar duct and the twenty or so alveoli which open on to it and cover it.

The alveolus can be described as a spherical segment with a diameter of $0 \cdot 28$ mm., depth of $0 \cdot 23$ mm., and volume of $1 \cdot 05 \times 10^{-5}$ ml. (Weibel, 1963); or by flattening two opposite sides for a better fit longitudinally, it can be described as a segment of a cylinder.

Region 27 is a simplifying distortion of the Weibel model made by Beeckmans and follows precedent. With a fictitious topology, it considers all alveoli as spheres placed at the end of the final duct of region 26, which is often called the alveolar sac.

A main purpose of this paper is to undo the standard oversimplification of the geometry of the alveolar space which considers it to be a system of smooth wall tubes leading to the alveoli, for both particle and gas transport. The alveolar duct together with its alveoli should be considered as a single spatial unit, the alveolar spatial unit, having interalveolar partitions. The different boundary conditions for flow velocity, aerosol concentration and gas concentration change the character of the solutions of the governing differential equations; some features of these changes are indicated next.

(1) With a smooth wall duct, velocity is zero at the boundary wall and the velocity profile is parabolic with central velocity twice average velocity. With the open duct, velocity at the open boundary is greater than zero and at the centre is less than twice average velocity, so that tidal flow has less penetration.

(2) With the smooth wall duct, aerosol concentration is zero at the boundary wall and diffusive transport will be radially outward at all times. With the open

duct aerosol concentration will build up at the open boundary, radially out-ward diffusive transport will be less during inhalation of aerosol, and during exhalation diffusive transport will be reversed, toward the centre axis from the alveoli, and aerosol will be dispersed axially during expiration.

(3) Now consider diffusion of an inert gas during breath-holding. With the smooth wall duct of these small dimensions and the high diffusivity of the gas, concentration will be effectively uniform in the cross-section and diffusive transport will be one-dimensional along the axis, governed by the true diffusive constant of the gas. With the open duct, axial transport is limited to the cross-section of the duct by the alveolar partitions, but gas has to diffuse radially to equilibrate with the alveoli, and this slows up axial diffusion in proportion to the ratio of the volume of the duct to the volume of the alveolar spatial unit.

All published theory on aerosol behaviour regards the respiratory tract as a series of filters—there are 27 of these in Beeckmans' model. Each region is supposed to remove a calculated fraction of the particles which reach it, independent of behaviour in the flow through preceding regions. Findeisen (1935) and Landahl (1950) reduced the number of regions by more than half by grouping. Brown and co-workers (1950) used two filters—one for anatomical dead space and one for alveolar space—to estimate gross regional deposition from the fractionated expired aerosol. Since the experimental technique of Altshuler and co-workers (1957) cannot be expected to resolve the details of the structure, Altshuler (1959) has considered the respiratory tract as a continuous tubular filter-bed with penetration characteristics varying with depth.

The manner in which aerosol deposition and penetration has been calculated in each element of the structural model is discussed in the following subsections.

Convective flow

Flow will be fully turbulent in part of the upper tract for sufficiently high respiratory rates, and for all usual respiratory patterns there will always be a portion of the respiratory tract in which flow is partially turbulent (above the deepest regions in which flow is always laminar). For the most part, the formalism proceeds as if there were steady piston flow, or as if there were Poiseuille flow (laminar with parabolic velocity profile), and without recogniz-ing the many difficult considerations that control the distribution of velocity.

It has often been stated that Poiseuille flow is prevalent in most of the lung—for example Davies (1967), that central axial velocity is nearly twice average velocity, and that particles snake down the centre of turning passageways to reach almost twice as far as would be obtained with uniform piston flow. But this is not a good description and may be misleading. The central streamline of one tube ends at a stagnation point on the leading edge of the wedge of the next branching. A boundary layer flow forms at the edge of the wedge, giving the velocity profile schematically illustrated in Fig. 2. This boundary layer increases in thickness until Poiseuille flow is fully developed after an inlet length which is even greater than Reynolds number × diameter/30, if we use

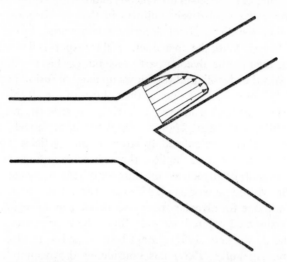

FIG. 2. Velocity distribution in the inlet length of a bronchus. It portrays a linear increase of velocity in the boundary layer merging with the semi-parabola of the entering distribution.

this expression for the uniform entry condition (Schlichting, 1968). At a steady 60 litres per minute, this means Poiseuille flow is fully developed only for regions below Region 12.

Fig. 3 illustrates that Poiseuille flow does not occur in the alveolar ducts, although the Reynolds number is very small. Since the duct is open to the alveoli, velocity will be greater than zero at the periphery of the duct, the velocity profile will be blunter than Poiseuille flow, and maximum velocity will be less than twice the average velocity. Furthermore, a vortex might be induced in the alveolus.

A large number of respirations per minute means a high frequency periodic flow, and this unsteady flow will have a considerable effect on flow stability in the upper passageways. As frequency increases and there is more fluid acceleration, the inertial effects dominate in the central core which then tends to move as a unit separated from the wall by a boundary layer (Schlichting, 1968).

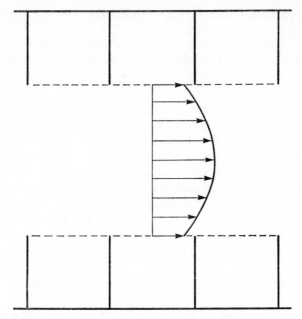

Fig. 3. Alveolar spatial unit. It shows a parabolic velocity
distribution in the duct with positive boundary velocity.

Irreversibility and convective mixing during flow are important factors
related to the separation of flow from the wall and vortex motion. They are
enhanced locally by the flexibility and curvature of the walls and on a larger
scale by the gross inhomogeneities in the expansion and contraction of the
lung structure.

Deposition

Deposition theory has not been accurate because of the complexities of
flow, surface geometry, and the joint action of diffusion, settling and inertial
displacement. To obtain a tractable theory, each region has been considered
as a separate and independent removal element and also in each region the
transport processes of diffusion, settling and inertial displacement are regarded
as mutually independent and additively superimposed on convective flow.
The simplifications are stated with various degrees of plausibility and generally
without rigorous inference from accurate assumptions. Some stand up under
close examination and some do not. In this section, we shall outline the major
considerations and indicate places where the analysis needs to be improved.

Pure impaction at a bifurcation has been calculated as a function of the
8*

distance perpendicular to the changed direction that a particle with the average approach velocity will be displaced because of its inertia. The fraction of particles impacted is determined by an empirical fit to data obtained from impaction in bent tubes (Landahl, 1950). However, a bent tube is probably a poor approximation to a bifurcation because the velocity distributions are very different in both inspiration and expiration. A more realistic derivation seems indicated. Also, the use of one angle to represent an average change of direction can be misleading because the dichotomy is irregular and in many cases one of the branches may continue in the same direction (Horsfield and Cumming, 1967).

Convective settling (during flow) and pure settling (during respiratory pause) have been handled by Beeckmans in a fairly straightforward manner, which may be sufficiently accurate. Neglected considerations are associated with the entering distributions of aerosol and velocity and with the distribution of the angle between the tube axis and the vertical. Because the tubes are short, pure settling may require more details of the geometry than have been considered.

Both convective diffusion for Poiseuille flow with uniform entry conditions and pure diffusion for tubes of infinite length and uniform initial concentration have exact solutions (Fuchs, 1964). Though the initial conditions are not uniform and flow is not steady, and the tubes have finite length, these solutions may be a satisfactory approximation for the smooth wall tubes in the bronchial tree. (Convective diffusion in the lower bronchial tree is being treated as a quasi-steady flow and non-steady concentration boundary-layer problem by Wang and Friedlander, 1968.)

However, the situation is radically different in the alveolar ducts. As stated earlier, neither the flow nor the concentration are zero at the boundary of the duct. The whole alveolar spatial unit with its complicated boundary needs to be treated numerically on a high-speed digital computer, as it cannot be solved analytically.

For pure diffusion during a respiratory pause or breath-holding, the end conditions at the branchings are also important, since the length of the duct is generally shorter than the diameter of the alveolar spatial unit (Fig. 3). It will probably suffice to require the end concentration gradients at a branching to be inversely proportional to total cross-sectional areas in the ducts, which matches exit and entry transport. Thus diffusion in the alveolar space may be represented by a linear series of alveolar spatial units with matching discontinuities at their junctions.

The situation is much simpler for pure diffusion of an inert gas, which is a good approximation to convective diffusion in the alveolar space since convective transport is here much less than diffusive transport. With an inert gas, concentrations are nearly uniform radially and diffusion is one-dimensional along the axis, but with an effective diffusion constant which is less than the true diffusion constant by a factor equal to the duct volume divided by the total volume of the alveolar spatial unit; and end gradients are related inversely to the total duct cross-sectional area times the true diffusion constant. This solution for pure diffusion in the alveolar space is the same as the solution for linear heat flow through a composite solid made up of parallel slabs with different conductivities and diffusivities and a reflector at one end (Carslaw and Jaeger, 1959). It will give considerably less diffusive mixing than the amounts that have been calculated by Rauwerda (1946) and Cumming and co-workers (1966).

These removal processes have been combined as if they were independent actions. Thus, if F_i, F_s, F_d denote the deposition fractions for impaction, convective settling, and convective diffusion in a single element, then the combined deposition fraction has been taken as $1 - (1 - F_i)(1 - F_s)(1 - F_d)$. This is not generally accurate, however, and lacks supporting reasoning. In the one case for which an exact solution has been obtained, particles suspended in a stationary fluid between parallel plane surfaces, it was shown by Wang, Altshuler and Palmes (1968) that deposition is better approximated by the larger of the two pure depositions—pure diffusion or pure settling—than by combining them in the above manner as if they were independent probabilities.

It is worth repeating that it is important to match entry conditions with previous exit conditions. Deposition efficiencies in the different removal elements are also not independent.

Aerosol mixing

Aerosol mixing or aerosol dispersion is the combined effect of convective mixing, diffusion, settling and inertial displacement. An oversimplified treatment has been given by Altshuler and co-workers (1959) and Altshuler (1959, 1961) which was used by Beeckmans (1965a). However, the mixing function adopted by Beeckmans is a pragmatic one with little empirical or theoretical basis and neglects the fact that aerosol mixing is different from convective mixing and does depend on the removal mechanisms. The problem needs improved analysis.

Aerosol mixing is particularly important for calculating the deposition of the more stable particles because the concentration of an aerosol builds up in lung air over a period of several breaths (Altshuler *et al.*, 1959). Experiments with resting subjects breathing the stable sizes indicate that about 25 per cent of the deposited particles had been suspended in the respiratory tract for more than one breath (Altshuler, 1961). Beeckmans (1965a) found that it was necessary to incorporate mixing in order to predict a size for minimum deposition that agreed with experimental results. Single-breath experiments are discussed in the next section.

AEROSOL DISPERSION IN FORCED EXPIRATION SINGLE BREATHS

This section discusses work done with William A. Briscoe of Columbia University (Altshuler and Briscoe, 1961). Aerosol dispersion has been examined in single-breath experiments using aerosols of 0·5 μm. diameter

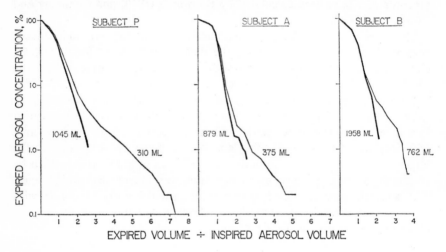

FIG. 4. Aerosol distribution in the forced expiration of a single aerosol breath. Curves are labelled with the volume of inspired aerosol.

which are approximate tracers of the gas motion. Respired aerosol concentration and volume were measured continuously during inspiration followed by forced expiration. We have done two types of such experiments: in one, aerosol was uniformly distributed throughout the inspiration; in the other, aerosol was inhaled as a small bolus—that is, a pulse followed by clean air. The measured distribution of aerosol in the expiration is an expression of longitudinal or axial aerosol dispersion which is due in part to convective mixing (turbulence, non-random vortex motion, and other aspects of irreversibility of flow) and in part to diffusion and settling.

Fig. 4 shows the concentration of aerosol in the forced expiration after a single complete aerosol inspiration for three subjects, each with a small and large inspired volume. Expired concentration is plotted on a logarithmic scale against expiratory volume expressed as a multiple of inhaled volume. Recovery was about 95 per cent for the small inhalations and 85 per cent for the large, in contrast to the results of Muir (1967) who recovered 100 per cent and 93 per cent for similar sized inhalations in a comparable experiment. For each subject there is close coincidence in the curves while expired volume is less than that inspired, but for the latter part of the expiration the curve for the larger inhalation is slightly but consistently below the curve for the smaller —the semilogarithmic plot being used to exaggerate and clearly exhibit this feature.

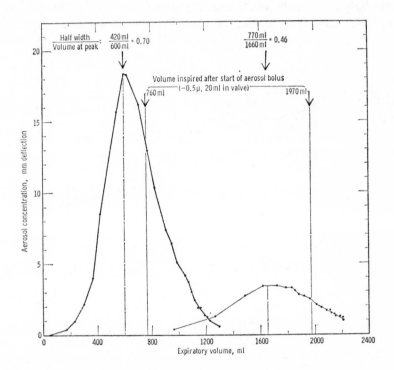

Fig. 5. Aerosol distribution in the forced expiration after a small aerosol bolus has been inspired, followed by clean air.

Fig. 5 shows the concentration of aerosol in the forced expiration after the inspiration of an aerosol bolus followed by clean air in two experiments, with clean air volumes of 760 ml. and 1,970 ml. The technique did not resolve the inspired pulse, and the expired concentration is given in an arbitrary unit not related to the amount inspired. This technique measures aerosol dispersion in its greatest accessible detail. The ratio of half-width (i.e. difference between volumes at which concentration is half maximum) to volume at peak concentration should be a useful index. The volume at peak concentration is seen to be less than the inspired volume and more aerosol is expired after the volume at peak concentration, as is consistent with diffusive transport from alveoli to duct during expiratory flow.

It is a challenge to develop the proper theoretical understanding of mixing or dispersion of aerosols in the respiratory tract and interpret such experimental data in terms of the basic physiological and physical parameters involved, particularly to evaluate pure convective mixing. With velocities no greater than that occurring in resting breathing, rough calculations suggest that

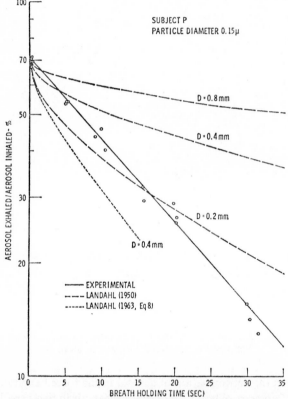

Fig. 6. Aerosol recovery against time of breath-holding. Experimental values are compared with calculations using the Landahl equations for initial uniform distribution in smooth wall tubes of diameter *D*. (From Palmes, Altshuler and Nelson, 1967.)

diffusion and settling of particles may contribute more to aerosol mixing than convective mixing.

Another type of single-breath aerosol experiment is being exploited by my colleague E. D. Palmes. The subject expires twice the inspired volume of aerosol, one or two bag-in-the-box systems being used to collect and measure aerosol and respired volumes, with a preselected and varied period of breath-holding between the two dynamic phases. Inspired volume is sufficiently great for most of the aerosol to penetrate beyond the anatomical dead space into the alveolar space. Experiments have been conducted with $0\cdot15$ μm.-diameter particles in which displacement is dominantly by diffusion and with $0\cdot75$ μm.-particles for which settling dominates. A main finding is that the recovery of aerosol decreases exponentially with time of breath-holding up to about 30 seconds. The rate of deposition during breath-holding is regarded as an index of an average dimension in the alveolar space in life.

Fig. 6 from Palmes, Altshuler and Nelson (1967) shows data for the smaller particles related to the theory for the smooth wall tube given by Landahl. The data are inconsistent with the supposition that the aerosol near its average concentration is close to the wall at the start of breath-holding, since this would mean that for small time t, diffusive deposition would vary as $\sqrt{t}$, and deposition rate as $1/\sqrt{t}$, which would imply a relatively high rate of deposition for small breath-holding times. The same characteristic exponential decrease with breath-holding was found for the larger, $0\cdot75$ μm. particles for which settling dominates. These data are inconsistent with the concept of a protective sheath of clean air in the duct around an inner core of tidal aerosol since there would then be a relatively small rate of removal for small breath-holding times while particles were falling through the protective sheath. The consistent linearity of the semilogarithmic plots for all sizes is compatible with a fairly uniform distribution of the aerosol in the cross-section of the open alveolar duct at the start of breath-holding.

Experiments have been done varying only the lung volume at which the breath was held (Palmes, Marrero and Altshuler, 1966). The deposition rate depended more sensitively on lung volume than is expected under homogeneous expansion; that is, more than on the two-thirds power of lung volume, representing surface area. This is positive evidence of structural inhomogeneity and introduces another poorly understood complexity into the situation.

As the purpose of these experiments is to assess an average dimension of the alveolar spatial units in life, it is important to obtain a suitable theory for these observations.

SUMMARY

The behaviour of airborne particles in the human respiratory tract is critically reviewed in relation to regional deposition and the study of pulmonary function. Since experimental studies are necessarily indirect, theoretical analysis is required. Major features of existing theory are examined, deficiencies are pointed out, and suggestions for future work are made.

Although deposition results have been useful, and consistent because of large uncertainties, some aspects have been oversimplified and some treated without sufficient justification. The situation calls for more rigorous treatment of individual features and their incorporation into a computer programme which relates their effects to the rest of the system. Evaluation of convective mixing and pulmonary dimensions in life also presents challenges for theoretical work.

The alveolar duct and its alveoli need to be treated as a single spatial unit with partitions. The smooth wall model of the duct imposes the wrong boundary conditions which distort flow, radial particle diffusion and axial gas diffusion.

Acknowledgements

This work was supported by Grant No. UI-00461 from the National Center for Urban and Industrial Health and is part of a Center programme supported by the Division of Environmental Health Sciences, National Institutes of Health, Grant No. ES-00260. Its background includes discussions with my colleagues N. Nelson, E. D. Palmes, R. E. Albert and C. S. Wang; the oral presentations of W. A. Briscoe, Y. C. Fung, P. G. Saffman, S. K. Friedlander, E. D. Palmes and W. D. Rannie at a conference on Gas Flow and Particle Transport in the Lung held at California Institute of Technology in January, 1968; and studies of aerosol physiology at the Institute of Environmental Medicine that were initiated almost two decades ago by N. Nelson and have received special attention in this review.

REFERENCES

ALBERT, R. E., LIPPMANN, M., SPIEGELMAN, J., LIUZZI, A., and NELSON, N. (1967a). *Archs envir. Hlth*, **14**, 10–15.
ALBERT, R. E., LIPPMANN, M., SPIEGELMAN, J., STREHLOW, C., BRISCOE, W., WOLFSON, P., and NELSON, N. (1967b). In *Inhaled Particles and Vapours II*, pp. 361–378, ed. Davies, C. N. Oxford and New York: Pergamon.
ALTSHULER, B. (1959). *Bull. math. Biophys.*, **21**, 257–270.
ALTSHULER, B. (1961). In *Inhaled Particles and Vapours*, pp. 47–53, ed. Davies, C. N. Oxford and New York: Pergamon.
ALTSHULER, B., and BRISCOE, W. A. (1961). In *The Intrapulmonary Distribution of Gases and Aerosols*, Appendices III and IV. Report for U.S.P.H.S. Grant No. RG-5587, N.Y.U. Institute of Industrial Medicine.
ALTSHULER, B., NELSON, N., and KUSCHNER, M. (1964). *Hlth Phys.*, **10**, 1137–1161.

ALTSHULER, B., PALMES, E. D., and NELSON, N. (1967). In *Inhaled Particles and Vapours II*, pp. 323–337, ed. Davies, C. N. Oxford and New York: Pergamon.
ALTSHULER, B., PALMES, E. D., YARMUS, L., and NELSON, N. (1959). *J. appl. Physiol.*, 14, 321–327.
ALTSHULER, B., YARMUS, L., PALMES, E. D., and NELSON, N. (1957). *A.M.A. Archs ind. Hlth*, 15, 293–303.
BEECKMANS, J. M. (1965a). *Can. J. Physiol. Pharmac.*, 43, 157–172.
BEECKMANS, J. M. (1965b). *Ann. occup. Hyg.*, 8, 221–231.
BROWN, J. H., COOK, K. M., NEY, F. G., and HATCH, T. (1950). *Am. J. publ. Hlth*, 40, 450–458.
CARSLAW, H. S., and JAEGER, J. C. (1959). *Conduction of Heat in Solids*, 2nd edn., p. 319. London: Oxford University Press.
CUMMING, G., CRANK, J., HORSFIELD, K., and PARKER, I. (1966). *Resp. Physiol.*, 1, 58–74.
DAVIES, C. N. (1964). *Ann. occup. Hyg.*, 7, 169–183.
DAVIES, C. N. (1967). In *Assessment of Airborne Radioactivity*, pp. 3–22. Vienna: International Atomic Energy Agency.
DOLLFUSS, R. E., MILIC-EMILI, J., and BATES, D. V. (1967). *Resp. Physiol.*, 2, 234–246.
FINDEISEN, W. (1935). *Pflügers Arch. ges. Physiol.*, 236, 367–379.
FUCHS, N. A. (1964). *The Mechanics of Aerosols*. New York: Macmillan and Oxford: Pergamon.
GLAZIER, J. B., HUGHES, J. M. B., MALONEY, J. E., and WEST, J. B. (1967). *J. appl. Physiol.*, 23, 694–705.
HATCH, T. F., and GROSS, P. (1964). *Pulmonary Deposition and Retention of Inhaled Aerosols*. New York: Academic Press.
HORSFIELD, K., and CUMMING, G. (1967). *Bull. math. Biophys.*, 29, 245–259.
HORSFIELD, K., and CUMMING, G. (1968). *J. appl. Physiol.*, 24, 373–383.
LANDAHL, H. D. (1950). *Bull. math. Biophys.*, 12, 43–56.
LANDAHL, H. D. (1963). *Bull. math. Biophys.*, 25, 29–39.
LANDAHL, H. D., TRACEWELL, T. N., and LASSEN, W. H. (1951). *A.M.A. Archs ind. Hyg.*, 3, 359–366.
LANDAHL, H. D., TRACEWELL, T. N., and LASSEN, W. H. (1952). *A.M.A. Archs ind. Hyg.*, 6, 508–511.
LIPPMANN, M., and ALBERT, R. E. (1968). *Am. ind. Hyg. Ass. J.*, in press.
MUIR, D. C. F. (1967). *J. appl. Physiol.*, 23, 210–214.
PALMES, E. D., ALTSHULER, B., and NELSON, N. (1967). In *Inhaled Particles and Vapours II*, pp. 339–349, ed. Davies, C. N. Oxford and New York: Pergamon.
PALMES, E. D., MARRERO, H. M., and ALTSHULER, B. (1966). *Physiologist, Wash.*, 9, 261.
RAUWERDA, P. E. (1946). *Unequal ventilation of different parts of the lung and determination of cardiac output*. Thesis, Groningen University.
SCHLICHTING, H. (1968). *Boundary-Layer Theory*, 6th edn. New York: McGraw-Hill.
TASK GROUP ON LUNG DYNAMICS (1966). *Hlth Phys.*, 12, 173–207.
WANG, C. S., ALTSHULER, B., and PALMES, E. D. (1968). *J. Colloid Interface Sci.*, 26, 41–44.
WANG, C. S., and FRIEDLANDER, S. K. (1968). *Envir. Sci. Technol.*, submitted.
WEIBEL, E. R. (1963). *Morphometry of the Human Lung*. Berlin: Springer and New York: Academic Press.

DISCUSSION

Philip: What boundary conditions at the surface do you use in analysing deposition by diffusion due to Brownian motion? Do you take a zero concentration condition, with everything arriving at the surface deposited? Is reflection not involved?

Altshuler: Reflection does not appear to happen. When a particle hits the wall it stays there.

Owen: May I follow that up by asking Dr. Altshuler for his views on the problem of a particle diffusing under Brownian motion towards the wall and at the same time being in a Poiseuille flow? Because in such a flow a particle must lag behind the fluid, and accordingly suffer a force which tends to be directed towards the axis of the tube. Have you any idea of the relative magnitudes of the particle mobility due to Brownian diffusion and that due to this lag effect; and is it possible for certain particles under certain conditions not to be able to reach the wall at all, because of such shear forces?

Altshuler: It is my understanding that this is very small compared to other displacements, but I have not looked at it independently.

Burton: Does the charge on the particles affect their deposition? I am thinking of the greater deposition of charged particles on synthetic materials.

Altshuler: Charge is generally considered to have a very small effect on the rate of deposition. It would be more important for very small particles, of diameter $0 \cdot 1$ μm. or less.

Muir: May I ask about the single-breath experiments? Whether you inhale a single breath of aerosol or a slug, the shape of the aerosol concentration curve in the subsequent exhalation does not depend on the duration of the breath. The one factor that governs it is the depth of inhalation. As the depth of inhalation increases the dispersion is that much greater. This seems to make it unlikely that dispersion is related to the movement of the particles themselves, certainly using $0 \cdot 5$ μm. diameter particles, and those are the largest I have used. We thought the dispersion could not be due to turbulence because we know that the Reynolds numbers are much too low in the fine airways of the lung. Then we thought in terms of unequal time constants. This is not very likely in the normal lung, however. Have you any suggestions of what is governing the shape of this curve? What makes the flow non-reversible, because that is really what we are looking at?

Altshuler: We have done some rough calculations of the contribution to dispersion by gravity and Brownian motion which indicate that they do play a significant role. But a proper description of axial dispersion is lacking in this field and I do not have one.

Muir: But have you found it to be time dependent or independent?

Altshuler: We have not done this. I would expect axial dispersion to be time dependent.

Mason: May I go back to the question of reflection of particles? Your idea that there is no reflection is perhaps not very realistic. I assume that the aerosol particles are liquid; then whether or not they are reflected will depend to a large extent on the spreading coefficient of the fluid composing the particle on the particular surface you are talking about. From my experience of coalescence and wetting I would question your assumption.

Altshuler: Both solid and liquid particles are expected to stick for these sizes and conditions. Your experience probably concerned much larger sizes and quite different conditions. Our own experiments have used triphenyl phosphate in the form of supercooled liquid droplets.

Burton: You have not stated whether the *absolute* percentage deposition agrees with prediction, using reasonable parameters. This should indicate whether the assumption of no reflection is a good one.

Altshuler: It is difficult to make comparisons. There is rough agreement in expired concentrations under certain conditions which is better at some sizes and worse at others. (See, for example, Landahl, H. D. [1950]. *Bull. math. Biophys.*, **12**, 43–56 and Landahl, H. D., Tracewell, T. N., and Lassen, W. H. [1951]. *A.M.A. Archs ind. Hyg.*, **3**, 359–366; [1952]. *Ibid.*, **6**, 508–511.)

Philip: But are you really matching parameters?

Altshuler: There are too many undetermined parameters for a simple matching statement. Although there is rough agreement in expired concentrations, predictive values of regional deposition could still be wrong.

Cumming: Dr. Altshuler made the very valid point that the calculations of deposition depend on the model of the lung used. We suggest that a useful model is obtained by counting up, not down, the lung branches. If you look at a cast of the human lung where all the airways have been pruned off at diameters of 750 μm., there is no apparent symmetry at all. In some pathways the end branch at 750 μm. will be reached very quickly, after relatively few branchings, whereas the end branch of another pathway is a great distance away and comes after many more branchings. If you are looking for airways at, say, the tenth generation, in one pathway it may never be reached, in another it may be an airway of 3 mm. diameter, and in other areas it may be down to a few hundred micrometres. We therefore suggest that it would be simpler to count upwards from below, and then all generations are of the same size. But in man it is technically impossible to do this. To get round this we have devised a suggested nomenclature for the airways according to diameter, and we think this gives a more relevant description (see Table I).

TABLE I (Cumming)

SUGGESTED NOMENCLATURE FOR AIRWAYS

Function	Distribution of gas by mass flow			Gas mixing and exchange
Descriptive term	Central airways	Resistance airways	Peripheral airways	Acinus
Anatomical structure	Trachea to BPS branch	BPS branch to small bronchi	Small bronchi to TB	RB and AD
Diameter (mm.)	5·0 and greater	2·0—5·0	0·5—2·0	0·3—0·5
Generation, counting up	20—30	10—20	0—10	—

Abbreviations: BPS = Bronchopulmonary segment
                TB = Terminal bronchiole
                RB = Respiratory bronchiole
                AD = Alveolar duct

In particular it takes account of the fact that, as Professor Mead mentioned, the lung is an asymmetrical structure; any analysis which considers it to be a symmetrical structure may be open to some error.

Altshuler: I agree that asymmetry should be considered. This superimposes more complexity on all the difficulties of the symmetrical model.

Philip: I am interested in Dr. Altshuler's ideas on the velocity distribution in the alveolar ducts, with the suggestion of induced vortices in the alveoli. I take it that he envisages this as Stokes flow (low Reynolds number flow), and I doubt if there will be vortices. Sometimes we tend to carry our intuitions over from high Reynolds number flow where we should not. The appropriate intuition here may be that viscous dissipation (or mean square velocity gradient) is minimized. This would suggest that the streamlines simply fill the whole cross-section as efficiently as possible, and that there is no reverse flow.

Saffman: For a shallow cavity, I think Dr. Philip is quite correct and you would not get the vortex, but if it is a sufficiently deep cavity you would get a vortex at the bottom of the cavity. The vortex would however be rather weak. A numerical solution of the problem would not be hard, and one could also do an experiment, because the geometry is very simple. That would be the easiest way to settle the question.

Davies: These cavities (the alveoli) in man are only about 150 μm. in diameter; in the regions below the respiratory bronchioles, where the alveolation is dense, flow is extremely small and gas exchange is entirely by molecular diffusion. Gas flow is quite irrelevant to it. I support the view that movement in the cavities is of no significance, as regards either gas flow or the deposition of aerosol particles.

Burton: In your experiments in man, how much difference in deposition is there between the horizontal and vertical postures? Or is the geometry such that it would make no difference to the sedimentation factor which way up you were?

Altshuler: We have not done this. A difference in posture will change dimensions in the alveolar space and there will be less change in the conducting airways. The effect then may be greatest for the most stable sizes.

Caro: We recently heard from Dr. J. Milic-Emili of McGill University a revival of the idea that some terminal parts of the airways may be closed off at normal lung volumes. If this is correct, does it provide an opportunity for particles entering these regions to be deposited there?

Mead: It would appear that in young, healthy individuals at ordinary resting end-expiration there is no evidence that any airways are closed off. In older individuals, certainly, and in *any* individual breathing to lower lung volumes, there is evidence of airway closure, and in such cases it must be highly important in studies such as Dr. Altshuler and Dr. Muir do to specify the depths of the breath involved. If the inspiration is initiated from a volume below F.R.C. in healthy individuals, you will preferentially get particles to the upper part of the lung first because the lower region, which is the smaller region, is closed off. Only in later inspirations would these regions receive particles. On the other hand, on expiration, the emptying would be more uniform. So that there is certainly not a reversible process of the distribution of ventilation in a lung over a large breath, in any individual, of whatever age, and with increasing age this is easier to demonstrate at progressively higher lung volumes. This is probably a very important matter to control.

Muir: I found no effect in normal individuals of variation in lung volume when doing single-breath aerosol curves; if you take an inspiration of half a litre of aerosol, at high lung volume or low, the shape of the exhaled aerosol concentration curve is the same.

Altshuler: In breath-holding you see these effects. Recovery of particles is very dependent on lung volume.

Cumming: I agree with Professor Mead that there is no evidence that in a normal human being any part of the lung is closed off, at ordinary lung volumes. Certainly there is evidence of lesser ventilation to the lower lobes but I don't know whether they are closed off. Perhaps this lesser ventilation might explain the greater deposition at lower lung volume, because if little ventilation goes to the bottom and a great deal goes to the upper lobes, the distance to which the interface reaches in the upper lobe is much further than normal. In the first experiment certainly the respiratory bronchioles, the first half of the alveolated ducts, are covered by bulk flow, but the distal ones are not, and the further bulk flow goes, the more likely deposition is to occur.

TURBULENT FLOW AND PARTICLE DEPOSITION IN THE TRACHEA

P. R. Owen

Department of Aeronautics, Imperial College of Science and Technology, London

AT vigorous levels of breathing, such that the rate of intake of air is greater than about 35 l. min.$^{-1}$, the Reynolds number of the flow in the trachea, based on its diameter and mean velocity, exceeds 2,500: a value at which, according to the classical experiments of Reynolds (1883), the motion in a long, straight pipe, in the absence of any special precautions to ensure a smooth flow at its entry, would be turbulent.

While the trachea is reasonably straight, it is not long, extending only to some seven or eight diameters before branching into the main bronchi. It follows that the flow in it is of the "entry" type, characterized by a boundary layer on the wall that gradually encroaches on the central stream. Nonetheless, Reynolds' observations, which were confined to the so-called fully developed flow that is formed after the boundary layer has reached the axis of the pipe, are open to the interpretation that the process of transition to turbulence is initiated in the entry flow, and we accordingly may expect part of the boundary layer on the wall of the trachea to be turbulent. That this part might occupy a substantial proportion of the length of the trachea is further suggested by the probable presence of highly disturbed flow conditions at its entry. Thus, the air entering the trachea by way of the larynx is presumed to take the form of a turbulent jet, the attachment of which to the wall of the infraglottic cavity gives rise to the boundary layer. Generated in those circumstances, the boundary layer is unlikely to exhibit much laminar flow while the stream outside it, in the central region of the pipe, remains turbulent and thereby capable of both disturbing and energetically sustaining it. Such a condition, according to the arguments in the next section, may be expected to be fulfilled when the Reynolds number of the tracheal flow is greater than about 3,000.

If the above, essentially qualitative, argument is accepted and it is agreed that, for flow rates of approximately 40 l. min.$^{-1}$ and above, the boundary layer on the wall of the trachea is predominantly turbulent, at least in that phase of inhalation during which the flow may be regarded as steady, two questions present themselves. First, how far into the respiratory system does

236

the turbulence persist? Secondly, if the inspired air is dust-laden, can the turbulence lead to a profuse deposition of solid particles on the tracheal wall, thus rendering them accessible to removal by ciliary action?

In an attempt to answer those questions, we shall first examine the decay of turbulence in a pipe at Reynolds numbers less than the critical, representative of the flow in generations of airways distant from the trachea. Then the theory of particle deposition from a turbulent airstream will be reconsidered. Next, the effect on the rate of particle deposition of the transport of water vapour from the tracheal wall to the drier inspired air will be estimated. Finally, the possibility of non-hygroscopic particles increasing their size, as a result of water vapour condensing on them during their migration from the central, cooler, unsaturated region of air flow to the warmer, saturated tracheal wall, will be studied.

In brief, it will be demonstrated that the turbulence generated in the trachea may persist as far as the segmental bronchi and perhaps slightly beyond, but that in the upper part of the system, including the trachea and possibly the main bronchi, the radial flow induced by evaporation from the walls of the airways when the air is breathed in through the mouth is sufficiently powerful to inhibit strongly the rate of deposition of the smaller particles (defined as those dependent on Brownian diffusion for their ultimate transport to the wall, and typically less than 1 μm. in diameter). Larger particles, on which the effect of Brownian diffusion is inappreciable, are not impeded by the evaporative flow. At the same time, the humidification of the inspired airstream does not appear to lead to any significant change in size of those particles transported to the wall, through water condensing on their surfaces.

It may therefore be concluded that, in spite of the apparently vigorous mechanism for particle deposition provided by the turbulent flow accompanying rapid inhalation, the upper part of the respiratory tract does not act as an efficient filter to the small particles, which may accordingly be deposited in the deeper parts of the system. In such parts, the secondary flows generated at branches offer an effective fluid dynamical mechanism for promoting deposition, by concentrating particles towards one side of the airway and, by means of the increase in the frictional stress there, facilitating the passage of those particles towards the wall.

DECAY OF TURBULENCE IN THE BRONCHI

Under unexceptional inlet conditions and at a Reynolds number of around 3,000, some ten or more diameters are (theoretically) required for a fully developed flow to be established in a smooth pipe (Latzko, 1921). But the entrance to the trachea provides a special case, since the flow through the glottic aperture presumably detaches from the vocal cords,† forming a jet at whose periphery turbulence is generated. The turbulence then spreads both inwards across the jet and outwards to the wall, on which a boundary layer is formed downstream of the line of attachment of the jet to the surface of the infraglottic cavity, in the manner shown in the highly idealized sketch of Fig. 1.

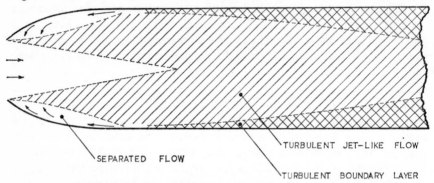

SEPARATED   FLOW

TURBULENT   JET–LIKE   FLOW

TURBULENT   BOUNDARY   LAYER

FIG. 1. A conjectural pattern of flow in the upper part of the trachea at inspired airflow rates exceeding 40 l. min.$^{-1}$

The subsequent growth of the boundary layer is influenced by the turbulent, sheared, jet-like flow in the central part of the trachea and, on that account, is more rapid than that occurring when the central stream is uniform. In certain respects the physical situation resembles that studied by Panofsky and Townsend (1964) in relation to the effect on the atmospheric wind profile of an abrupt change in terrain. They found that the wind profile was influenced within a wedge-shaped region which, far from the discontinuity, was inclined to the surface at an angle of about 6°. In the trachea, the boundary of the wedge-shaped region may be interpreted as the interface between the central jet and the portion of the flow directly affected by the wall: that is to say, the boundary layer, which accordingly would reach the axis of the trachea in some five or six diameters. Naturally, such a result can be treated as only roughly indicative of events in the trachea, but it suggests that the flow at the lower end, where the trachea branches into the main bronchi, cannot be far from fully developed.

As the flow proceeds down the airways its Reynolds number falls, as shown in Table I. The values of velocity and Reynolds number were calculated and kindly supplied to the writer by Dr. R. C. Schroter who based them on average

† An assumption that is commented on at the end of this section.

values of the airway dimensions, as given by Weibel (1963), in each generation of the bronchial tree.

TABLE I

VARIATION OF REYNOLDS NUMBER AND VELOCITY IN THE UPPER AIRWAYS

INSPIRED VOLUME FLOW, 40 l. min.$^{-1}$

Generation	Length/diameter	Velocity cm. sec.$^{-1}$	Reynolds number
Trachea	6·7	263	3,100
Main bronchi	4·0	286	2,290
Lobar bronchi	2·3	314	1,710
Segmental bronchi	1·3	334	1,230

It is evident that at the flow rate of 40 l. min.$^{-1}$, whereas the Reynolds number in the trachea is large enough to sustain a turbulent flow, it is below the critical level in each subsequent branch.

The form of decay law followed by the turbulence may be inferred from an approximate energy equation in which the rate of change of turbulent energy is equated to the difference between the rate of production of energy and its rate of dissipation. Accordingly, if q^2 is a typical turbulent fluctuation in mean square, with components $\overline{u_1'^2}$, $\overline{u_2'^2}$ and $\overline{u_3'^2}$ in the axial (x), radial (r), and circumferential directions respectively, the energy equation becomes

$$\frac{1}{2}\frac{\partial q^2}{\partial t} = \overline{u_1' u_2'}\frac{\partial U}{\partial r} - \varepsilon$$

where ε is the rate of energy dissipation per unit mass of fluid and U is the axial velocity in the mean flow.

Except very close to the wall, an order of magnitude estimate of $\partial U/\partial r$ gives $\partial U/\partial r \sim u_\tau/a$, where a is the radius of the pipe and u_τ is the friction velocity defined by $\rho u_\tau^2 = \tau_0$, in which ρ is the density of the fluid and τ_0 the shearing stress it exerts on the wall.

Also, following Townsend (1956), it may be assumed that

$$\overline{u_1' u_2'} = a_0 q^2$$

a_0 being a constant of order 10^{-1}.

In order to estimate the magnitude of the dissipation term it may be supposed that the small turbulent eddies responsible for the ultimate degradation of the kinetic energy are locally isotropic, in which case

$$\varepsilon = 15\nu \overline{\left(\frac{\partial u_1'}{\partial x}\right)^2} \sim a_2 \frac{\nu q^2}{a^2}$$

where ν is the kinematic viscosity of the fluid and a_2 is a constant of order 10.

In casting the dissipation term into the above form we have made the crucial assumption that in the decay process the energetic turbulent eddies are bounded in size by the walls of the pipe and therefore exhibit a typical dimension comparable with the pipe radius. In consequence, the decay may be expected to follow in time, or distance, a different law from that obeyed by an unbounded field of decaying homogeneous turbulence in which the length scale of the energetic eddies increases as the decay proceeds.

If the turbulence is convected with the mean flow,

$$\frac{\partial q^2}{\partial t} = \bar{U}\frac{\partial q^2}{\partial x}$$

where $\bar{U}$ is the mean axial velocity averaged across the pipe. Consequently, the energy equation may be written

$$\frac{dw}{d\xi} = 2a_1 w - 4a_2 w/R \qquad (1)$$

where $w = q/\bar{U}$, $\xi = x/d$, d is the pipe diameter and R is the Reynolds number, $\bar{U}d/v$; $a_1 = a_0 (u_\tau/\bar{U})$ and is of order 10^{-2}.

(1) is integrated to give

$$w/w_0 = \exp\{(2a_1 - 4a_2/R)(\xi - \xi_0)\} \qquad (2)$$

in which w_0 is the initial value of w at $\xi = \xi_0$.

The exponential law of decay appears to agree quite well with the measurements of decaying turbulence in a pipe made by Sibulkin (1962). His observed

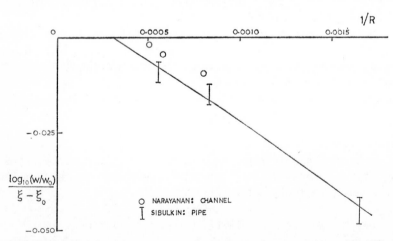

FIG. 2. The decay of turbulence in a pipe and channel at subcritical Reynolds numbers.

values of w (on the axis of the pipe) are incorporated in Fig. 2, where $(\xi - \xi_0)^{-1}\log_{10}(w/w_0)$ is plotted against $1/R$. From the straight line drawn through the experimental points it appears that $a_1 = 0\cdot011$ and $a_2 = 17\cdot9$: values which conform, in order of magnitude, to the estimates made above.

The results of more recent work by Narayanan (1968) are also shown in Fig. 2. They apply to the decaying turbulent flow in a channel. Again, the exponential form of decay appears to be obeyed although, not unexpectedly, the constants in (2) are different from those applicable to a pipe. Narayanan also estimated the integral scale of the turbulence and found, as argued above, that it was comparable with the lateral dimension of the flow.

We now apply (2) piecemeal to the bronchial tree, with an allowance made by means of Batchelor's (1953) theory for the change in turbulent energy accompanying the (assumed rapid) contraction of the flow at a bifurcation. At an inspired volume flow of 40 l. min.$^{-1}$, in the segmental bronchi where the Reynolds number falls to 1,230 (see Table I) the value of w has diminished only to roughly half its value at the end of the trachea.

In generations of airways deeper than the segmental bronchi a marked decrease in Reynolds number occurs and the rate of decay of the turbulence becomes greatly enhanced.

It appears, therefore, that if turbulence is generated in the trachea, its subsequent decay in the bronchi is initially slow. (At inspired flow rates greater than 40 l. min.$^{-1}$ it would be even slower.)

In arriving at this conclusion we have ignored an important feature of the flow: namely the swirling secondary motions created at branch junctions. Their effect on the turbulence is difficult to assess, although it is possible that a secondary flow might assist the decay, tending to concentrate the region of turbulent energy production towards one side of the branch and to distribute that energy by convection over the remaining extensive regions of the flow, where it is dissipated. That must, however, be treated as a conjecture. Another conjecture, implicit in the argument about the conditions at entry to the trachea, concerns the extent to which the glottic slit distends to admit rapid flow into the trachea. The assumption has been made that the distension, at any rate when the volume flow of inspired air is 40 l. min.$^{-1}$, is not sufficient to prevent separation from the vocal cords, for if it were, and the downstream flow were initially laminar, the blockage area presented by the cords would have to be less than about 10 per cent of the cross-sectional area of the trachea: and that, from the anatomical information available, seems to be unlikely. However, the possibility of an unseparated flow through the glottic slit must be allowed for, in which case transition to turbulence would occur in the boundary layer on the tracheal wall at a larger Reynolds number than 3,000 and full development of the pipe-flow would not be achieved within the trachea. In those circumstances, the rate of decay of the turbulence previously calculated is likely to be an underestimate, but the conclusions reached in the remainder of the paper are unaffected, except that the lowest rate of inspired airflow to which they apply would be greater than 40 l. min.$^{-1}$

PARTICLE DEPOSITION

The presumed existence of a turbulent flow in the trachea, confined mainly to the boundary layer on its wall, implies a powerful mechanism for assisting deposition of particles that may be present in the inspired air.

In general, the transport of fine, solid particles from a turbulent gas stream to an adjoining surface is achieved principally by turbulent diffusion, in which the particles acquire a motion in response to the fluctuating gas velocities in their immediate neighbourhood. But very close to the wall, within the so-called viscous sub-layer, the turbulent fluctuations are evanescent and some additional process is required to enable a particle to achieve the final motion needed to make an impact with the wall. For larger particles, not susceptible of any significant Brownian diffusion, it has been argued by Friedlander and Johnstone (1957), Owen (1960) and Davies (1966a) that projection towards the wall occurs as a result of the action of turbulent eddies outside the viscous sub-layer. We shall briefly reconsider this view later. Smaller particles, on the other hand, are capable of traversing the viscous sub-layer by means (largely) of Brownian diffusion (Davies, 1966b). Very broadly speaking, the distinction between the two mechanisms emerges at a particle diameter of the order of a micrometre.

Regarding the larger particles, it appears that the projection theory is difficult to reconcile with the requirement that, in order to respond fully to the turbulent fluctuations just outside the viscous sub-layer, the relaxation time of a particle must be shorter than the lifetime of the eddy in which it is entangled; yet to traverse the neighbouring viscous sub-layer unimpeded, its relaxation time must be longer than the characteristic times of the eddies there. In order to overcome this difficulty a different mechanism is proposed. The revised argument is based on the hypothesis that particles are *convected* to the wall from the region of energetic turbulent motion outside the viscous sub-layer by the occasional eddy that encroaches on it, as sketched in a much simplified way in Fig. 3. Such an eddy may occur in response to the sporadic violent eruption from the viscous sub-layer observed by Kline and co-workers (1967) or simply as a chance event. The region adjacent to the wall, in which particle convection is dominant, is distinguished from that further from the wall, in which turbulent diffusion is dominant, by the condition that in the former region the relaxation time of the particle is equal to or greater than the characteristic eddy time. If we take account of the variety of eddy sizes available to perform the convection, as well as the particle's sluggish response to the turbulent velocity, and use the fact that the measurements of Laufer (1954) in the flow outside the viscous sub-layer are consistent with the component of turbulent velocity normal to the wall, in root mean square, increasing

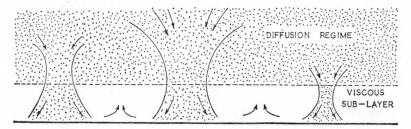

Fig. 3. Rough sketch of the assumed eddy system responsible for the convection of particles to a wall. The main flow is normal to the plane of the paper.

with distance from the wall like its one-third power, we can show that the number N of particles deposited in unit time on unit area of the wall from a stream in which the concentration of particles by number is ψ_0 is given by

$$N = k u_\tau \psi_0 \sigma^2 \qquad (3)$$

Here k is a constant, estimated to be of order 10^{-4} in magnitude, u_τ is the friction velocity, and

$$\sigma = u_\tau^2 \tau^* / \nu$$

σ is a measure of the ratio of the relaxation time of a particle, τ^*, to the characteristic time of an eddy in the viscous sub-layer and is related to the particle and flow properties by

$$\sigma = \frac{1}{18} \frac{\rho_p}{\rho} \left(\frac{u_\tau d}{\nu} \right)^2$$

in which ρ and ρ_p are respectively the densities of the gas and of the particulate material, and d is the particle diameter.

Although obtained according to a different set of physical assumptions, (3) is similar to the equation for the particle flux derived by Friedlander and Johnstone (1957); it is not therefore surprising that with a suitable choice of the constant k, $2\cdot 8 \times 10^{-4}$, (3) can be fitted to their measurements, as shown

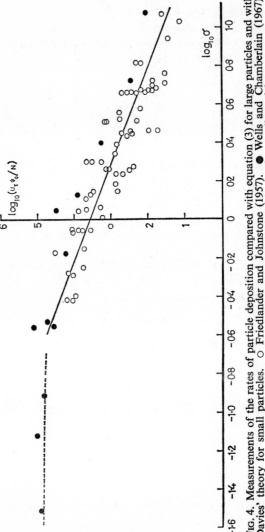

Fig. 4. Measurements of the rates of particle deposition compared with equation (3) for large particles and with Davies' theory for small particles. ○ Friedlander and Johnstone (1957). ● Wells and Chamberlain (1967). ——— $N/u_\tau \psi_0 = 2.8 \times 10^{-4} \sigma^2$. ---- Davies' (1966b) theory for small particles.

in Fig. 4. That figure also contains some more recent deposition measurements by Wells and Chamberlain (1967).

There is an important restriction on (3), for it evidently cannot be valid for indefinitely small values of σ (nor for values in excess of about ten, but for a different reason which need not concern us here). This is because, as σ is reduced, the diffusion regime progressively approaches the viscous sub-layer, a region of uniformly small turbulent eddies and characteristic times. Once the boundary between the diffusion and convection regimes reaches the edge of the viscous sub-layer any further reduction in σ, for a given value of the particle concentration (which is distributed very nearly uniformly throughout the diffusion regime), cannot lead to a change in the deposition rate. Moreover, that deposition rate must persist even when the particle size, hence σ, becomes so small that Brownian diffusion provides the dominant means of transporting particles across the viscous sub-layer.

The residual deposition rate for small values of σ can be estimated by matching the solutions for large particles, where the final stage of the transport is accomplished convectively, and for small particles (less than 1 μm.) where it is achieved principally through Brownian diffusion. A solution in the latter case has been given by Davies (1966b) and can be written

$$N = u_\tau \, \psi_0 \, Df(z) \cdot \frac{1}{v\lambda} \qquad (4)$$

where D is the Brownian diffusivity, $\lambda = (D/bv)^{1/2}$, $z = \frac{1}{2}(u_\tau d/v)\lambda^{-1}$ and

$$f(z) = \left\{ \frac{\pi}{2\sqrt{3}} - \frac{1}{6}\log\left[\frac{(1+z)^2}{(1-z+z^2)}\right] - \frac{1}{\sqrt{3}}\tan^{-1}\left(\frac{2z-1}{\sqrt{3}}\right) \right\}^{-1}$$

b is the constant appearing in the assumed law of variation of the eddy viscosity in the viscous sub-layer with distance, y, from the wall: namely $bv(yu_\tau/v)^3$. Its value is here taken to be 10^{-3}.†

A consideration of (3) and (4) in the light of the experimental results of Wells and Chamberlain (1967), which covered both small and effectively large particles, suggests that the residual deposition rate, n_0, for small σ is roughly 3×10^{-6}.

In ordinary circumstances such a small value of n_0, which must be added to the right of (4), hardly disturbs Davies' solution; but it is significant in the case of a wet, evaporating surface, which we shall examine in the next section.

† We have worked out the equivalent of equation (4) on the basis of a variation of the eddy viscosity with distance from the wall like $(yu_\tau/v)^n$, where n can take values between 2 and 3. The best, and only acceptable, agreement with the experimental results of Wells and Chamberlain (1967) is obtained by setting n equal to 3.

DEPOSITION ON TO AN EVAPORATING SURFACE: APPLICATION TO THE TRACHEA

If the mucous lining to the trachea can be regarded as saturated with water at body temperature whereas the inspired air, if drawn in through the mouth, as during the inhalation of tobacco smoke, is saturated at some lower temperature, evaporation must take place from the tracheal wall across the boundary layer and continue, possibly into the bronchi, until the airstream is uniformly humidified.

The motion of the water vapour away from the wall induces a similar motion in the air, whose velocity in the neighbourhood of the wall can be shown to be

$$v_0 = \frac{m_a}{m_w} \frac{G}{\rho} \tag{5}$$

where m_a and m_w are respectively the molecular weights of air and water, ρ is the air density and G the mass rate of evaporation of the water from unit area of the wall.

G may be roughly estimated by using Reynolds' analogy between the turbulent transport of momentum and matter as, for example, explained by Owen and Ormerod (1954) with the result

$$G = \frac{u_\tau^2}{U}(\rho_{s1} - \rho_{s0}) \tag{6}$$

in which U is the air velocity in the central part of the trachea, ρ_{s0} the density of the water vapour there and ρ_{s1} the corresponding density at the wall.

Inserting in (6) the values of ρ_{s0} and ρ_{s1} appropriate to saturation at temperatures of 20°c and 37°c (thus ignoring any change in temperature that occurs upstream of the trachea, which may be permissible for mouth breathing) we obtain from (5)

$$\frac{v_0}{u_\tau} = 3 \cdot 4 \times 10^{-2} \frac{u_\tau}{U} \tag{7}$$

Since, typically, u_τ/U is around $1/20$, (7) becomes

$$v_0/u_\tau \approx 10^{-3}$$

Evidently the radial flow induced by the evaporation is very small; at an inspired flow rate of 40 l. min.$^{-1}$ it amounts to a velocity of about $0 \cdot 1$ mm. sec.$^{-1}$ Nonetheless, it is not small compared with, and may indeed be much larger than, the velocities of migration of small particles across the viscous

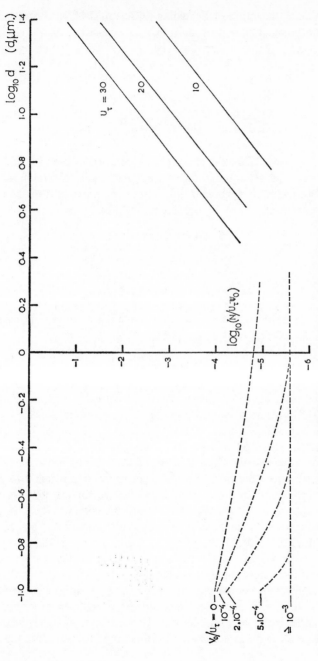

Fig. 5. Estimated rates of particle deposition in the trachea.

9

sub-layer under the action of Brownian diffusion. In fact, were it not for the existence of the residual deposition rate, n_0, discussed in the previous section, all particles below 1 μm. in size would be prevented from reaching the tracheal surface.

Taking account of the term n_0, as well as the velocity v_0, the equation for the transport of particles across the viscous sub-layer is

$$N - n_0 = (by_\tau^3 + D/\nu) u_\tau \frac{d\psi}{dy_\tau} - v_0 \psi \tag{8}$$

in which $y_\tau = yu_\tau/\nu$. When the particle concentration at the edge of the viscous sub-layer, $y_\tau = 5$, is set equal to ψ_0, its value in the central stream (an equality very closely assured by turbulent diffusion in the outer part of the boundary layer, provided that $v_0/u_\tau \ll 1$), the integral of (8) is

$$N - n_0 = v_0 \psi_0 (e^\zeta - 1)^{-1} \tag{9}$$

where

$$\zeta = \frac{v_0}{u_\tau} \cdot \frac{\lambda\nu}{D} \cdot \frac{1}{f(z)}$$

in which λ, D, z and $f(z)$ have the same meanings as in (4). For sufficiently small d, $z \approx 0$ and $f(z)$ can be approximated by

$$f(z) \approx \frac{2\pi}{3\sqrt{3}} - z$$

For larger particles, insensitive to Brownian diffusion, a value of v_0 as small as $10^{-3} u_\tau$ can have no appreciable effect on their rate of deposition, because the eddies responsible for the final, convective stage of the transport to the wall possess velocities of order u_τ.

The rate of deposition of particles in the trachea has been calculated from (3) and (9) for a number of values of u_τ, corresponding roughly to flow rates of from 40 l. min.$^{-1}$ to 100 l. min.$^{-1}$, as well as for evaporative velocities ranging from zero to $10^{-3} u_\tau$ and greater, and is shown in Fig. 5. The density of the particulate material is assumed to be 1,800 times that of air. The straight lines on the right of the figure apply to the larger particles, whose rates of deposition are governed by (3), whereas the lower broken curves are appropriate to particles undergoing Brownian diffusion.

It is clear from the figure that an evaporative motion near the wall, such that $v_0/u_\tau \approx 10^{-3}$, will decrease markedly the deposition of particles under 1 μm. (at least as far as a diameter of 10^{-1} μm.; smaller particles still can participate so strongly in a Brownian diffusion as to overcome the repulsive effect of the radial flow at the wall), thus weakening the effectiveness of the trachea as a fine particle filter. However, the small particles, in traversing the boundary layer from a region of low specific humidity to one of higher, might collect so much water by condensation on their surfaces as to be converted to large particles. We shall study, and reject, that possibility in the next section.

THE CONDENSATION OF WATER VAPOUR ON TO NON-HYGROSCOPIC PARTICLES

Condensation can occur on a particle if the concentration of water vapour in its vicinity is higher than that at its surface, a condition that can in turn be satisfied in a saturated atmosphere only if the temperature of the particle is lower than that of its immediate surroundings. In traversing the boundary layer on the tracheal wall a particle moves not merely into a region of higher humidity but into one of higher temperature. In addition, water vapour condensing on its surface contributes its latent heat to the particle, so that it is not at all obvious that the particle can maintain a sufficiently large temperature difference from its environment for appreciable condensation to occur.

In order to resolve the problem, we first of all note that the mass flux of vapour from a gas containing a mass concentration c of water to a small, wet, spherical particle, of radius a, at whose surface the water vapour concentration is c_1, can be shown to be

$$G = \{4\pi aj(c - c_1)\}\left\{1 + \frac{2-\alpha}{\alpha}\left(\frac{j}{\nu}\right)\left(\frac{L}{a}\right)\left(\frac{m_w}{m_a}\right)^{1/2}\right\}^{-1} \tag{10}$$

Here j is the diffusivity of water vapour in air, m_w and m_a, as previously defined, are the respective molecular weights of water and air, α is an accommodation coefficient which according to Oswatitsch (1942) and Fuchs (1959) is equal to $0 \cdot 03$, and L is the molecular mean free path in the gas (which enters into the equation to enable particles of radii not necessarily very large compared with the mean free path to be considered).

An equation analogous to (10) may be derived for the heat transfer Q into a particle at a temperature T_1 from a gas at temperature T. It is

$$Q = \{4\pi aK(T - T_1)\}\left\{1 + \frac{2-\beta}{\beta}\left(\frac{2\gamma}{\gamma+1}\right)\frac{1}{\bar{\sigma}}\left(\frac{L}{a}\right)\right\}^{-1}$$

$$= 4\pi aK(T - T_1)B \tag{11}$$

K is the thermal conductivity of air, γ the ratio of its specific heats, $\bar{\sigma}$ the Prandtl number, equal to $0 \cdot 72$, and β a thermal accommodation coefficient whose value is likely to be of order unity for a non-hygroscopic surface.

In addition, heat is transferred into the particle at a rate Gh_L, where h_L is the latent heat of condensation of a unit mass of water vapour.

Equation (10) may be put into a more convenient form by writing

$$c - c_1 = \frac{m_w}{\bar{R}} \left\{ \frac{p_s(T)}{T} - \frac{p_s(T_1)}{T_1} \right\} \tag{12}$$

in which p_s is the vapour pressure of water and $\bar{R}$ the gas constant, $8 \cdot 31 \times 10^7$ erg. °c^{-1}. If the temperature difference $(T_0 - T_1)$ is small,

$$\frac{p_s(T)}{T} - \frac{p_s(T_1)}{T_1} \approx (T - T_1) \frac{d}{dT} \left(\frac{p_s}{T} \right)$$

$$= (T - T_1) \frac{p_s(T)}{T^2} \left(\frac{m_w h_L}{\bar{R}T} - 1 \right) \tag{13}$$

where use has been made of the Clausius-Clapeyron equation

$$\frac{dp_s}{dT} = \frac{m_w h_L p_s}{\bar{R}T^2}$$

Consequently

$$G = 4\pi a j (T - T_1) H(T) \tag{14}$$

where

$$H(T) = p_s(T) m_w \{(m_w h_L / \bar{R}T - 1)\} \left\{ 1 + \frac{2 - \alpha}{\alpha} \left(\frac{j}{\nu} \right) \left(\frac{L}{a} \right) \left(\frac{m_w}{m_a} \right)^{1/2} \right\}^{-1}$$

Since the total rate of heat transfer into the particle is $Gh_L + Q$, that quantity must equal the time rate of change of $mc_d T_1$, c_d being the specific heat of the particulate material and m its mass (the contribution to the heat capacity of the particle from its liquid sheath is ignored). It follows that the difference in temperature between the particle and its surroundings at time t is proportional to

$$\exp\{-(4\pi a/mc_d)[jH(T)h_L + BK]t\}$$

so that the quantity

$$t^* = (mc_d/4\pi a)\{jH(T)h_L^- + BK\}^{-1} \tag{15}$$

describes a thermal relaxation time which a particle requires in order to adjust its temperature from that of one environment to that of another.

Now consider a particle engaged in a turbulent diffusion in the y-direction through a gas whose temperature T is a function of y, the distance from the surface on to which it is ultimately deposited. The particle, in its travel, samples many gas temperatures and but for the fact that it has a preferred direction of drift towards the surface $y = 0$, would acquire on the average at each value of y the gas temperature $T(y)$. However, the effect of a turbulent excursion in the y-direction with velocity v' is a lag between the particle temperature and the gas temperature by an amount $v' t^* dT/dy$. If there are on average ψ particles in a unit volume at the level y and of these ψ' engage in a vertical turbulent excursion, the mean temperature lag experienced by the particles is

$$\frac{1}{\psi} \overline{v' \psi'} \, t^* \frac{dT}{dy}$$

But the quantity $\overline{v' \psi'}$ is equal to (minus) the net rate of particle transport across the flow towards the surface $y = 0$. Hence the temperature lag, averaged among the particles at any level y, is

$$\overline{(T - T_1)} = -\frac{N}{\psi} t^* \frac{dT}{dy}$$

and, from (14), the corresponding rate of increase in the mass of a particle is

$$\frac{dm}{dt} = -4\pi a j N t^* H(\bar{T}) \frac{1}{\psi} \frac{dT}{dy} \qquad (16)$$

in which for simplicity $H(\bar{T})$ is calculated at some temperature $\bar{T}$ of the gas between its extremes.

As N/ψ is the average velocity of migration towards the surface, (16) becomes

$$\frac{dm}{dy} = -4\pi a j t^* H(\bar{T}) \frac{dT}{dy}$$

which, by integration and the use of (15), gives for the fractional change in mass

$$\frac{\Delta m}{m} = c_d (T_a - T_0) \{ h_L + BK/jH(\bar{T}) \}^{-1} \qquad (17)$$

T_0 is the temperature of the stream outside the boundary layer and T_a that near the surface, but outside the viscous sub-layer.

For the inspired flow through the trachea, $(T - T_a)$ is of the order of $10°$ c. According to (17), the change in particle mass is of the order of 1 per cent, which is negligibly small.

SUMMARY

At inspired flow rates of 40 l. min.$^{-1}$ and greater, the boundary layer on the tracheal wall is largely turbulent. If in addition it may be supposed that the air entering the trachea separates from the vocal cords, it is argued that almost fully developed turbulent pipe flow exists at the lower end of the trachea, the subsequent decay of which is slow and may not be complete even within the segmental bronchi.

The existence of turbulence in the trachea, and the powerful mechanism for solid particle deposition it normally provides, might imply that the trachea acts as a particle filter, thereby protecting the deeper parts of the respiratory tract from impact. Such an argument would be effective but for the fact that, during mouth breathing at any rate, the trachea acts as a humidifier to the inspired air. The normal rate of evaporation from the tracheal wall leads to a radial motion sufficient to impede the deposition of all but the finest (less than $0 \cdot 1$ μm.) and coarsest (greater than 1 μm.) particles on to the tracheal wall.

The possibility that, in traversing the boundary layer, particles collect water and consequently increase in size is rejected.

REFERENCES

BATCHELOR, G. K. (1953). *The Theory of Homogeneous Turbulence.* London: Cambridge University Press.

DAVIES, C. N. (1966*a*). *Proc. R. Soc. A*, **289**, 235–246.

DAVIES, C. N. (1966*b*). *Proc. R. Soc. A*, **290**, 557–562.

FRIEDLANDER, S. K., and JOHNSTONE, H. F. (1957). *Ind. Engng Chem.*, **49**, 1151–1156.

FUCHS, N. A. (1959). *Evaporation and Droplet Growth in Gaseous Media.* Oxford: Pergamon Press.

KLINE, S. J., REYNOLDS, W. C., SCHRAUB, F. A., and RUNSTADLER, P. W. (1967). *J. Fluid Mech.*, **4**, 741–773.

LATZKO, H. (1921). *Zeit. angew. Math. Mech.*, **1**, 277–280.

LAUFER, J. (1954). *Natn. Advis. Comm. Aeronaut. Technol. Note* 2954.

NARAYANAN, M. A. B. (1968). *J. Fluid Mech.*, **31**, 609–623.

OSWATITSCH, K. (1942). *Zeit. angew. Math. Mech.*, **22**, 1–14.

OWEN, P. R. (1960). In *Aerodynamic Capture of Particles*, pp. 8–25, ed. Richardson, E. G., and Morgan, B. B. Oxford: Pergamon Press.

OWEN, P. R., and ORMEROD, A. O. (1954). *Rep. Memo. aeronaut. Res. Comm. (Coun.)*, 2875.

PANOFSKY, H. A., and TOWNSEND, A. A. (1964). *Q. Jl R. met. Soc.*, **90**, 147–155.

REYNOLDS, O. (1883). *Phil. Trans. R. Soc.*, **174**, 935–982.

SIBULKIN, M. (1962). *Physics Fluids*, **5**, 280–284.

TOWNSEND, A. A. (1956). *The Structure of Turbulent Shear Flow.* London: Cambridge University Press.

WEIBEL, E. R. (1963). *Morphometry of the Human Lung.* Berlin: Springer.

WELLS, A. C., and CHAMBERLAIN, A. C. (1967). *Br. J. appl. Phys.*, **18**, 1793–1799.

DISCUSSION

Davies: If we accept Professor Owen's figures for inhalation, we have to remember that when ordinary, moderately dry air is inhaled it cools the surface and removes moisture as it sweeps through the trachea; in the course of moving down towards lower regions of the lung the air becomes very nearly saturated (but not quite, because it is in equilibrium with isotonic solution) and then, on the way up again, it gives some moisture and heat back to the upper parts of the respiratory tract. So that whereas particles will be projected slightly away from the surface on the way in, particles of fairly penetrating sizes (between $0 \cdot 2$ and $1 \cdot 0$ μm.) will receive a reciprocal impulsion towards the surface on the way out. The work of A. C. Chamberlain and E. D. Dyson ([1955]. *A.E.R.E. HP/R* 1737, Harwell) using radon and thoron emanation—experiments from which the water problem was absent—roughly bears out molecular diffusion theory for these tiny particles.

On the question of evaporation and its effect on particle deposition, calculation indicates that the growth of particles during the penetration of the trachea is small; in the case of tobacco smoke it appears that you have not necessarily to inhale *deeply*, but to carry the tobacco smoke down into the larger passages of the respiratory tract and hold it there for about 3 or 4 seconds to get the full degree of growth and to equilibrate it with the isotonic solution at about $99 \cdot 3$ per cent relative humidity. The work of L. Dautrebande and W. Walkenhorst ([1961]. In *Inhaled Particles and Vapours*, pp. 110–120, ed. Davies, C. N. Oxford: Pergamon Press) indicates that small inhaled particles of sodium chloride contribute to this humidity.

Burton: During the war we studied the evaporation and humidity relations in the respiratory tract of dogs. We were interested in whether breathing air at $-40°$ F compared to $+40°$ F (Armstrong, H. G., Burton, A. C., and Hall, G. E. [1958]. *J. Aviat. Med.*, **29**, 593) made any difference to the temperature of the lungs. The results showed that there is remarkably good air conditioning regarding *humidity* before air reaches the neck, and I doubt if any moisture is added to the inspired air, at normal breathing rates (I don't know about very high breathing rates), below the level of the thyroid. There is really very complete equilibration of the water vapour before that.

Owen: This is a point I did try to seek data on, but unfortunately almost all I could find were really applicable to nose breathing where the humidification you describe certainly occurs. I should have thought that the less tortuous path taken by the air during mouth breathing would lead to a less complete humidification.

In any case, you will notice that Fig. 5 (p. 247) presents estimates of the deposition rates for various magnitudes of the evaporative velocity. Even when that velocity is $5 \times 10^{-4} u_\tau$, such as would occur when the air entering the trachea was saturated at a temperature only about 2° c lower than the body temperature, deposition of particles in the size range $0 \cdot 2$–$2 \cdot 0$ μm. is strongly inhibited.*

Burton: Temperature equilibration occurs even sooner than equilibration of water vapour; there is no difference in the temperatures in the respiratory tract when the dog is breathing air at $-40°$ F or at $+40°$ F, below the level of the thyroid. This was an anaesthetized dog, not intubated, so I suppose it was breathing through the mouth.

Cumming: The inadequacy of the trachea to act as a humidifier is exemplified very clearly by the behaviour of a patient with a tracheostomy, in which the nasopharynx is therefore eliminated; it is common for the trachea to dry out and to encrust.

Professor Owen, did you say that the developed turbulence in the trachea decays more rapidly as a result of the branching in the early segments, but that branching in later segments produces secondary flow?

Owen: That is what I was implying, although secondary flows are present in both cases, but the argument is a rather vague one and I am not certain of it. I believe that if a secondary motion is set up in a turbulent flow and if that flow is decaying, the secondary motions may assist the decay.

Davies: I like the idea of the adventitious eddy; I was surprised when I first worked out the theory of turbulent deposition that such sensitivity was shown to conditions extremely near the surface; it has been confirmed experimentally by A. C. Wells and A. C. Chamberlain ([1967]. *Br. J. appl. Phys.* **18**, 1793–1799) that a surprisingly small degree of roughness on the surface has a very large influence. There is no doubt that the occasional impact on the surface of the adventitious eddy would have a very important effect.

Saffman: May I ask Professor Owen how much his results depend upon his particular model of the viscous sub-layer, as that unfortunately is the part of turbulent flow about which we know the least? I find it a little difficult to reconcile his Fig. 3 (p. 243) with the observations by S. J. Kline and his

---

* *Note added in proof:* Professor Lighthill has drawn attention to the work of Dr. H. E. Lewis at the National Institute for Medical Research, Hampstead. He has used schlieren cine-photography to study the pattern of airflow around the human body, and has demonstrated that a layer of air about 1 cm. thick is convected up the front surface of the body when erect. This layer is closely attached to the surface of the skin; when it reaches the mouth or nose some of this air is inspired and this accounts for about 10 to 15 per cent of the tidal volume, the rest coming from the ambient air. This 10 to 15 per cent will have been at least partially humidified during its passage over the skin.—Eds.

colleagues ([1967]. *J. Fluid Mech.*, **30**, 741–773) on the way the viscous sub-layer interacts with the flow outside it.

Owen: I have taken Kline's work into account, and it was largely his observations which suggested the model I put forward—that is to say, rapid eruptions outwards accompanied by slower motions towards the wall.

Saffman: The motion towards the wall would be rather slow so that particles would really move with the fluid? I thought you were assuming that the particles were not moving with the fluid as it approached the wall.

Owen: They do not necessarily move with the fluid because the fluid itself may also be decelerated quite rapidly as it approaches the wall.

Philip: Professor Owen, I take it that your theory of deposition involves this rule that everything that arrives at the wall stays on the wall?

Owen: Yes.

PULMONARY CAPILLARY FLOW, DIFFUSION VENTILATION AND GAS EXCHANGE

JOHN B. WEST, JON B. GLAZIER, JOHN M. B. HUGHES AND
JOHN E. MALONEY

Department of Medicine, Royal Postgraduate Medical School, London

CAPILLARY MORPHOLOGY AND BLOOD VOLUME

FOR several years we have been interested in the effect of gravity on the distribution of blood flow in the lung. Recently we have studied the regional differences of capillary blood volume and capillary morphology which result from the increase in vascular pressures down the lung.

The measurements were made on excised perfused dog lungs which were rapidly frozen by flooding with liquid freon cooled to about −150°C (Glazier *et al.*, 1969). Staub and Storey (1962) showed in this way that the outer few millimetres of tissue could be fixed within a few seconds with no measurable distortion. The tissue was then freeze-dried, and sections 2 μm. thick were stained and mounted for microscopic examination.

Three types of measurements were made: the number of red blood cells per unit length of septum, the mean width of the capillaries, and the proportion of the septum occupied by red blood cells. In a series of lungs, the effects of changing vascular and alveolar pressures were studied with particular attention to the relationship of downstream pressure to alveolar pressure; that is, venous pressure was set lower than alveolar pressure (Zone II) or higher (Zone III).

RED BLOOD CELLS PER UNIT LENGTH OF SEPTUM

When pulmonary arterial pressure was less than alveolar pressure (Zone I), there were less than 0·5 red blood cells per 10 μm. of septum. We have

---

FIG. 1. Photomicrographs of sections of dog lungs rapidly frozen while being perfused at various vascular pressures. Sections are 2 μm. thick. A shows the appearance when arterial pressure was 24 cm. less than alveolar pressure (high Zone I). In B, arterial pressure was 5 cm. water higher than alveolar pressure but venous pressure was much lower (Zone II). In C, both arterial and venous pressures were about 44 cm. water higher than alveolar pressure (Zone III). D shows a high-power view of distended capillaries low in Zone III where the capillary pressure was 88 cm. water higher than alveolar pressure. (From Glazier *et al.*, 1969, with permission of the *Journal of Applied Physiology*.)

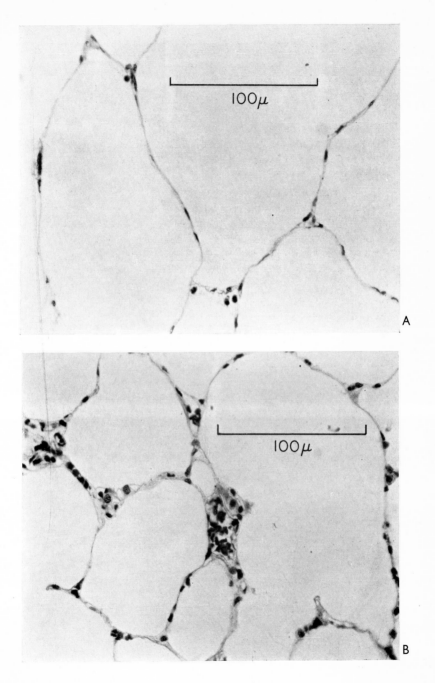

A

B

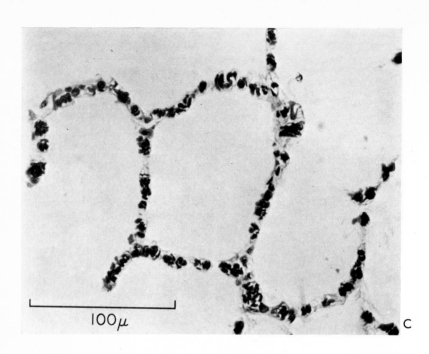

C

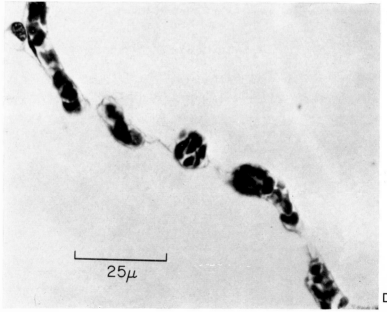

D

previously found that under these conditions, a zone of no blood flow can be demonstrated using radioactive xenon (West, Dollery and Naimark, 1964). The mean capillary width was only 2·3 μm., and the characteristically thin alveolar septa can be seen in Fig. 1A. There was evidence that the trapped red blood cells high in this zone were compressed and elongated since their average length along the septum (5·39 ± 0·12 μm.) exceeded their maximum dimensions in the fully open capillaries low in Zone III (see below).

The numbers of red blood cells increased rapidly as pulmonary arterial pressure was raised above alveolar pressure. Fig. 2 shows an almost linear

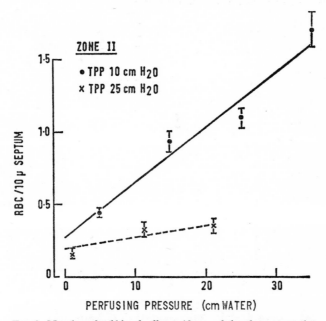

FIG. 2. Number of red blood cells per 10 μm. of alveolar septum plotted against distance down Zone II. Since arterial pressure rises at the rate of about 1 cm. water per cm. distance, the abscissa is here shown as perfusing pressure (in relation to alveolar pressure). Venous pressure was low. Measurements are shown at transpulmonary pressures (TPP) of 10 and 25 cm. water. Note the rapid increase in red cell concentration down the lung and the great reduction which occurred when lung volume was increased.

increase in red blood cells per 10 μm. of septum with distance down Zone II, which accords with the rapid increase in blood flow down this zone. The typically patchy opening up of the capillaries is seen in Fig. 1B where the perfusing pressure was 5 cm. water above alveolar pressure. Some septa still contained no red blood cells whereas others had strings of erythrocytes (see below).

Red cell density also increased down Zone III but less rapidly than down Zone II. Nine of the lungs which were frozen under Zone III conditions had an arterial–venous pressure difference of 4 cm. water or less. Thus if we take the capillary pressure to be halfway between arterial and venous pressures, we cannot be in error by more than 2 cm. water. Accordingly the number of red blood cells has been plotted against capillary pressure in Fig. 3. Note that under these conditions, the red blood cell concentration becomes a manometer of pulmonary capillary pressure.

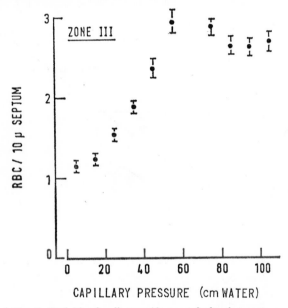

Fig. 3. Red blood cells per 10 μm. of alveolar septum plotted against distance down Zone III. Since the arterial–venous pressure was small (less than 1 cm. water in six lungs and not more than 4 cm. water in the other three), the abscissa can be labelled capillary pressure with little error. Note the rapid increase in red cell concentration with capillary pressure up to about 50 cm. water but the little subsequent change.

Fig. 3 shows that the number of red blood cells increased quickly up to a capillary pressure of about 50 cm. water but there was then no further change. The appearance when the capillary pressure was 44 cm. water is shown in Fig. 1c. The mean of the red blood cell counts for capillary pressures over the range 50–105 cm. water was 2·8 (standard deviation 0·1), which presumably represents the maximum red blood cell concentration attainable in the dog lung. This corresponds to about 14 red blood cells per average septum.

CAPILLARY WIDTH

This was measured by projecting film strips on to a screen, the final magnification being 4,500. The mean width of the capillaries was obtained by

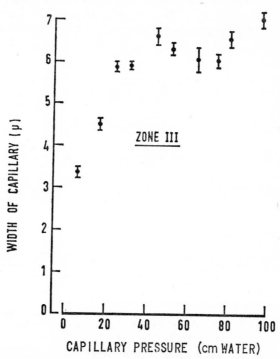

FIG. 4. Mean capillary width plotted against distance down Zone III. Again the abscissa has been marked capillary pressure, as in Fig. 3. Note the increase in width up to a capillary pressure of about 50 cm. water but no consistent change at higher pressures.

averaging measurements made at 10 μm. intervals along the septa. Measurements were only made if an open capillary was present, as indicated by a red blood cell. Thus mean width is with respect to distance in this context.

The mean width increased from 2·3 μm. high in Zone I to 6·5 μm. low in Zone III. As Fig. 4 shows, capillary width increased rapidly with capillary pressures up to about 50 cm. water but there was no further consistent change. An example of the appearance of the vessels is shown in Fig. 1D, where the bulging into the alveolar spaces can be clearly seen. Although the mean width with respect to the distance along the septum under these conditions was about 6·5 μm., maximum capillary diameters of 10 μm. were frequently encountered, the greatest being 13 μm. Blood cells lying two or three abreast were often seen (Fig. 1D). In Zone III, the red blood cells tended to move with their long axes directed perpendicular to the alveolar septum, as has been described in other capillaries. In a series of measurements made on lung frozen with a capillary pressure of 44 cm. water, the red cells had an average dimension along the septum of $3·16 \pm 0·11$ μm., whereas at right angles to the septum the dimension was $4·42 \pm 0·08$ μm. ($P < 0·001$).

In the past physiologists have sometimes disputed whether the pulmonary capillaries do or do not bulge into the alveolar spaces. The answer, not

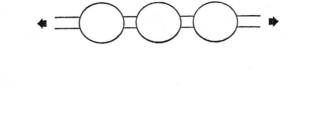

Fig. 5. Diagram to explain the reduction in red cell concentration and capillary width at high lung inflations. This is attributed to the direct effect of increased tension in the alveolar walls which flattens the capillaries and thus reduces their volume.

surprisingly, is that it depends on the capillary pressure; when this is low, they do not bulge (Figs. 1A and B) but when it is high, they do (Fig. 1D).

Does the increase in capillary width mean that pulmonary capillaries "distend"? If by distend we mean an increase in cross-sectional area of the vessels, the answer is clearly yes. If, however, we mean an increase in the perimeter of the vessels, these measurements give no information on this point. It may be that the capillaries increase in volume somewhat like a plastic bag does when it is inflated from the collapsed state; a considerable increase in volume is possible before the wall is stretched.

EFFECT OF LUNG INFLATION

We were surprised to find that increasing the transpulmonary pressure from 10 to 25 cm. water caused a striking reduction in the number of red blood cells and the capillary width. This was not due to the higher alveolar pressure squeezing blood out of the capillaries because the comparison was made at the same vascular–alveolar pressure differences. An example is shown in Fig. 2 where at a perfusing pressure of 20 cm. water and transpulmonary pressure of 25 cm. water, the red blood cell density was less than half that found at a transpulmonary pressure of 10 cm. water. Under Zone III conditions where the capillary pressure was known, it was found that over capillary pressures ranging from 0 to 40 cm. water, the number of red blood cells and capillary width were reduced, as if the capillary pressure was some 20 cm. lower.

We believe that this reduction in capillary blood volume must be attributed to the direct effect of increased tension in the alveolar walls causing flattening

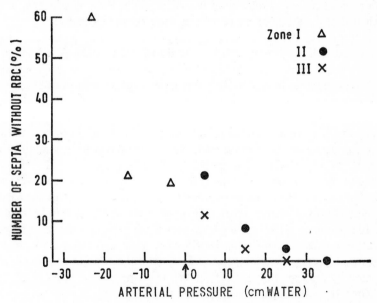

FIG. 6. Number of alveolar septa at various levels in the lung which contained no red blood cells and therefore presumably no open capillaries. The abscissa shows arterial pressure in relation to alveolar pressure (arrow). Note that even when arterial pressure exceeded alveolar pressure by up to 25 cm. water, some septa had no red blood cells when the venous pressure was low (Zone II). When venous pressure exceeded alveolar pressure (Zone III), an arterial pressure of 15 cm. water was not sufficient to open all the capillaries.

of the capillaries and a consequent reduction in their volume (Fig. 5). The increase in pulmonary vascular resistance which occurs at high lung inflations is well-known (Roos *et al.*, 1961) and is presumably caused by the same mechanism. The larger extra-alveolar vessels are unlikely to be responsible because they are pulled open during lung inflation (Howell *et al.*, 1961) though they are thought to explain the high vascular resistance at very low states of lung inflation and the critical closing pressure which has been demonstrated in the collapsed lung (West, Dollery and Heard, 1965).

CAPILLARY OPENING PRESSURES

The patchy filling of the pulmonary capillary bed has already been referred to, and an example can be seen in Fig. 1B. Fig. 6 shows that with perfusing pressure of 25 cm. water under Zone II conditions, nearly 10 per cent of the alveolar septa contained no red blood cells. Even in Zone III with a capillary pressure of 15 cm. water, some of the capillaries had not opened up. In addition to whole septa remaining bloodless under these conditions, it was also clear that the filling of the remaining septa was often uneven.

The reason why the pulmonary capillary bed opens up so unevenly is not fully understood, but it may well have to do with the "sheet flow" nature of the circulation (Fung and Sobin, 1968). The capillaries are sometimes regarded as pipes but in reality the bed is more like a thin sheet of blood with intervening posts (Fig. 7), so that an enormous number of parallel channels are available. Intuitively, it is not surprising that a bed like this opens up in a patchy fashion. In any biological situation, there is bound to be a path of least resistance where flow occurs first. The unevenness will be magnified if a minimum pressure difference is required before flow occurs at all, owing for example to the yield stress of blood (Merrill *et al.*, 1963), although this is very small. Perhaps too the pressure required to force red cells through the narrow channels which exist when the perfusing pressure is very low should be included here. In addition, it is likely that a large part of the resistance in the pulmonary circulation resides in the capillaries (Fowler, West and Pain, 1966) so that the perfusing pressure available for opening up the vessels will be considerably dissipated by the time that part of the bed near the venous outlet is reached.

In Zone III conditions, it is surprising that with both inflow and outflow pressures in the region of 15 cm. water, some parts of the bed are not open, though the proportion of vessels that behave in this way is small. We are reluctant to invoke active tension in the walls of the small vessels to explain this until we understand the physical forces more clearly. It is unlikely that critical closing pressures in the "arteriolar" vessels (of say 100 μm. diameter or

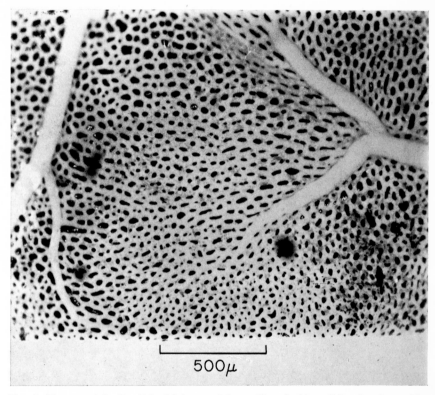

500μ

FIG. 7. Photograph by Dr. John Maloney of the capillary bed in a living frog lung. The frog was pithed, the thorax opened, and contrast material injected into the pulmonary artery. Note the enormous number of parallel channels resulting in a "sheet-flow" type of circulation.

[To face page 262

more) are responsible because the unevenness of filling occurs within septa (as well as between septa) and therefore presumably within the area of supply of a single large vessel. In addition, the unevenness occurs in the presence of a raised venous pressure, which cannot be explained unless critical closing pressures in the venules are also postulated.

SITE OF VASCULAR RESISTANCE

We have shown that the number of red blood cells per unit length of alveolar septum can be used as a capillary manometer if the "calibration" measurements are done at a low arterial–venous pressure difference (Fig. 3). Such a mano-meter can be used to determine the capillary pressure in lungs perfused at high flow rates under Zone III conditions with large arterial–venous pressure differences, and thus to deduce the chief site of vascular resistance.

Fig. 8 shows the results of measurements on four lungs; two were perfused forwards (artery to vein) and two in the reverse direction. It appears that for both directions of flow, the number of red blood cells at any level was such that the capillary bed was "seeing" the upstream or perfusing pressure. For

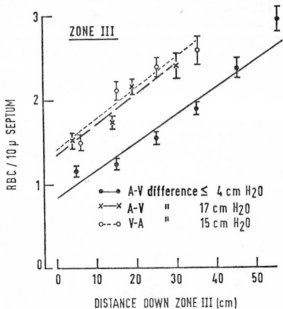

Fig. 8. The effect of a large arterial–venous pressure difference (forward flow) and venous–arterial pressure difference (reverse flow) on the red blood cell concentration. In both cases, the capillaries appear to be "seeing" a pressure which is close to upstream pressure (see text for details). (From Glazier *et al.*, 1969, with permission of *The Journal of Applied Physiology*.)

example, in the lungs perfused forwards where the arterial–venous pressure difference was 17 cm. water, the red blood cell density at any level was the same as that at a point 17 cm. lower in the "calibration" lungs where the arterial–venous difference was small (less than 1 cm. water in six lungs and less than 4 cm. water in three more).

This intriguing finding that none of the perfusing pressure is lost in the vessels upstream of the capillaries is in accord with previous work from this laboratory (Fowler, West and Pain, 1966) showing that much of the resistance to flow lies in the vessels exposed to alveolar pressure. However, since both forward and backward perfused lungs show a similar pattern, one is left wondering where the pressure from artery to vein (or vein to artery) is lost. The paradox may perhaps be explained by uneven filling of the capillary bed. If, on the one hand, most of the pressure is dissipated in the capillaries, and on the other the portions of the bed near the supplying vessel which are exposed to the highest pressures have a much higher concentration of red cells than the low-pressure downstream regions, the red cell count could be heavily biased by the upstream pressure. However, we have insufficient data yet to decide whether this is a feasible explanation.

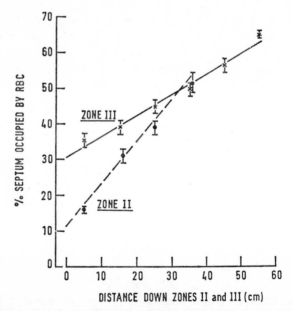

FIG. 9. Percentage of alveolar septum occupied by red blood cells in Zones II and III. The steepness of the slope chiefly reflects the opening of previously closed vessels. This graph shows the striking effect of a small rise in venous pressure on the number of vessels open when the perfusing pressure is low. It also suggests that recruitment of vessels is more important in Zone II than Zone III.

A related topic is the site of the vascular waterfall in the lung. It is now generally accepted that when pulmonary venous pressure is less than alveolar pressure, collapse occurs somewhere in the vessels exposed to alveolar pressure and flow becomes independent of venous pressure (Permutt, Bromberger-Barnea and Bane, 1962). The site of collapse when the lung is operating under these Zone II or Starling resistor conditions is not known. In the past, the collapse point has often been assumed to occur at the extreme downstream end of the collapsible vessels because this is where the collapse initially occurs in rubber tube models operating under similar conditions. The present measurements provide some evidence on this point.

Fig. 9 shows the percentage of the alveolar septum occupied by red blood cells at various levels in lungs operating in both Zone II and Zone III conditions. These results were obtained by following along individual septa and noting at 5 μm. intervals whether a red blood cell was present or not. This measurement is dominated by the number of vessels open, so that the graph implies that the number of capillaries open high in Zone III is very much greater than that high in Zone II. Since the only difference between the two situations is whether the venous pressure is above or below alveolar pressure, it appears that merely raising venous pressure above alveolar pressure under these conditions is sufficient to open up many capillaries. We take this as evidence that the collapse in Zone II conditions occurs throughout much of the capillary mesh, not just at the downstream end.

RECRUITMENT OR DISTENSION IN THE CAPILLARY BED

It is possible to use the three principal measurements—red blood cells per unit length of septum, capillary width, and percentage of septum occupied by red blood cells—to evaluate the roles of distension of already opened capillaries and recruitment of unopened capillaries in the increase in blood volume as capillary pressure is raised. (Note that by distension we mean an increase in the cross-sectional area of the capillaries, and we do not necessarily imply any increase in the perimeter of the vessel by stretching of the vessel wall.) The first measurement is an indication of the total capillary red blood cell volume. The second measurement depends solely on the expansion of capillaries, while the third is related partly to the opening of new capillaries and partly to the distension of existing capillaries in so far as they distend along the septum. We have squared the measured mean capillary width at each level in order to determine the increase in capillary area that occurs solely from the expansion of already open capillaries, on the assumption that the capillaries expand along the septa to the same extent as they expand at right angles to it.

The results are presented in Fig. 10. The magnitude of the increase in red

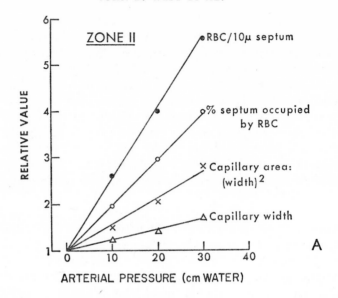

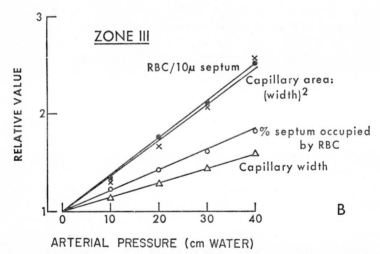

FIG. 10. Analysis of the relative importance of recruitment and distension in Zones II and III, based on the three measurements: red blood cell concentration, capillary width, and percentage septum containing red blood cells. Capillary width has been squared to indicate the increase in capillary area due to expansion of already open vessels. A shows that about half of the increase in red blood cell number is due to recruitment of new vessels down Zone II. B shows that the increase down Zone III can be almost entirely explained by the distension of already open vessels. (From Glazier *et al.*, 1969, with permission of *The Journal of Applied Physiology*.)

blood cell concentration depends on the increase in total capillary area. If all of the increase in capillary area could be explained by expansion of already open vessels the line for capillary area (width^2) would lie on the line for red blood cells per 10 μm. of septum; whereas if there were no expansion of already open vessels, the line for width^2 would run along the abscissa. Furthermore, on the assumption that already open vessels expand along the alveolar septum to the same extent as into the alveolar space, we may subtract the line for capillary width from the line for the percentage of septum occupied by red blood cells to indicate how much of the increase in percentage of septum occupied by red blood cells is due solely to the opening up of previously closed capillaries.

In Zone II the increase in width^2—that is, capillary distension—accounts for approximately half of the total increase in capillary area while the percentage of septum occupied by red blood cells minus capillary width—that is, capillary recruitment—accounts for the remaining increase in area. In Zone III the situation is strikingly different. Here capillary distension (width^2) accounts for the whole of the increase in the number of red blood cells per 10 μm. of septum. Furthermore the increase in the percentage of septum occupied by red blood cells is almost completely explained by the increase in capillary width. Thus expansion of already open vessels is the principal mechanism accounting for the increase in red blood cell volume as capillary pressure increases. This analysis suggests that most capillaries are already open in Zone III, whereas recruitment of new vessels is an important mechanism under Zone II conditions.

DIFFUSION VENTILATION IN TERMINAL AIR SPACES

I now wish to turn to the pattern of blood flow in the respiratory lung unit as a whole, but to introduce this it is necessary to look briefly at the diffusion of gas along the peripheral airways. It is generally accepted that fresh inspired gas does not reach the alveoli by bulk flow but that the inspired front only reaches the smaller airways, perhaps the terminal bronchioles. The rest of the distance to the blood–gas barrier is covered by molecular diffusion and ordinarily the diffusion rate of gas is so high and the distance so small that almost complete equilibration occurs rapidly. Nevertheless, a small concentration gradient down the terminal lung unit remains even in the normal lung, as was clearly recognized by Krogh and Lindhard (1917). In disease, the differences of concentration may remain much larger.

The dominant role of diffusion in the ventilation of the peripheral regions is clearly shown during liquid breathing where the diffusion rates of gases are reduced by a factor of 10^5 or so. Fig. 11 shows data obtained using radioactive xenon-133 in an excised dog lung breathing saline. When the expiration was made immediately after inspiration, the expired concentration of xenon (as a percentage of the inspired concentration) fell continuously as more saline was exhaled. The late expired saline had a relatively low xenon concentration because the inspired gas did not have time to complete the equilibration process by diffusion within the alveolar gas. By contrast, the exhalation after three

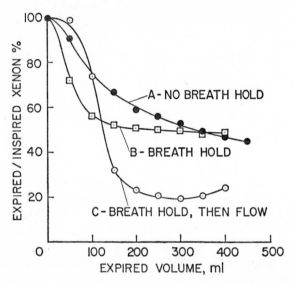

FIG. 11. Expired xenon concentration (as a percentage of inspired) in a saline-filled excised dog lung. Note that when the exhalation was made after 3 minutes of breath-holding, the xenon concentration in the expired alveolar saline was substantially uniform. However, when the exhalation occurred immediately after inspiration, the concentration fell continuously, indicating that diffusion equilibration within the alveolar saline was not complete. The expiration made after 3 minutes of breath-holding and a subsequent short period of perfusion shows a rise in concentration at the end of expiration, indicating relatively poor perfusion of the alveoli deepest in the lung.

minutes of breath-holding showed an almost uniform concentration of xenon in the expired alveolar gas after the dead space in the large airways had been washed out. Similar patterns have been found using radioactive oxygen and carbon dioxide. Even more striking differences with increasing periods of breath-holding could be demonstrated using iodine-labelled albumin in saline as a tracer, since this molecule is large and diffuses correspondingly more slowly (West et al., 1965). Studies with aerosols and gases of different molecular weights have been described by other participants in this symposium and they, too, emphasize the importance of gaseous diffusion in the mixing of gas in the lung.

Pattern of blood flow in the terminal lung unit

The incompleteness of diffusion equilibration within the gas of the respiratory portions of the lung (stratified inhomogeneity) can be looked upon as a type of ventilatory inequality, in that the alveoli nearest the mouth (proximal alveoli) receive more fresh inspired gas than those deeper in the lung (distal alveoli). Since the relations between ventilation and blood flow determine the amount of gas exchange which occurs in any part of the lung, the question arises of whether the pattern of blood flow in the respiratory units is well or poorly suited to this uneven ventilation.

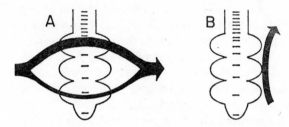

FIG. 12. Two possible ways in which the lung could minimize the impairment of gas exchange which would otherwise result from the failure of diffusion equilibration in the terminal air spaces. In A, blood flow per unit volume is higher in the proximal (near the mouth) than distal alveoli. In B, a "counter-current" scheme is shown which would actually exploit the concentration gradient in the air spaces. Gas flows distally by diffusion against the general trend of blood flow. Preliminary data suggest that A exists but that its effect on overall gas exchange is small. (Note that a single alveolar duct is shown for simplicity only; the model extends over several ducts.)

Fig. 12 shows two ways in which the lung could minimize the impairment of gas exchange which would otherwise result from the concentration gradient in the terminal air spaces. In Fig. 12A the blood flow per unit volume of the proximal alveoli is higher than that of the distal alveoli. Evidence for this has been obtained by Wagner, McRae and Read (1967), who injected iodine-labelled macro-aggregated albumin into rats and showed that the peripheral parts of the secondary lobules near the pleural surface of the lung contained less radioactivity than the more centrally located regions.

Fig. 12B shows a possible pattern of blood flow which would not only reduce the effects of the uneven ventilation on gas exchange but would actually exploit it. In this model, the general trend of blood flow within the respiratory tissue is from distal to proximal alveoli. As a result, the blood leaving the alveolated regions "sees" a concentration of inspired gas which is higher than the average value in the alveoli. Such an arrangement could give a higher oxygen partial pressure in pulmonary venous blood than in mean alveolar gas. This arrangement is analogous to the "counter-current" mode of flow in the fish gill, described by Van Dam (1938). The directions of flow of water over the gill surface and of blood through the gill capillary of the trout are such that the blood leaving the gill is exposed to the fresh water entering the gill. In this way, the partial pressure of oxygen in the blood draining from the gill approaches that of inspired rather than expired water with an enormous advantage in the efficiency of gas transfer.

Recently Dr. Maloney and I have been studying gas exchange in saline-filled excised dog lungs in an attempt to determine whether any special pattern of blood flow exists in the respiratory tissue, and if so, whether this results in a more efficient transfer of inspired gas to the pulmonary venous blood. Liquid breathing was used because we wanted to exaggerate the normal diffusion gradient in the terminal air spaces, and radioactive xenon-133 was selected to measure gas transfer because its large molecule diffuses relatively slowly in the airways and it is a convenient tracer to detect. The preliminary results indicate that the proximal alveoli are better perfused in relation to their volume than the distal alveoli. Fig. 11 shows an example of the pattern of expired xenon which supports this assertion. After a single inhalation of xenon in saline followed by a breath-hold of three minutes to allow diffusion equilibration in the alveolar regions to take place, the lung was perfused for about 45 seconds and then allowed to exhale. It can be seen that the concentration of expired xenon first fell and then increased towards the end of expiration. This indicates that the alveoli which contributed the last expired gas had been less depleted of xenon than those which exhaled earlier, which means that the distal alveoli were relatively poorly perfused in relation to their volume. This is consistent with the model shown in Fig. 12A.

Does the matching of the distribution of blood flow along the terminal air spaces to the uneven ventilation caused by incomplete diffusion equilibration significantly facilitate gas exchange in the lung? We have been trying to answer this by measuring the xenon concentration in pulmonary venous blood in the presence and absence of a diffusion gradient of xenon in the air spaces. On the one hand, the lung is perfused immediately after an inhalation of xenon when we know that a concentration difference between proximal and distal alveoli exists, and on the other, perfusion is begun after a 3-minute breath-holding period when we know diffusion equilibration in the alveolar gas is virtually complete. The peak venous concentrations in both instances are compared. As yet we have not been able to detect any consistent difference between the two measurements and can only say that if a difference exists, it must be small. This negative finding also suggests that the lung does not have a "counter-current" mechanism as shown in Fig. 12B to any appreciable extent.

SUMMARY

Capillary morphology and blood volume were studied in perfused excised dog lungs rapidly frozen with liquid freon. The number of red blood cells per unit length of septum, mean width of capillaries and percentage of septum occupied by red blood cells were measured in freeze-dried sections.

When alveolar pressure exceeded arterial pressure, less than $0 \cdot 5$ red cells were seen per 10 μm. of septum and capillary width was only $2 \cdot 3$ μm. As capillary pressure was increased up to 50 cm. water, both measurements rose rapidly but there were no further changes with pressures up to 100 cm. water. At high lung volumes, both red cell density and capillary width were greatly reduced, presumably because of increased tension in the capillary walls. Recruitment of new vessels was the predominant mechanism to account for the increase in red cell concentration down Zone II whereas expansion of already open capillaries was more important in Zone III.

Diffusion mixing of inspired xenon in the alveolar spaces was demonstrated in excised dog lungs ventilated with saline where the rate of diffusion of the gas was very slow. As a consequence, the alveoli deepest in the lung were relatively poorly ventilated. By perfusing the lungs and measuring the transfer of radioactive xenon, it was possible to show that these distal alveoli were also relatively poorly perfused. However, any beneficial effect on overall gas transfer was very small.

REFERENCES

FOWLER, K. T., WEST, J. B., and PAIN, M. C. F. (1966). *Resp. Physiol.*, **1**, 88–98.
FUNG, Y. C. B., and SOBIN, S. S. (1968). *Fedn Proc. Fedn Am. Socs exp. Biol.*, **27**, 578.
GLAZIER, J. B., HUGHES, J. M. B., MALONEY, J. E., and WEST, J. B. (1969). *J. appl. Physiol.*, **26**, in press.
HOWELL, J. B. L., PERMUTT, S., PROCTER, D. F., and RILEY, R. L. (1961). *J. appl. Physiol.*, **16**, 71–76.
KROGH, M., and LINDHARD, J. (1917). *J. Physiol., Lond.*, **51**, 59–90.
MERRILL, E. W., GILLILAND, E. R., COKELET, G., SHIN, H., BRITTEN, A., and WELLS, R. E. (1963). *Biophys. J.*, **3**, 199–213.
PERMUTT, S., BROMBERGER-BARNEA, B., and BANE, H. N. (1962). *Med. Thorac.*, **19**, 239–260.
ROOS, A., THOMAS, L. J., NAGEL, E. L., and PROMMAS, D. C. (1961). *J. appl. Physiol.*, **16**, 77–84.
STAUB, N. C., and STOREY, W. F. (1962). *J. appl. Physiol.*, **17**, 381–390.
VAN DAM, L. (1938). *On the Utilization of Oxygen and Regulation of Breathing in Some Aquatic Animals.* Groningen: Drukkerij "Volharding".

WAGNER, P., MCRAE, J., and READ, J. (1967). *J. appl. Physiol.*, **22**, 1115–1123.
WEST, J. B., DOLLERY, C. T., and HEARD, B. E. (1965). *Circulation Res.*, **17**, 191–206.
WEST, J. B., DOLLERY, C. T., MATTHEWS, C. M. E., and ZARDINI, P. (1965). *J. appl. Physiol.*, **20**, 1107–1117.
WEST, J. B., DOLLERY, C. T., and NAIMARK, A. (1964). *J. appl. Physiol.*, **19**, 713–724.

DISCUSSION

Caro: In your studies using the pulmonary capillary as a manometer, you seemed in some cases to be measuring the number of red blood cells per unit length of septum under more or less static conditions, whereas other measurements were made during blood flow. You were therefore comparing a static haematocrit with a dynamic haematocrit. Flow might reduce the haematocrit in these small vessels by perhaps 10–15 per cent.

West: That is true, and we have tried to assess this error by making those measurements on two sets of lungs. Four of the nine lungs used for the capillary manometer experiments were quick frozen while blood was flowing, the arterio-venous difference being about 4 cm. of water. In the other five there was no flow. There was no consistent difference in the results between the two groups.

Cumming: In your estimations of the percentage of septum occupied by red cells (Fig. 9, p. 264), in Zone III conditions where the capillaries are fairly well distended the percentage never reached 100, but this presumably would be expected if we view the capillary network as a syncytium with holes in it, because you are very likely to cut through some of the holes? Also you would expect relatively more of the distended capillaries to be collapsed at the septal junctions.

West: The highest value found for the proportion of septa occupied by red blood cells was between 60 and 70 per cent. We would not expect to find a value of 100 because the alveolar wall is not covered by a continuous sheet of blood.

Burton: I had thought that in the lung the average capillary width was invariably greater than the diameter of the red cell, but from your measurements under certain conditions it seems that the average is considerably less, so the red cells must be going through the capillaries in a deformed shape in some conditions? What we have heard about lubrication theory from Professor Lighthill therefore may not really apply throughout the lung, and while some capillaries are big enough for one or even two or three red cells to pass, would you say that on average they are not as wide as the red cells themselves?

West: This is certainly true at low perfusion pressures. In lungs which may be 30 cm. high and therefore have a difference of capillary pressure of 30 cm. water from top to bottom, the red blood cells at the top may be squashed, whereas at the bottom they may have plenty of room to flow.

Burton: In general, then, the picture of red cells distorted into an overall sausage shape may be the more typical picture of the circulating red cell, in the lung capillaries; certainly in peripheral capillaries of the systemic circulation this is true. It is interesting that Auguste Krogh showed in his classical book drawings of capillaries with red cells just as you have shown (Krogh, A. [1922]. *The Anatomy and Physiology of Capillaries*, chapter 1. New Haven: Yale University Press).

Caro: Can you determine from your sections whether just an occasional capillary here or there is open or whether the response is characteristic of a larger unit or area? You might see this if you cut serial sections across an alveolus, for example.

West: We can say that this patchiness of opening occurs within septa as well as between septa. We were interested in this because it has been suggested by S. Permutt, for example (personal communication), that the lung may have a good deal of tone in some of the upstream arterioles and this may be responsible for patchy filling. However I do not believe that the appearance we see is compatible with that idea, because we see patchiness which must be within the field of supply of a single large vessel, being only a few micrometres away.

Burton: You showed (Fig. 7, p. 262) a capillary bed in a frog lung and suggested that we should think of it as a sheet of blood interrupted by welded buttons, so to speak, but this seems entirely different from your pictures of the mammalian lung where the capillaries are so thin. Are the two pictures compatible?

West: The frog lung capillary bed is seen in plan in Fig. 7; this is a view looking on to the wall of an alveolus. Our sections of dog lung are cuts across that view. So I think they are compatible. In fact, Fig. 7 is not so dissimilar from the pictures that Weibel and others too have published, from man. All the capillaries in Fig. 7 are presumably full, because it was taken at a high perfusion pressure.

Cumming: That would be a fairly good representation of the capillary bed in the normal human lung.

Saffman: These two pictures of the pulmonary microcirculation as an assembly of tubes and as a system of sheets which are spot-welded together at certain points may look very different but from the hydrodynamic point of view the gross behaviour would be very similar. In both cases the flow would probably be proportional to the pressure gradient, and the diffusion properties and mixing are unlikely to be very different.

Burton: When you watch with a microscope through a thoracic window the microcirculation in the capillary of the mammalian lung, you have the same impression as from watching the frog's web, that flow goes one way, then stops and goes the other way; in the network it is not at all one-way flow.

Caro: Professor Lighthill recently discussed the fluid mechanics of the so-called physiological waterfall in the microcirculation. He threw out of court the idea that the losses across the orifice, which is supposed to form as a result of vessel compression, are in any way determined by fluid inertia, since the Reynolds numbers are so low.

Saffman: As Professor Stuart mentioned earlier (p. 135), at very low Reynolds numbers acceleration, which is essentially an inertial effect, can be ignored completely in calculations.

Caro: It is a viscous loss across the orifice rather than an inertial one.

West: The notion of a loss across an orifice like this is then valid? Certainly this is how the lung circulation behaves; that is to say, in conditions where alveolar pressure exceeds venous pressure, flow is independent of venous pressure.

Burton: It seems to me that the term "waterfall" is a very misleading one for this situation, because the energetics and kinetics of an actual waterfall seem to have no relation to this feature of the pulmonary circulation. It can be most misleading for physicists, for example. It would be useful to devise a more descriptive term.

Renkin: The historical precedent is, I think, for the term "sluice". This was used by Bannister and Torrance in 1960, before the Baltimore group published (Bannister, J., and Torrance, R. W. [1960]. *Q. Jl exp. Physiol.*, **45**, 352–367).

Caro: But this is physically unacceptable too, because again it implies an inertial force.

Mead: Surely "waterfall" antedates "sluice"; Duomarco used the term in the early fifties (Duomarco, J. L., and Rimini, R. [1954]. *Am. J. Physiol.*, **178**, 215–220).

Cumming: Would "Starling resistor flow" be acceptable?

Caro: The implication is of a viscous loss.

Burton: I like the word "pinch", because that is what happens!

Stuart: There is another use for that term in a quite different kind of plasma physics!

Caro: I prefer the term "collapse" because it carries no overtones regarding the fluid mechanics. One could thus have collapse mechanism and collapse pressure.

Mead: Collapse implies complete closure, but complete closure is not necessary.

Burton: Would "obstruction by collapse" be more specific, which would avoid the implication of total collapse?

Cumming: The disadvantage of "obstruction by collapse" is that there could be confusion with the following situation in the airways. When a bronchitic person breathes out, his airways become narrow or partially collapsed, and this leads to airway obstruction, but this is in no way a waterfall effect. It results from the raised intrapleural pressure which causes the apposition of the sides. It occurs in bronchitics but can be imitated by a normal person who makes a wheezing expiration.

Caro (added in proof): The term "Starling regulator", though requiring the use of two words, recommends itself. The eponym is appropriate and there is no restriction as to the mechanics.

West: Professor Burton, may I ask you about the behaviour of flow under these conditions; what about pushing red blood cells through one of these Starling resistors? We are looking for reasons why flow may be inherently unstable in this capillary mesh; how much pressure would it take to push a red blood cell through a tube with a diameter when full of, say, 7 μm. when the tube is being squashed by a pressure of, say, 2 cm. water?

Burton: Prothero made a series of measurements pushing blood through micropipette tips (you can go up to 20 per cent haematocrit only) and under the microscope it was still a hundred times the Reynolds number of physiological capillary flow for a single capillary (Prothero, J. W., and Burton, A. C. [1962]. *Biophys. J.*, **2**, 199–212). He obtained pressure–flow relations, and by doing this with saline and with blood plasma he measured the effective relative viscosity. The question is, if we are to apply Poiseuille's Law, what viscosity should we use? It turns out that it is the viscosity of plasma, and so the contribution of the energy required to deform and push the cell through, and the friction with the wall, sliding through because of lubrication, must be quite negligible. I do not understand how this can be; perhaps the energy of deformation is recovered when the cell springs out again.

West: I was thinking more of a collapsible tube.

Burton: I would predict that if the diameter of the tube is less than 3·7 μm. the cells are trapped; this is the size which a normal population of human red cell shapes and volumes could go through without increase of area.

Renkin: In the frog mesentery, when intermittence of capillary flow is produced by the opening and closing of one particular precapillary sphincter, flow frequently stops when a red cell gets stuck in the sphincter, which is like a narrow cylindrical tube (see Zweifach, B. W. [1939]. *Anat. Rec.*, **73**, 475–495). You can often see the red cell sticking out of the sphincter at each end; at some specific diameter the red cell seems to be stopped, and as soon as the sphincter relaxes slightly, flow starts again and the cell comes through. The pressure squeezes the red cell out to a length of 40–50 μm. Red cells are normally about 22 μm. long in the frog, but they are nucleated, so this may make their physical properties rather different from mammalian red blood cells. However, the relation of the cell size to capillary size is about the same as in mammals; the mesenteric capillaries are barely wide enough for a red cell to go through. Have you any idea how much force it takes to move a frog's red cell through a small opening?

Burton: I know nothing about the frog red cell membrane; its mechanical properties might be quite different, and the shape is not so determined; it is not "geometrical".

DIFFUSIVE AND CONVECTIVE MOVEMENT OF GAS IN THE LUNG

L. E. FARHI

Department of Physiology, State University of New York, Buffalo, New York

BECAUSE so much of our understanding of pulmonary gas exchange is based upon the concept of "mean alveolar gas", a mythical gas present in *all* parts of *all* the respiratory elements *all* the time, it is of utmost importance to examine to what extent these assumptions of constancy in time, of regional uniformity and of homogeneity within each pulmonary lobule correspond to what occurs in fact.

Obviously, since ventilation is a cyclic phenomenon in which no carbon dioxide can be vented to the atmosphere during inspiration and no oxygen can be taken up from the environment during expiration, changes in alveolar composition, synchronous with the respiratory movements, must take place. The calculations of Rahn and Fenn (1955) indicate that in the normal resting man, mean alveolar oxygen tension may vary from 98 to 101 mm. Hg while carbon dioxide pressure would fluctuate between 38 and 40 mm. Hg. That uniform gas composition in different areas of the lung is at best a simplifying assumption has been apparent for several years, following reports by Martin, Cline and Marshall (1953), Martin and Young (1957) and Rahn and others (1956) that gas exchange in the different lobes of man and dog is not identical, a finding consistent with the more recent description of unequal vertical gradients for ventilation and perfusion in the lung (Ball *et al.*, 1962; West, Dollery and Hugh-Jones, 1962).

The last assumption, that of uniform gas composition within the respiratory lobule, has proved more resistant to investigation and criticism. More than a 100 years ago, Gréhant (1862) noted that if a subject inspired a breath of hydrogen, the hydrogen fractions in two successive samples of the expired gas were not identical. The timing of the samples was open to criticism but similar results were later obtained by Krogh and Lindhard (1917) using a valid technique. These authors thought that their data indicated inhomogeneity within the terminal respiratory units. The possible occurrence of such a phenomenon was discussed for several years before Rauwerda's celebrated thesis (Rauwerda, 1946), in which he indicated that the dimensions of the

277

respiratory lobule were such that diffusive mixing of its contents should be rapid enough to lead to a homogeneous gas composition within an extremely short time. This view has generally prevailed, and in his recent exhaustive review, Bouhuys (1964) reflected a quasi-unanimous opinion when he stated that "It is now generally believed that gas mixing by diffusion alone within small lung units is rapid enough to eliminate any gas concentration difference within a period of time that is short compared to the duration of the inspiration. This view is based mainly on observations and theoretical calculations by Rauwerda." The belief that any variation in the concentration of expired alveolar gas was due only to regional differences was further strengthened by several important contributions. In 1956, the effects of possible regional differences in mechanical properties of the lung on effective ventilation were admirably described in a joint paper by two groups of investigators (Otis *et al.*, 1956). When Milic-Emili and his collaborators (1966) demonstrated that in the normal lung volume range the compliance of the different lung regions is not identical, the case for regional inhomogeneity (and by inference against diffusive inhomogeneity, also called stratified inhomogeneity) seemed complete.

However, during the last few years, several independent reports have indicated that although regional inhomogeneity is certainly present and at times considerable, some findings could be explained best—or only—on the basis of stratified inhomogeneity, and the object of the present paper is to summarize and discuss some of this recent information.

EVIDENCE IN FAVOUR OF STRATIFIED INHOMOGENEITY

A substantial amount of the evidence on uneven distribution of inspired gas is based on single-breath techniques in which the subject inhales once a gas of abnormal composition. This gas may contain only one or more of the species present in air but in a different amount (such as 100 per cent oxygen) or it may include one or more elements which are not part of the normal atmosphere. This abnormal mixture may constitute the whole inspiration or part of it. After a preselected breath-holding time, expiration follows and during that time gas composition and expired flow or volume are recorded. The best known single-breath test is probably that described by Fowler (1948), in which the inspired gas is 100 per cent oxygen and the gas monitored during expiration is nitrogen. After elimination of the gas contained in the dead space, all the gas appearing at the mouth must come from the alveoli. In the curve describing gas concentration against expired volume, the corresponding part of the tracing is usually designated as the alveolar plateau. Even in normal subjects, the plateau shows a progressive change in gas composition which is commonly ascribed to inhomogeneity in the ratio of inspired volume to pre-existing alveolar volume.

Before we can discuss the type of unevenness in distribution of ventilation that may be responsible for the slope of the plateau, it is proper to point out that although the solubility of nitrogen (and that of the various tracer gases used to study this distribution) in blood is so small that there is no direct effect of lung perfusion, the indirect effect of pulmonary blood flow may be significant. This is possibly best demonstrated by considering alveoli which are relatively overperfused and in which the oxygen uptake from the alveolar gas far exceeds the carbon dioxide output. As a result, the gas phase shrinks and the relatively insoluble gases, which are not exchanged, are concentrated.

It is also important to bear in mind that there is little doubt that the inspired gas reaches by convective movement only the part of the respiratory element that is nearer the bronchiole. This has been well documented by experiments in which the subject inhales an aerosol (Altshuler et al., 1959; Cumming et al., 1967). The droplets have such a low rate of diffusion that they are transported only by airflow and can be used as a tracer of mass transport. The question here is only whether respiratory gases then diffuse to the periphery at a rate such that equilibrium occurs extremely rapidly or whether the diffusion process is slow enough to be demonstrable. The arguments against the accepted concept of near-instantaneous diffusion fall into three main categories.

Critique of sequential emptying theory

The sloping alveolar plateau normally encountered in the single-breath test is usually attributed to a combination of two factors. Because of regional differences in certain characteristics of the lung, more of the test gas may reach certain areas. If during the following expiration discrepancies in mechanical properties lead to a situation where the less ventilated regions contribute more to the last part of expiration, the composition of the mixed gas appearing at the mouth must change. The two requirements for this explanation, low ventilation and phase lag, can be coupled since an increase in time constant would cause both (Otis et al., 1956). Because compliance is one of the determinants of time constant, Milic-Emili's findings of a regional, gravity-dependent gradient in compliance (Milic-Emili et al., 1966) has lent credence to this view.

However, Mead (1969) has indicated that the time constants of the different alveolar pathways are indeed different but are all very short in relation to the breathing period, and consequently distribution of ventilation depends

10

normally only on distribution of compliance. The data of Milic-Emili and co-workers (1966) shows that although compliance varies in different parts of the lung, it is maintained at a fixed value in each area as long as the lung volume is in its normal range. There is therefore no theoretical reason to postulate *a priori* that sequential emptying *must* occur.

Sikand, Cerretelli and Farhi (1966) have recently described the results of their investigation on the cause of the slope of the alveolar plateau. In order to eliminate the indirect effects of pulmonary blood flow they modified Fowler's technique by using a mixture of 20 per cent oxygen in argon as the

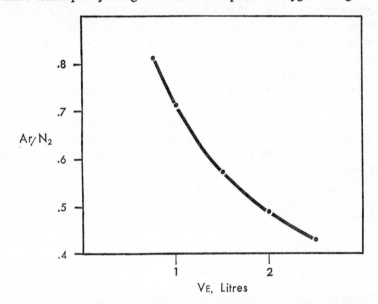

FIG. 1. Argon-nitrogen ratio in the expired gas (V_E) following a single inspiration of 20 per cent oxygen in argon. The data are taken from the work of Sikand, Cerretelli and Farhi (1966). The argon/nitrogen ratio, which is very close to the ratio of inspired to alveolar volume, drops from 0·81 at 750 ml. to 0·46 at 2,500 ml. These figures are compatible with sequential emptying only if the average ventilation per unit volume of the elements corresponding to the first figure is double that of the alveoli contributing to the end of expiration. For discussion see text.

inspired gas. These authors reasoned that change in gas volume due to inequality between oxygen and carbon dioxide exchange with the circulation should affect all insoluble gases in proportion to their concentration and expressed their results in terms of the argon/nitrogen ratio, thus cancelling the possible error.

Fig. 1 gives the argon/nitrogen ratio as a function of the cumulative expired volume. Analysis of this curve in terms of sequential emptying leads to two incompatible statements. Since argon represents the contribution of the test breath to the expired gas while nitrogen indicates the volume of the alveolar gas to which the inspired gas was added, the changes in the argon/nitrogen ratio must parallel changes in the ratio of ventilation per unit volume of the elements contributing to a certain aliquot of the expired gas. West's calculations (West, 1962), based on figures for distribution of ventilation obtained by the radio-active gases technique, show that ventilation per unit volume doubles from the top of the lungs to the bottom part. Since this is the magnitude of the change in argon/nitrogen in Fig. 1, the latter can be explained in terms of sequential emptying only by assuming that the gas expired at 750 ml. originates practically entirely in the lung bases, while the gas volume appearing at 2,500 ml. must represent very selectively gas from the uppermost areas. A corollary statement is that the 750-ml. specimen comes from a region in which the oxygen tension before the test breath was 89 mm. Hg, while the 2,500-ml. aliquot corresponds to a PO_2 of 132 mm. Hg. Sikand and his associates monitored the expired gas composition in terms of oxygen and carbon dioxide as well as argon and nitrogen, which allowed them to calculate the PO_2 before the test breath in the compartment corresponding to each expired aliquot. They found a mean value of 105, with a range of 103 to 108 mm. Hg. Because of this minor change in oxygen tension, some degree of sequential emptying cannot be ruled out, but it is well below what would have been required to explain entirely the argon/nitrogen curve. This statement can safely be made even when corrections for possible inequalities in regional anatomical dead space are introduced.

Farber, working in the same laboratory some years later, was also unable to demonstrate sequential emptying using a different and very sensitive technique (Farber, 1968). The subject was required to breathe 100 per cent oxygen until most of the nitrogen was washed out of his lungs, rebreathe rapidly in a bag containing 20 per cent argon, 20 per cent oxygen and 60 per cent nitrous oxide and then breathe out, while argon was being monitored. The initial rebreathing was introduced to obtain a uniform gas composition in the lungs at the beginning of the expiration. In the areas where blood flow per unit volume is great, the lung volume should decrease very rapidly because both oxygen and the very soluble nitrous oxide are taken up and this must result in a sizeable vertical gradient of argon (which will be present in a much higher amount in the well-perfused elements) as expiration proceeds. In spite of the magnification of the perfusion effect by the addition of nitrous oxide, the expiratory argon curve did not show any clear evidence of sequential emptying.

Studies based on inert gases of different diffusivities

Because the conclusions of Sikand, Cerretelli and Farhi (1966) and of Farber (1968) rely on the absence of perfusion effects, they may be considered as indirect evidence. Fortunately, single-breath techniques also yield a different type of data, the most recent of which has been elegantly presented by Cumming and co-workers (1967) who, like Georg and co-workers two years earlier (Georg *et al.*, 1965), based their investigation on the premise that gases of low molecular weight have a faster rate of diffusion. Consequently, following inspiration, gases of smaller molecular weight should reach the most remote portions of the lobule earlier. The subjects for these experiments inhaled a gas mixture containing both neon (atomic weight 20) and sulphur hexafluoride (molecular weight 146). In a system in which diffusion is very rapid, the concentration of each of these gases may be different in the various regions of the lung if regional inhomogeneity is present. In any area, however, all tracer gases must represent the same fraction of their respective inspired concentration, since they have been identically diluted. In other words, the

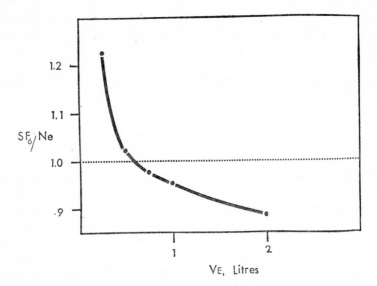

FIG. 2. Sulphur hexafluoride–neon ratio in the expired gas following a single inspiration of a mixture containing these gases. The data are taken from the work of Cumming and co-workers (1967). If the only inhomogeneity present in the lung was regional, the ratio of sulphur hexafluoride (expressed as the percentage of inspired sulphur hexafluoride) to neon (expressed similarly) should remain unity throughout expiration. The actual curve indicates that diffusion of neon to the periphery is measurably faster than that of sulphur hexafluoride.

relative fraction of sulphur hexafluoride (that is, the fraction in reference to the inspired fraction) must be the same as that of neon and the ratio of these two relative fractions must be unity, regardless of the ventilation per unit volume. Since this ratio would be uniform throughout the lung, it should also appear in all elements of the expired gas, irrespective of the proportion in which dead space gas, gas from well-ventilated alveoli and gas from poorly ventilated alveoli are mixed. The actual findings are shown in Fig. 2, in which changes in expired gas composition during expiration are plotted, the abscissa giving the cumulative expired volume and the ordinate indicating the ratio just described. Obviously the experimental results do not conform to the pattern discussed above, in which only regional inhomogeneity is present, but can well be explained on the basis of stratified inhomogeneity. In the early part of the expired gas, representing gas from the central parts of the respiratory elements, the ratio is high, showing that more of the lighter gas has left this volume, while in the later part of the expiration, the low ratio indicates that less of the heavy gas has reached more remote parts of the respiratory unit. The experiments described by Georg and his associates (Georg et al., 1965) were essentially similar, the main differences being that these authors took serial samples and that the effects of breath-holding time are not reported. In these studies, the ratio sulphur hexafluoride/helium drops to 1 at expired volumes between $0 \cdot 8$ and $1 \cdot 5$ litres.

Effects of breath-holding

If the sloping alveolar plateau is due to stratified inhomogeneity it should be greatly reduced and possibly abolished if the breath is held for a sufficiently long time. A decrease in the slope of the expired nitrogen following a single breath of 100 per cent oxygen after breath-holding or prolonged expiration has indeed been reported and served as an argument against Rauwerda's conclusions (Roos, Dahlstrom and Murphy, 1955; Kjellmer, Sandqvist and Berglund, 1959), but because the effects of perfusion—which are magnified in this type of manoeuvre—are not taken into account, they are open to some criticism, which cannot be applied to some of the more recent work.

Sikand, Cerretelli and Farhi (1966) found that the ratio of argon to nitrogen expired after an inspiration of argon became progressively more uniform as the breath was held for periods extending up to 20 seconds (Fig. 3A), and felt that the pattern of change was indicative of diffusive mixing inside the respiratory elements as well as between the "alveolar volume" and dead space. The experiments of Cumming and co-workers (1967) show that the expired sulphur hexafluoride/neon ratio was still uneven after 5 seconds of breath-holding, but had stabilized at $0 \cdot 995 \pm 0 \cdot 005$ after 30 seconds (Fig. 3B).

Because values for breath-holding times between 5 and 30 seconds are not given, it is difficult to compare these figures exactly to those of Sikand, Cerretelli and Farhi, although it appears that the rate of readjustment is much faster and certainly more complete in Cumming's data. It is of interest to note that Read, whose very elegant approach cannot be discussed here (Read, 1966), also found that after holding the breath for 20 seconds the expired argon plateau (argon being the test gas) still presents a residual slope.

A very ingenious differentiation of the effect of time on regional and stratified inhomogeneity was recently given by Farber (1968) who described how breath-holding affects the cardiogenic oscillations. These are periodic changes in the composition of the expired gas, synchronous with the heart beat (Fowler, 1951), and have been shown to be dependent on the pulsatile blood flow in the lung (Dahlstrom, Murphy and Roos, 1954; Langer, Bornstein and Fishman, 1960). They have been attributed by Fowler and Read (1961) to the fact that the cardiac cycle causes rapid alterations in lung volume which are quantitatively different in the upper and lower parts of the lung. The result is a transient shift in the relative contribution of the lung apex and base to the expired gas, causing the "ripples" often seen on the alveolar plateau. Farber was able to obtain cardiogenic oscillations with the subjects holding their breath for varied periods of time and showed that breath-holding for 60 seconds always decreased the slope of the plateau significantly although the magnitude of the cardiac oscillations had not diminished (Fig. 4). If the amplitude of the oscillations is an indication of the regional differences in concentration, this finding leads again to the conclusion that the major part of the alveolar plateau slope must indeed be due to stratified inhomogeneity.

Although there is general agreement that the slope of the nitrogen plateau after the inspiration of 100 per cent oxygen decreases with breath-holding, sometimes drastically, there is no doubt that in nearly all cases a residual slope is still present after as much as 60 seconds. This probably indicates that sequential emptying contributes to the slope of the plateau, to an extent that is minor but demonstrable after diffusion equilibrium has been reached. A strong argument in favour of this point of view can be derived from the data of Cumming and co-workers (1967), whose results indicate that after 30 seconds although the ratio of sulphur hexafluoride to neon—which cannot be affected by sequential emptying—has become uniform throughout the alveolar plateau,

FIG. 3. Influence of breath-holding time on the slope of the alveolar plateau. In both figures breath-holding time, in seconds, is the abscissa. The change in argon/nitrogen from Sikand, Cerretelli and Farhi (1966) and Cumming and co-workers (1967) at different expired volumes (indicated to the left of the curves) is shown in Figures A and B respectively. The reason for the secondary rise in argon/nitrogen is described by Sikand. For discussion see text.

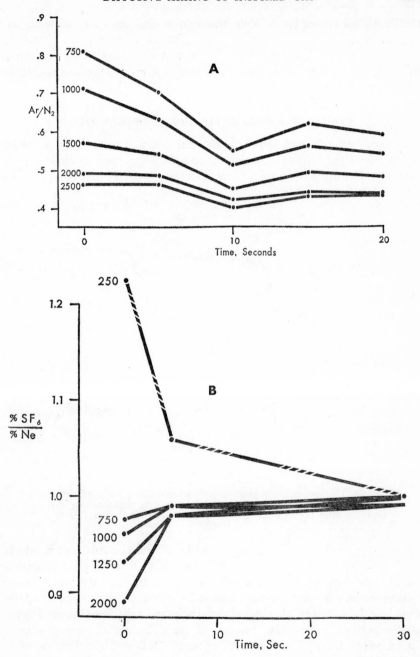

the individual curves for sulphur hexafluoride and neon still show an un-
disputable slope. In a similar way, the data of Kjellmer, Sandqvist and
Berglund (1959) show that the slope of the nitrogen plateau after the inspiration
of 100 per cent oxygen decreases rapidly for 5 seconds and remains essentially
unchanged thereafter.

LUNG MODELS BASED ON STRATIFIED INHOMOGENEITY

Sikand, Cerretelli and Farhi (1966) described a simple analogue model
which would yield the same argon/nitrogen ratios as they obtained experimentally. It consists of an anatomical dead space leading into a compartment

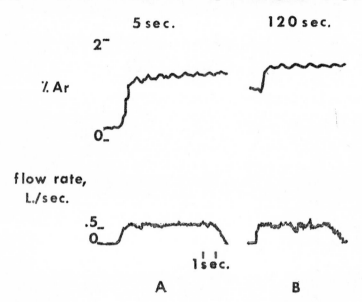

Fig. 4. Changes in cardiogenic oscillations with time. For explanation
see text. Curve A was obtained after 5 seconds of breath-holding and
curve B after 120 seconds. (Reproduced, by permission, from Farber,
1968.)

ventilated by addition of inspired gas and a second compartment in which
gas is renewed only by diffusion. Diffusive mixing between dead space and
the first compartment has a half-time of 5 seconds, while the half-time for
mixing between the two compartments is 2·4 seconds. The central compartment loses inspired gas into the peripheral zone and gains from the dead space
as breath-holding proceeds. Because of the difference of time constants,
there is an initial drop in the argon/nitrogen ratio, followed by a slight increase.

Cumming and co-workers (1966) described a much more sophisticated model. It consists of a hollow segment of a sphere, with a bronchial opening at the apex, a central region ventilated by convective flow and a peripheral area in which the inspired gas diffuses. The dimensions of this spherical segment closely approximate those of the lung lobule. A computer programme allows the prediction of changes in gas composition as a function of time.

A more recent model (T. Sasaki and Farhi, unpublished) incorporates some of the features of each of the preceding analogues. Like that described by Sikand, it is made up of discrete compartments in series, in which mixing takes place during inspiration, but the volumes of these now conform to definite anatomical elements, an idea taken from Cumming's paper. This model (Fig. 5), which can easily be simulated with an analogue computer of modest capability, presents two major advantages, the first being that it takes into account the diffusion that occurs while inspiration is proceeding. The importance of this factor becomes apparent when one considers that normal inspiration or inspiration of a sizeable volume of test gas may last approximately 2 seconds and that Cumming's experiments (Fig. 3B) show that the difference in the ratio of sulphur hexafluoride to neon between expired volumes of 750 ml. and 2,000 ml. drops from its initial value of 9 per cent to only 1 per cent in 5 seconds. In addition, the model can be expanded to take into account the "stratification" in perfusion of the lung lobule which has been described recently (Read, 1966; Wagner, McRae and Read, 1967), in order to simulate the behaviour of soluble tracer gases. The results obtained with this model (Fig. 6) are in good general agreement with the experimental data of Sikand, Cerretelli and Farhi and Cumming and co-workers.

In all these models the gas composition in the lung lobule is influenced significantly by diffusion of gas in and out of the tracheo-bronchial tree. A decrease in the measured anatomical dead space with breath-holding has indeed been shown several years ago (Fowler, 1948) and Roos, Dahlstrom and Murphy (1955) demonstrated conclusively that this was due to diffusion, and indicated that in 5 seconds of breath-holding the dead space could contribute as much as 200 ml. of inspired gas to the alveoli.

CONVECTIVE TRANSPORT AND DIFFUSIVE TRANSPORT

One of the limitations in the use of any of the models described above is that they require knowledge of the volume ventilated by bulk flow. This volume determines the size of the central compartment in Sikand's model and Sasaki's, and the position of the interface in Cumming's analogue. It is therefore important to determine whether for a given lung and given tidal

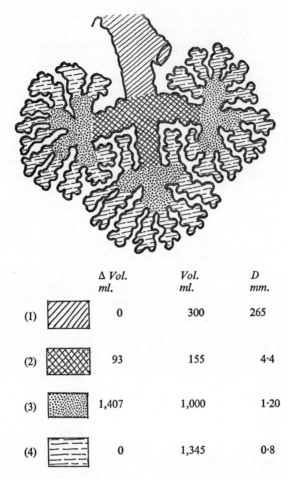

		Δ Vol. ml.	Vol. ml.	D mm.
(1)		0	300	265
(2)		93	155	4·4
(3)		1,407	1,000	1·20
(4)		0	1,345	0·8

FIG. 5. Anatomical basis for the model of Sasaki and Farhi. The schematic drawing of a secondary lobule is adapted from Miller (1950). The four compartments in series, taken from Weibel (1963), are (1) the conductive zone (i.e. the anatomical dead space to the peripheral end of the terminal bronchioles), (2) the respiratory bronchioles, (3) the alveolar ducts, and (4) the alveolar sacs. The volume of each compartment is shown below the diagram. D is the distance, in mm., from one end of the compartment to the other. Δ Vol. indicates the increase in volume after an inspiration of 1,500 ml. In reality, the terminal compartment does indeed expand, but is ventilated only by diffusion. In order to show this, the inspiratory volume of this compartment has been included in that of the alveolar ducts.

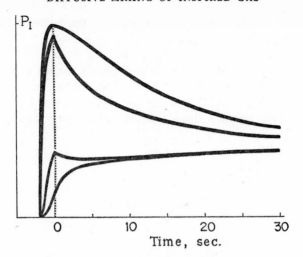

FIG. 6. Behaviour of an inspired tracer gas in the model of Sasaki and Farhi. The four curves indicate the change in partial pressure of an inspired tracer gas (the inspired tension of that gas, P_I, is given for reference) during inspiration and breath-holding, in each of the four compartments shown in Fig. 5; the curves are in the same order from top to bottom as the four compartments. It is assumed that the subject inspires 1,500 ml. of the test mixture at the rate of 750 ml./sec. Note that at zero breath-holding time (dotted vertical line) there is a significant amount of tracer gas in the alveolar sacs.

volumes the extent of effective bulk flow remains identical under all conditions.

An indirect answer to this question can be obtained by comparing the model presented by Cumming and co-workers with that described by Kylstra, Paganelli and Lanphier (1966) to explain the results they had obtained on dogs. These animals were "ventilated" with normal saline and serial samples of the expired liquid were collected and analysed for oxygen and carbon dioxide. Mathematical treatment of the results led to the description of a spherical model having a radius of less than 1 mm.—that is to say, 25 times smaller than that which Cumming uses to simulate his data. Since this staggering difference cannot be explained on the basis of species difference, it becomes tempting to hypothesize that the increased turbulence associated with the density of water leads to much more extensive mixing in the centre of the lobule. One of the objections that can be raised to this comparison is that Cumming's data deal with insoluble gases on which lung perfusion has little direct effect, while Kylstra's results pertain to oxygen and carbon dioxide and are therefore closely bound to blood flow. The recent findings of Read

(1966) and Wagner, McRae and Read (1967) indicating an uneven distribution of perfusion in the lung lobule may imply that Kylstra's model should be confirmed by experiments with inert gases of low solubility.

This criticism cannot be applied to the work of Cruz, Lanphier and Farhi (1968) who repeated the experiments of Sikand and his collaborators on human subjects at 1 and 7 atmospheres and whose results showed that the increase in ambient pressure significantly reduced the initial slope of the argon/nitrogen

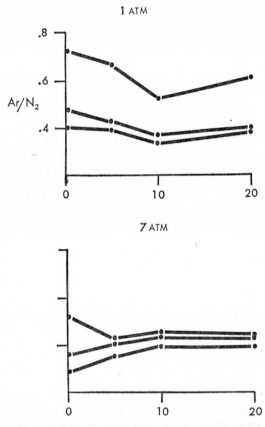

FIG. 7. Effects of gas density on the slope of the alveolar plateau. The results are taken from the work of Cruz, Lanphier and Farhi (1968). The curves correspond to expired volumes of 750, 2,000 and 4,500 ml. The initial mixing, as shown by the vertical distance between the curves at zero breath-holding time, seems improved at 7 atmospheres. In these conditions the effects of breath-holding are less marked.

curve (Fig. 7). Under the same conditions, the effects of breath-holding on the alveolar plateau were definitely less marked than at 1 atmosphere. Such changes can readily be explained on the basis of improvement in bulk mixing coupled with a reduced rate of diffusion, both changes being possibly due to the increased density of the inspired gas.

The importance of bulk mixing was shown in an entirely different manner by Cerretelli, Kylstra and Farhi (unpublished) who investigated whether the large size of the gas exchange unit in the turtle lung (about 100 times larger than mammalian lungs) would cause an increase in the diffusion gradient. In their experiments, a motor-driven syringe was used to force a known volume of argon into the lung of the turtle through a tracheal cannula and to withdraw alveolar gas after a preset breath-holding time. Part of the expired gas was drawn continuously in a mass spectrometer and did not reveal the expected increase in stratified inhomogeneity. A similar experiment in which the turtle lung was replaced by a syringe having approximately the same dimensions showed that in this system there was a definite inhomogeneity which persisted for several seconds during "breath-holding". A clue to the possible reason for the near-homogeneous gas composition in the turtle lung was obtained using an air-dried turtle lung. The central part of the lung was cut open and the tracheal end was jammed into the syringe opening. Ventilation of the syringe through the tracheo-bronchial tree greatly reduced the degree of inhomogeneity.

The experimental evidence of turbulent mixing in the central part of the lobule contradicts a number of theoretical calculations. It will therefore be of considerable interest to extend the data of Cruz, Lanphier and Farhi (1968) and to reconcile this with the predicted behaviour of the inspired gas mass. It is obvious that if this mixing occurs, its increase in situations where the subject is breathing a denser gas may be instrumental in offsetting the decrease in diffusivity that might occur at the same time.

SUMMARY

Recent evidence that gas diffusion within the respiratory lobule is not as rapid as usually postulated is reviewed and discussed. The idea that at the end of inspiration there exists a measurable concentration gradient from the bronchiolar opening to the alveolar wall is supported by experiments which demonstrate the following three points. First, the slope of the alveolar plateau during a single-breath test cannot be explained on the basis of regional inhomogeneity and sequential emptying. In addition, when the test breath contains tracer gases of different diffusivity, the relative changes in their concentration during expiration can be explained only on the basis of diffusion. Finally, the rapid change in slope of the alveolar plateau must also be due to intralobular diffusion. This process is accompanied by considerable mixing with the gas initially contained in the dead space. The central volume in which the inspired gas mixes by convective movement can be influenced by the physical characteristics of the inspired medium.

REFERENCES

ALTSHULER, B., PALMES, E. D., YARMUS, L., and NELSON, N. (1959). *J. appl. Physiol.*, **14**, 321–327.

BALL, W. C., STEWART, P. B., NEWSHAM, L. G. S., and BATES, D. V. (1962). *J. clin. Invest.*, **41**, 519–531.

BOUHUYS, A. (1964). In *Handbook of Physiology, Section 3: Respiration*, vol. I, pp. 715–733, ed. Fenn, W. O., and Rahn, H. Washington, D.C.: American Physiological Society.

CRUZ, J. C., LANPHIER, E. H., and FARHI, L. E. (1968). *Proc. XXIVth int. Congr. Physiol. Sci.*, **7**, 97.

CUMMING, G., CRANK, J., HORSFIELD, K., and PARKER, I. (1966). *Resp. Physiol.*, **1**, 58–74.

CUMMING, G., HORSFIELD, K., JONES, J. G., and MUIR, D. C. F. (1967). *Resp. Physiol.*, **2**, 386–398.

DAHLSTROM, H., MURPHY, J. P., and ROOS, A. (1954). *J. appl. Physiol.*, **7**, 335–339.

FARBER, J. P. (1968). *Study of regional emptying of the lung with soluble inert gas.* Ph.D. Dissertation, State University of New York, Buffalo.

FOWLER, K. T., and READ, J. (1961). *J. appl. Physiol.*, **16**, 863–868.

FOWLER, W. S. (1948). *Am. J. Physiol.*, **154**, 405–416.

FOWLER, W. S. (1951). *Am. J. med. Sci.*, **222**, 602.

GEORG, J., LASSEN, N. A., MELLEMGAARD, K., and VINTHER, A. (1965). *Clin. Sci.*, **29**, 525–532.

GRÉHANT, N. (1862). *C. r. hebd. Séanc. Acad. Sci., Paris*, **55**, 278–280.

KJELLMER, I., SANDQVIST, L., and BERGLUND, E. (1959). *J. appl. Physiol.*, **14**, 105–108,

KROGH, A., and LINDHARD, J. (1917). *J. Physiol., Lond.*, **51**, 59–90.

KYLSTRA, J. A., PAGANELLI, C. V., and LANPHIER, E. H. (1966). *J. appl. Physiol.*, **21**, 177–184.

LANGER, G. A., BORNSTEIN, D. L., and FISHMAN, A. P. (1960). *J. appl. Physiol.*, **15**, 855–862.

MARTIN, C. J., CLINE, F., and MARSHALL, H. (1953). *J. clin. Invest.*, **32**, 617–621.

MARTIN, C. J., and YOUNG, A. C. (1957). *J. appl. Physiol.*, **11**, 371–376.

MEAD, J. (1969). This volume, pp. 204–209.

MILIC-EMILI, J., HENDERSON, J. A. M., DOLOVICH, M. B., TROP, D., and KANEKO, K. (1966). *J. appl. Physiol.*, **21**, 749–759.

MILLER, W. S. (1950). *The Lung.* Springfield, Ill.: Thomas.

OTIS, A. B., MCKERROW, C. B., BARTLETT, R. A., MEAD, J., MCILROY, M. B., SELVERSTONE, N. J., and RADFORD, E. P., Jr. (1956). *J. appl. Physiol.*, **8**, 427–443.

RAHN, H., and FENN, W. O. (1955). *A graphical analysis of the alveolar gas exchange— the O_2—CO_2 diagram.* Washington, D.C.: American Physiological Society.

Rahn, H., Sadoul, P., Farhi, L. E., and Shapiro, J. (1956). *J. appl. Physiol.*, **8**, 417–426.

Rauwerda, P. E. (1946). *Unequal ventilation of different parts of the lung.* (Dissertation.) Groningen: University of Groningen Press.

Read, J. (1966). *J. appl. Physiol.*, **21**, 1521–1531.

Roos, A., Dahlstrom, H., and Murphy, J. P. (1955). *J. appl. Physiol.*, **7**, 645–659.

Sikand, R., Cerretelli, P., and Farhi, L. E. (1966). *J. appl. Physiol.*, **21**, 1331–1337.

Wagner, P., McRae, J., and Read, J. (1967). *J. appl. Physiol.*, **22**, 1115–1123.

Weibel, E. R. (1963). *Morphometry of the Human Lung.* New York: Academic Press.

West, J. B. (1962). *J. appl. Physiol.*, **17**, 893–898.

West, J. B., Dollery, C. T., and Hugh-Jones, P. (1962). *Ciba Fdn Symp. on Pulmonary Structure and Function*, pp. 159–175. London: Churchill.

DISCUSSION

Caro: What is the relative diffusivity of sulphur hexafluoride and neon?

Farhi: The relative diffusivity is 2·8. Georg and co-workers ([1965]. *Clin. Sci.*, **29**, 525–532) took this even further by giving sulphur hexafluoride and helium, which gives a much larger range. I did not report on their results because they did not discuss the breath-holding effect.

Mead: Would one expect with such differences between helium and sulphur hexafluoride that the time-course of wash-out for those two gases would be dissimilar in normal lungs?

Cumming: Yes. The rate of wash-out is more rapid using helium than using sulphur hexafluoride.

Caro: Dr. Farhi, I do not see why a change of density should affect mixing in your scheme of things.

Farhi: I could speculate on that. In the model that I showed there were several mixing compartments, and we stopped arbitrarily at four. If one accepts that denser gases will create a different pattern of turbulence, mixing may be pushed further in certain conditions than in others.

Caro: So you are taking account of the big airways (that is, those where turbulence may occur) influencing what happens in the peripheral parts of the lung. Do the conducting airways really influence this?

Farhi: Our results substantiate the fact that breathing air at one atmosphere gives the equivalent of having mixing up to a certain point and then diffusion; with a more dense gas mixing will proceed further down and so there will be a shorter diffusing path. This is why the initial mixing appears better at seven atmospheres, but the time effects are not as pronounced as with the more dense gas.

Owen: Do you mean that after taking account of the difference in the diffusivities there is a separate density effect? That seems surprising.

Farhi: Diffusivities will not make much difference to these calculations; the effect is small in comparison to that of density.

Altshuler: I would expect more turbulence with the heavier gas. This would arise in the upper airways.

Cumming: We are dealing with a point 2 mm. from the end of the alveolar duct.

Altshuler: But we are concerned with an interface that starts at the mouth and proceeds through the airways.

Farhi: The last 2 mm. are what is necessary to explain the results obtained with a gas density of one, and therefore may not apply to a denser gas. This is corroborated to a certain extent by the fact that if instead of going from air at one atmosphere to air at seven atmospheres you take the liquid breathing experiments, you move much further even than that, and with a denser liquid, you go still further.

Philip: Dr. Farhi, is this density effect completely separable from a straight Reynolds number effect?

Farhi: I can't answer that.

Philip: By density you mean that inertia is more important than viscosity?

Farhi: I would say turbulence, which would bring me back to the Reynolds number.

Philip: I wonder whether there is some way of bringing experimental work with different gases back to a common basis by, say, varying the rate at which things are happening and seeing whether there is a consistent story when some suitable Reynolds number, or perhaps also Péclet number, is made constant. One might in this way test whether or not the process is largely determined by the fluid mechanics.

Farhi: One possibility is to repeat the experiments at one and seven atmospheres with an aerosol which would be an index of bulk mixing. I understand that Dr. Altshuler does not completely agree with that but it might indicate that we have more turbulence and mixing in one condition than in the other.

Mead: Dr. West appeared to be able to demonstrate real differences in concentration in time in a fluid-filled lung in which we have heard that the diffusion was some five orders of magnitude slower than in air. But if one takes away five orders of magnitude one is not left with much in a gas-filled lung, and it is hard to believe that any meaningful diffusion gradients can exist in a gas-filled lung on the basis of that observation. Have you tried to predict gaseous diffusion from your own measurements on the fluid-filled lung, Dr. West?

West: I have not done this, but I understand that that is what Dr. Farhi is thinking of—a comparison of the liquid-filled and air-filled lung.

Farhi: My point is that in comparing the liquid-filled and air-filled lung, one must take into account that in the latter the pattern of bulk mixing is very different and brings the inspired gas much nearer the most remote parts of the respiratory elements.

Stuart: I am confused about what Dr. Farhi means on this matter of density. Are you thinking of the sort of phenomenon called Rayleigh-Taylor instability, in which there are two fluids of different densities separated by an interface, with an acceleration normal to the interface, which may or may not be due to gravity? If the acceleration is from the lighter to the heavier fluid, there is a mixing stimulated by the density difference.

Farhi: No: I was referring more to something which would be an increase in the Reynolds number which would therefore lead to more turbulent mixing.

Davies: This word turbulence is being rather over-worked! When you reach tubes which are smaller than, say, 4 mm. the turbulence in the upper stages has already done its job and you need not worry about turbulence any more. But we must remember that the density of the gas brings in an effect on Reynolds number, and Reynolds number produces other things besides turbulence. In the tubes between the ones 4 or 5 mm. in diameter and the very tiny ones (below $0 \cdot 5$ mm.) deep down in the lung, there is a transition not from turbulent flow but from laminar flow with inertia to laminar flow without inertia. To go back to Dr. Philip's paper (pp. 25–44), when there is laminar flow without inertia there will be perfect recapitulation of the inhaled flow during exhalation; but where the Reynolds number is so high that although still far away from turbulence, the inertial effect is important, this recapitulation fails. The physiological concept of an interface between flow and diffusion is very much more complicated than Dr. West has made out, because you have to bring in the multiplicity of paraboloids and the tremendous complexity of interfaces generated by the numerous branches in the lung. When you raise the gas density and bring in inertial terms (without any turbulence; still with laminar flow in all these branching regions), you will affect the level of the interfaces; here is where the complexity arises.

Farhi: This is certainly more palatable to most people than dealing with turbulence so far down the airways.

Philip: I agree with Dr. Davies. The difference between a Reynolds number of $0 \cdot 5$ and one of 5 could make a spectacular difference in the amount of recovery.

Caro: Dr. Altshuler, do we conclude that it needs quite a lot of breath-holding time to get a particle into the alveolar sacs?

Altshuler: I identify your "alveolar sac" with the "terminal duct" in the scheme I used. The size of the tidal volume controls whether or not particles reach the terminal duct, and in order to penetrate that far, it needs to be comparable to the interior volume of the passageways, that is, the conductive and transitory zones of Weibel ([1963]. *Morphometry of the Human Lung.* Berlin: Springer and New York: Academic Press) (see Table I of my paper, p. 219).

Lassen: Can anyone comment on the diffusion difficulties in diseased human lung, for instance in chronic bronchitis?

Cumming: We have looked at diffusion in people with chronic bronchitis in a variety of ways, first by comparing the slope of the expired gas in normal subjects and bronchitic patients; secondly by using a nodal analysis technique from the known anatomical deformation; and thirdly by giving a mixture of two gases and plotting the recoveries (unpublished observations).

All our evidence suggests that the dominant defect in chronic bronchitis is in gas exchange within the gas phase; in other words the difficulty in moving a molecule of oxygen from the atmosphere to the capillary blood lies in the inadequacy of mixing by gaseous diffusion within the airways.

Piiper: Dr. Farhi mentioned that the stratification theory propounded by Krogh and Linhard was discredited on the basis of theoretical calculations by Rauwerda, and now Dr. Farhi has very convincingly shown that there is stratification. What exactly was Rauwerda's error? Did he use a wrong model or did he put wrong dimensions into an appropriate model?

Cumming: Rauwerda's mathematics were unexceptionable; the trouble came with the primary assumptions on which he based his model. He chose to consider diffusion in the terminal acinus which has a length of 7 mm., and supposed that it was a closed tube in which an interface was established 2 mm. from the end: he then asked how quickly that would equilibrate. The answer was then very simple; the gradient was reduced to 16 per cent of the original in $0 \cdot 38$ seconds. But he knew that the lung is not a straight tube and could be represented better as a shell of a concentric sphere, also of length 7 mm. closed at either end. Analysis of this model gave similar results.

The trouble was that the lung cannot be represented by any *closed* object 7 mm. in length, because reflection and diffusion from both ends makes mixing very rapid. We tried to avoid this by considering the tube as 27 cm. long, that is, up to the mouth, but there were difficulties using analytic techniques. Analytic techniques applied to a more satisfactory model have been described (Cumming, G., Crank, J., Horsfield, K., and Parker, I. [1966]. *Resp. Physiol.*, **1,** 58). We have now done it using numerical techniques.

Altshuler: My paper includes consideration of stationary gas diffusion in the alveolar space and points out two dominant considerations. First, the air in the surrounding alveoli slows up axial diffusion in the duct by equilibrating radially with duct gases. Second, the increase (peripherally) in cross-sectional area at each bifurcation decreases the concentration gradients and so also the associated axial transport. The first decreases peripheral transport by a half to one-third, and the second decreases it by about a half; and thus there is a total reduction of almost an order of magnitude from that in the simple Rauwerda model.

Cumming: We have recently taken the dimensions of our normal human lung cast and have treated this as a heat diffusion problem (unpublished observations). We have used a method of nodal analysis, taking 80 nodes down every pathway and setting up the heat-transfer situation by a sequential analysis, taking the movement down the airways and then the immediate movement back up with no halt at the bottom. Thus we can calculate the concentration of gas at the lips. Over the alveolar plateau at normal lung volume this works out to about 8 per cent of nitrogen, which is very similar to what one sees in the normal single-breath nitrogen test.

Lassen: It would be a great help to physiologists if our theoretical colleagues were to provide ways of separating the two functions of diffusion and mass transport in a clearer way than by single-breath or breath-holding experiments. Ideally we would like to be able to give a number, which would perhaps be a distance, and to be able to say that a diffusion distance of two in a patient with respiratory disease is a good sign whereas a value of ten might be a bad sign. But we need a method of handling this complex system where both types of transport occur.

GENERAL DISCUSSION

A MATHEMATICAL TREATMENT OF DISPERSION IN FLOW THROUGH A BRANCHING TREE

Saffman: My contribution at this point is really a postscript on the question of dispersion through the bronchial tree. However, to make the problem amenable to elementary mathematical analysis one has to simplify so considerably that I have serious doubts whether the discussion will be very significant.

I have considered the following problem. Let us suppose one has a bronchial tree with uniform dichotomy. Suppose that at some time $t = 0$ you start breathing air containing some contaminant at a uniform rate; then at some later time t, where is the contaminant spread throughout the system? The method to be used is an application of some simple statistical ideas, and supposes that we know hydrodynamic details of the flow through each of the individual branches.

Let us call the various branching stages in the tree 1, 2, 3 . . . n. We assume that at any stage the individual branches are the same. Let us suppose that for any particular branch in stage n we know the function $p_n(t)$, which is the fraction of contaminant introduced at the entrance to this particular branch at time $t = 0$ that remains in the same branch at time t. This function $p_n(t)$ depends upon the mechanics of the flow through each branch; for Poiseuille flow through each branch, it can be written down immediately in terms of the length of the branch and the velocity; one can also take account of molecular diffusion and of deposition on the walls. For both laminar and turbulent flow through a straight pipe without deposition on walls, this function can be deduced from work by Sir Geoffrey Taylor ([1953]. *Proc. R. Soc. A*, **219**, 186; [1954]. *Ibid.*, **225**, 473) and others on axial diffusion in flow through a long straight pipe. If we assume that this function is known for each individual branch in the following way, we can construct for the whole bronchial tree a function giving us the distribution of the contaminating material.

The function $p_n(t)$ has the property that $p_n(0)$ is equal to one. We also suppose for simplicity that there is no reverse transport and material goes from the nth to the $n + 1$th branch, so that $p_n(t)$ decreases monotonically; $p_n(\infty)$ may be zero, or it may be greater than zero if contaminant is deposited, because in this case a finite amount stays in the branch for an infinite time. The negative derivative of $p_n(t)$, $h_n(t) = -dp_n/dt$, is proportional to the fraction of the material which leaves branch n in a time-interval of length dt; this function is well known in studies of tracer dilution techniques in flow through blood vessels where it is called the wash-out or tracer dilution curve, and most of what I say is in fact implicit in work by K. Zierler of Johns Hopkins ([1965]. *Fedn Proc. Fedn Am. Socs exp. Biol.*, **24**, 1085).

These functions are for a single branch; now consider the corresponding functions for the whole tree, denoted by $P_n(t)$ and $H_n(t)$. The quantity $H_n(t)dt$ is the fraction of material which entered the first branch at $t = 0$, leaving the nth branch of the tree in the time-interval from t to $t + dt$—that is, $H_n(t)$ is the wash-out function for the first n branches of the tree. It is almost obvious that $H_n(t)$ is the convolution of $h_1(t), h_2(t), \ldots . h_n(t)$; that is,

$$H_n(t) = h_1(t) * h_2(t) * h_3(t) \ldots . * h_n(t)$$

where

$$f(t) * g(t) = \int_0^t f(t')g(t-t')dt'$$

if we make the further assumption that the times spent by particles in successive branches are statistically independent. Thus, if all the individual $h_n(t)$ functions are known, $H_n(t)$ can be calculated. The calculation may be difficult analytically, but is child's play for a computer. The function $P_n(t)$, which is also the probability that a particle entering the first branch at time $t = 0$ is somewhere in the first n branches after time t, is given by

$$P_n(t) = 1 - \int_0^t H_n(t)dt$$

Given the function $H_n(t)$ we can answer the question: if at $t = 0$ a certain amount of material is injected at the entrance to the first branch, what fraction of it is in the first branch, or the second branch or the nth branch, at a later time? This is another function which I shall call $S_n(t)$; in statistical terms it is the probability that a particle goes from the entrance of the tree to the nth branch in time t. The function $S_n(t)$ is the difference between the fraction that enters and the fraction that leaves the nth stage in time t. Mathematically,

$$S_n(t) = P_n(t) - P_{n-1}(t)$$

or

$$\frac{dS_n}{dt} = H_{n-1}(t) - H_n(t)$$

In principle at least, one therefore knows the function $S_n(t)$, the fraction of incident material which has gone into the nth branch after time t.

We can extend this a little more. Suppose that one has a continuous input at a rate $Q(t)$ (>0) into the tree, so that in the time T, $\int_0^T Qdt$ enters; this can be any kind of contaminant, an aerosol or a tracer gas being convected along. Then the amount in the nth branch is the convolution integral of $Q(t)$ and the function $S_n(t)$, namely

$$\int_0^T Q(t) S_n(T-t) dt$$

So with a continuous injection one can also answer formally the question of dispersion and spread. The case of the material coming to a stage with no exit, say the Nth branch is the last, is covered by taking $p_N(t) = 1$.

By taking particular values of the functions $h_n(t)$ one can easily work out examples on how material spreads. I have been looking at the case of Poiseuille flow with no molecular diffusion, for which $p_n(t) = 1$ when $t < \frac{1}{2}\bar{t}_n$ and $p_n(t) = (\bar{t}_n/2t)^2$ for $t > \frac{1}{2}\bar{t}_n$, where $\bar{t}_n$ is the mean time spent in the nth branch.

This discussion is all very simple in principle, although the details may be quite hard and the determination of the $p_n(t)$ may be difficult. However, a big question-mark hangs over the two main assumptions: (1) that there are uniform dichotomies, and (2) that the motion in different branches is statistically independent—that is, that the amount of time a particle spends in one branch does not affect the amount of time it spends in the next branch. According to Dr. Cumming's remarks, the assumption of uniform dichotomy may not be good for the bronchial tree. The second assumption means that considerable mixing has to take place at the junction between branches, and this may be an unreasonable thing to suppose because a particle which takes a long time in one branch because, say, it is very close to the wall will tend to be close to the wall in the following branch and therefore the times will not be independent. This is a very big question-mark, unless we are dealing with flows at fairly large Reynolds numbers so that there is appreciable secondary motion and therefore mixing at the junctions. To take account of the statistical correlation between the times spent in one branch and the next, we get into more difficult mathematical problems in the field of Markov processes which are not so simple and somewhat harder to analyse.

Cumming: Is there any constraint on $p_n(t)$?

Saffman: It must be positive, equal to 1 at $t = 0$, and monotonic decreasing, all corresponding to forward transport. I think reverse transport could be done, but the theory would be much harder. If one assumes that motion in different branches is statistically independent, one can answer the question of what happens when the direction of flow in the tree is reversed and air is expelled. The assumption of uniform dichotomy can be dropped and asymmetry of the tree can be incorporated into the functions $p_n(t)$; however assumption (2) of statistical independence is then even more doubtful.

Philip: May I point out what seem to me some formidable obstacles to applying these ideas to the bronchial tree. Firstly, your specific discussion seems to apply only to steady, unidirectional flow. In the respiratory system the flow is oscillatory and the Taylor description of dispersion must be modified. (Appropriate references are given in my paper, pp. 25–44.) Secondly, the convection–diffusion interaction is profoundly influenced by the boundary conditions at the surface. When there is uptake at the surface, the mathematical structure of the problem is changed. The leading eigenfunction of the exact solution corresponds to a diffusion description in the no-uptake (classical Taylor) case, but this is no longer so when uptake (deposition) occurs, as in the bronchial tree. Thirdly, there are serious complications associated with entry behaviour both of flow and of dispersion, and there are a great number of entries in your system. In other words, it would seem that a lot of difficult and very interesting problems must be faced in studying the properties of your $p_n(t)$ for real, messy, situations.

Cumming: Professor Saffman, how do you propose to deal with $p_n(t)$ in an alveolar duct of diameter 300 μm. with holes leading out in five different directions? How do the exit holes along the alveolar ducts modify the situation?

Saffman: There are many difficult questions buried in the determination of $p_n(t)$. However, for many cases, I think one can make reasonable estimates by a variety of different methods.

Altshuler: These questions have to be handled separately; Professor Saffman is giving a framework for an overall situation and one has to look at each component to see if it is realistic.

CHAIRMEN'S CLOSING REMARKS

C. G. CARO

M. J. LIGHTHILL

ONLY outstanding impressions of this detailed and vigorous meeting can be recorded here. Early among these was our impression that physiologists and physical scientists seemed to succeed remarkably in making themselves usefully comprehensible to one another—and, dare it be suggested, in refining one another's understanding of physiology and mechanics. A very substantial slice of physiology was discussed. The ability to do this undoubtedly owed much to the presence of the physical scientists and to the diversity of their backgrounds. In physical terms coverage was immense, including velocities ranging from those characteristic of diffusional motion in liquids to near-sonic velocities in air, and dimensions from the molecular to log jams on the St. Lawrence, though the latter are of uncertain physiological relevance...!

In attempting a summary it seems appropriate to concentrate as much on problems and difficulties highlighted during the meeting (and constituting possible lines of future research) as on the formal papers. Among these problems is the explanation of the low pressures recorded in tissue spaces and the tremendous increase of fluid conductance encountered when this pressure is raised. The structure of tissue space is unclear, and as a result the complexity required of a model porous medium which would reasonably describe some of the features of tissue spaces is not clear either. The capillary pore is also in this area of uncertainty.

Predictably, much interest centred on the red blood cell, including its probable rotation (alternately under compression and tension) in a sheared flow. Its deformability, and the lubrication by plasma of its passage through capillaries, may prove an instructive field. Only the fittest of red cells seem able to survive their periodic forays through very narrow capillary channels. Theories there are, but why and how it is that the red cell is biconcave, seems still to be unanswered.

A conference of this sort emphasizes the bottlenecks which impede further study. One such is the lack, in certain instances, of accurate dimensional measurements. But the data now needed may have to be gathered by the physiologist rather than the anatomist, for it is experimental data, gathered under precisely specified physiological conditions, that are required. Physiologists who embark on such data-collecting expeditions, and who are as a result able to describe path lengths and branching area ratios in the airways or in vascular beds, are to be commended. Particularly when it is coupled with local mechanical studies, this type of information permits more precise treatment of systems and enormously enhances our understanding of them. Especial skill is displayed by the physiological anatomist when he is able to use capillaries, *in vivo*, as manometers and even to measure the local haematocrit.

The physiologist takes pleasure in obtaining experimental results with simple equipment that causes minimal disturbance. But the ability to do this, as in the study of the time-course of changes in the arterioles, depends substantially on assistance from the theoretician. Nonetheless, the physiologist welcomes advanced technology, especially when this is reinforced by detailed fluid mechanic theory which explains, for example, the motion of blood cells travelling in tubes of various sizes. In the same "vein", those who succeed in so refining an engineering technique as to make possible blood velocity measurements at different stations over the diameter of an artery, and in establishing unequivocally whether flow is laminar or turbulent, are also to be admired.

Studies of variation of input impedance with frequency throw very useful light on the modes of pulse propagation in arteries. The need for sophisticated treatment of such data is shown, however, by the accumulating evidence that the whole arterial system is one vast "inlet length".

Simplification of theory, another favourite pastime of the physiologist, is particularly satisfying when done with the consent of his more rigorous colleagues in the physical sciences. Thus it is an attractive concept that in the lung the effect on gas distribution of airway resistance may, under some conditions of breathing, be negligible by comparison with that of compliance. But again it is only departures from the predictions of simple theory that may reveal detailed behaviour. In this sense the aerodynamics of the airways would seem to have been insufficiently studied. There is now considerable interest in the transport and deposition of fine particles in the airways, and the influence of gas humidification is a tantalizing additional complication. In the bread and butter part of respiratory physiology, upper airways aerodynamics may influence alveolar gas exchange.

There can be little doubt that this meeting will add to physiological knowledge and, it seems likely, serve to extend relevant interdisciplinary collaboration. Nevertheless, it is appropriate for the participants to question whether and how, given another opportunity, they would wish to modify a future symposium. One possibility is that the assembly of physiologists and physical scientists should aim to probe a little more into the physics of active rather than passive processes. Another is that the meeting might concentrate on probing smaller areas to greater depth.

One task remains and that a most pleasurable one, of thanking Dr. Wolsten-holme and his staff for arranging this memorable meeting.

INDEX OF AUTHORS*

Numbers in bold type indicate a contribution in the form of a paper; numbers in plain type refer to contributions in the discussions.

*Author and subject indexes prepared by Mr. William Hill.

SUBJECT INDEX

Aerosols,
  behaviour in respiratory tract, 45,
    215–235
  deposition, 216, 223–225, 229
  during forced expiratory single
    breaths, 226–229, 232
  effect of gravity, 232–233
  effect of lung volume, 229, 235
  effect of posture, 234–235
  mixing, 225–226
  theoretical considerations, 217–226
  condensation of water vapour on,
    249–251
  convection to wall, 242–244
  deposition on evaporating surface,
    246–249, 253–254
  in alveolar sac, 295–296
  in trachea, 129, 236–255
  transport of, 279
  use in pulmonary function tests, 216
Airborne particles, *See Aerosols*
Alveolar ducts,
  deposition of aerosols in, 224
  gas flow in, 222
  time constants in, 279
  velocity destribution, 234
Alveolar membrane, interstitial fluid
  movement, 16, 17, 24
Alveolar plateau, slope of, 279, 280, 283,
  284, 290, 291
Alveolar sac, 288, 295–296
  See also Alveolar spatial unit
Alveolar septum, erythrocytes in, 265,
  267, 272
Alveolar spatial unit, 220–221, 269–271
Alveolar wall, increased tension, effect
  on capillaries, 261
Aorta,
  blood velocity in, 172, 180, 181, 183,
    184, 189, 195, 200, 202
  pressure in, 189
Aortic incompetence and stenosis, effect
  on blood velocity, 194, 196
Arterial branches, input impedance in,
  factors, 137
Arterial pressure, 142–146
  effect on erythrocytes in capillaries,
    257, 258
Arteries,
  blood velocity in, effect of heart
    lesions, 189, 192, 193, 196
  effect of turbulence, 191, 194, 196,
    200, 201
  experimental methods for study,
    173–180

Arteries—*contd.*
  blood velocity in—*contd.*
    in dogs, 180–188
    in man, 188–196
    laminar flow, 194–195, 200
  distensibility of, 142, 151
  effect of vasomotion on impedance,
    150
  elastic properties, 136–156
  non-linearity of, 150
  oscillatory flow in, 188
  resonance in, 147
  transition in, 172–202
  velocity distribution in, 172–202
    pulsatile, 186–188
Arteriolar sphincter, 101
Arterioles, pressures in, 103, 153
Atrial fibrillation, effect on blood
  velocity, 192
Axial concentration, of red cells, 87–91,
  127

Blood,
  rouleaux in, *See Rouleaux*
  viscosity of, 82–83, 128, 161
Blood flow,
  and lung volume, 281
  in arteries,
    secondary, 202
    turbulent, 191, 194, 196, 200, 201
  in capillaries, 51–52, 57, 70, 84,
    256–276
  in glass and plastic fibres, 130–135
  in terminal lung unit, 269–271
  post-congestion, 162, 164, 165
Blood pressure, raising of, 142–143
Blood velocity,
  in aorta, 172, 180, 181, 183, 184, 189,
    195, 200, 202
  in arteries, 172–202
    effect of heart lesions, 189, 192, 193,
      196
    effect of turbulence, 191, 194, 196
    in dogs, 180–188
    in man, 188–196
  measurement of, 173–180
Blood vessels
  See also Arteries, Capillaries etc.
  distensibility of, 138–146, 153, 154, 170
  optimum size, 70
  permeability of, 85
  pressure–flow relations, 153–171
    effect of posture, 169
    myogenic mechanism, 166–167
    vasodilatation and, 163–164

306

Printed by Spottiswoode, Ballantyne & Co. Ltd., London and Colchester.